ANNALS OF THE NEW YORK ACADEMY OF SCIENCES
Volume 279

THE GLASS TRANSITION AND THE NATURE OF THE GLASSY STATE

Edited by Martin Goldstein and Robert Simha

The New York Academy of Sciences
New York, New York
1976

Library of Congress Cataloging in Publication Data

Workshop on the Glass Transition and the Nature of the Glassy State, New York, 1975.
The glass transition and the nature of the glassy state.

(Annals of the New York Academy of Sciences; v. 279)
Sponsored by the New York Academy of Sciences.
1. Glass—Congresses. 2. Polymers and polymerization—Congresses. I. Goldstein, Martin, 1919– II. Simha, Robert, 1912– III. New York Academy of Sciences. IV. Title. V. Series: New York Academy of Sciences. Annals; v. 279.
Q11.N5 vol. 279 [TP845] 508′.1s [666′.1′042] 76-43100
ISBN 0-89072-053-3

SP
Printed in the United States of America
ISBN 0-89072-053-3

ANNALS OF THE NEW YORK ACADEMY OF SCIENCES

VOLUME 279

October 15, 1976

THE GLASS TRANSITION AND THE NATURE OF THE GLASSY STATE*

Editors and Workshop Chairmen

MARTIN GOLDSTEIN AND ROBERT SIMHA

CONTENTS

*This series of papers is the result of a workshop entitled Workshop on the Glass Transition and the Nature of the Glassy State, held by The New York Academy of Sciences on December 10–12, 1975.

Part IV. Cryogenic Anomalies

Part V. Structure of Amorphous Solids

Financial support was received from:

- DOW CHEMICAL U.S.A.
- THE MONSANTO COMPANY
- THE NATIONAL SCIENCE FOUNDATION
- PPG INDUSTRIES
- THE UNITED STATES ARMY RESEARCH OFFICE

INTRODUCTION

Martin Goldstein

Belfer Graduate School of Science
Yeshiva University
New York, New York 10033

Robert Simha

Department of Macromolecular Science
Case-Western Reserve University
Cleveland, Ohio 44106

The guiding purpose of this Workshop Conference was to focus on those features of glass behavior and glass properties that are shared by all chemical classes of glass-forming substances: inorganic oxides, chalcogenides, metal alloys, fused salts, organic polymers, and molecular liquids. In so doing, we hoped to bring together workers in different fields of glass research, representing different disciplines, for a fruitful exchange of ideas.

The affiliations of those attending, the extent of their participation in the discussions, and the opinions expressed by a number of the participants after the conference lead us to believe we succeeded. We hope the reader of these *Annals* will come to the same conclusion.

The Conference was divided up into five subtopics, each followed by a discussion period: Thermodynamic and Transport Properties of Liquids near the Glass Transition Temperature; The Glass Transition: Thermodynamic and Kinetic Aspects; Secondary Relaxations; Cryogenic Anomalies; and Structure of Amorphous Solids.

We want to express our gratitude to the speakers, session chairmen, discussants, and participants for their contributions, to The New York Academy of Sciences for sponsoring the Workshop and for handling the mechanical details of it so efficiently, and to the National Science Foundation, The U.S. Army Research Office, The Dow Chemical Company, the Monsanto Company, and PPG Industries for financial support.

CONFIGURATIONAL STATISTICAL THERMODYNAMICS OF POLYMER LIQUIDS*

Robert Simha

Department of Macromolecular Science
Case Western Reserve University
Cleveland, Ohio 44106

Introduction

A variety of descriptions of the glass transition process and the glassy state have been developed over the years. Some are more or less empirical in character. Others are based on molecular models or on certain postulates and the formalism of irreversible thermodynamics.

In dealing with this subject, our motivating concern and area of application have been polymer solids. It is hoped in the spirit of this conference, however, that one may inquire to what extent the general approach is pertinent for other types of glassy systems as well.

Our point of departure has been a liquid state theory of the equilibrium system. Two features of this theory have allowed us to proceed to the glass transition and to the glassy state. One is the quantitative success of the equation of state and of the corresponding compressional energy and entropy derived. Secondly, this is a parametric theory, that is, it operates with an ordering parameter that is determined as a function of the variables of state by the minimization of a configurational free energy. On this basis then one may continue to the glass and inquire into the behavior of this parameter along a liquid-glass boundary and in the glassy state. The question then arises to what extent a bridge between the melt and its glass or glasses can be formed by the functional dependence of this parameter in the two states. Clearly, such a quasiequilibrium approach can not provide, although it may be a starting point, for a treatment of retardation phenomena. We are dealing only with situations where viscoelastic relaxation is negligible or in other words, with the results of fast experiments.

The Liquid State

The basis and applications of the theory have been discussed on previous occasions.[1,2] The conceptual starting point is the cell model of Lennard-Jones and Devonshire,[3] who replace the fluctuating molecular field acting on a given unit by an average. This average in turn is defined by lattice sites, which define the surroundings of a given unit. Despite the well-known weaknesses of this model, its extension to chainmolecular fluids by Prigogine and his collaborators[4] has proven fruitful. The chain character of the constituent units is taken into account in two ways. First, by the connectivity of the lattice sites occupied by successive segments of the chain, as is familiar from the lattice theories of mixtures. Since we are

*This work was supported by the National Science Foundation.

dealing with thermal properties, there is also a dynamic factor. In monatomic and structurally simple molecular fluids there is a clear-cut separation of internal and external degrees of freedom. Only the latter matter for configurational properties or in other words, only soft modes, namely translations and external rotations are involved. For a chainmolecule, however, additional modes appear. Some of these, corresponding to bond stretching and bending motions, are clearly internal. The roles of internal bond rotations and of sidechain motions, on the other hand, are not clearly specifiable, because they may be the result of inter- *and* intra-molecular effects. A detailed evaluation of the partition function for other than idealized extremes or other than in the harmonic approximation is difficult and has never been offered; instead Prigogine's original proposal stands, which assigns a *fixed* number $3c$ of degrees of freedom to the chain. It need not be specified explicitly, except to recognize that it must increase with, and become proportional to the number of repeat units in the limit, since it will be absorbed in the definition of the scaling temperature. More will be said about this later.

Now lattice theories have the characteristic fault, particularly at elevated temperatures, of yielding too much order. We have modified the theory alluded to by the introduction of lattice vacancies into the configurational partition function. The number of these is specified as a function of volume and temperature by the minimization of the configurational Helmholtz free energy. We refer for details to Reference 1 and cite only the final results, expressed in reduced variables. The definitions of the scaling factors arise directly from the theory. We have

Equation of state:

$$\tilde{P}\tilde{V}/\tilde{T} = [1 - 2^{-1/6}y(y\tilde{V})^{-1/3}]^{-1} + (2y/\tilde{T})(y\tilde{V})^{-2}[1.011\,(y\tilde{V})^{-2} - 1.2045], \tag{1}$$

Internal energy:

$$\tilde{U} = (y/2)(y\tilde{V})^{-2}[1.011\,(y\tilde{V})^{-2} - 2.409], \tag{2}$$

Entropy:

$$\tilde{S} = -s/c[(1 - y)/y]\ln(1 - y) + 3\ln[(y\tilde{V})^{1/3} - 2^{-1/6}y] + \ln V^* + \text{const.}, \tag{3}$$

Extremum condition:

$$\begin{aligned}(s/3c)[1 + y^{-1}\ln(1 - y)] \\ = (y/6\tilde{T})(y\tilde{V})^{-2}[2.409 - 3.003\,(y\tilde{V})^{-2}] \\ + [2^{-1/6}y(y\tilde{V})^{-1/3} - 1/3][1 - 2^{-1/6}y(y\tilde{V})^{-1/3}]^{-1}.\end{aligned} \tag{4}$$

Here y is the fraction of occupied sites and the results are given in the limit of infinite chain length s. We note the appearance of the ratio $3c/s$, a characteristic flexibility parameter, viz., degrees of freedom per segment, which determines the value of y from Equation 4. Now the numerical values of the scaling parameters are obtained from a graphical or numerical superposition of experimental or computed isotherms and isobars. One may expect then to establish in this manner also appropriate values of $3c/s$ for different systems. This however does not turn out to be the case, since the isotherms and isobars computed for widely different values of this ratio are superimposable. An a priori specification is required and most reasonably attempted for simple compounds as the starting members of a homologous series whose equations of state can be analyzed. We will not concern

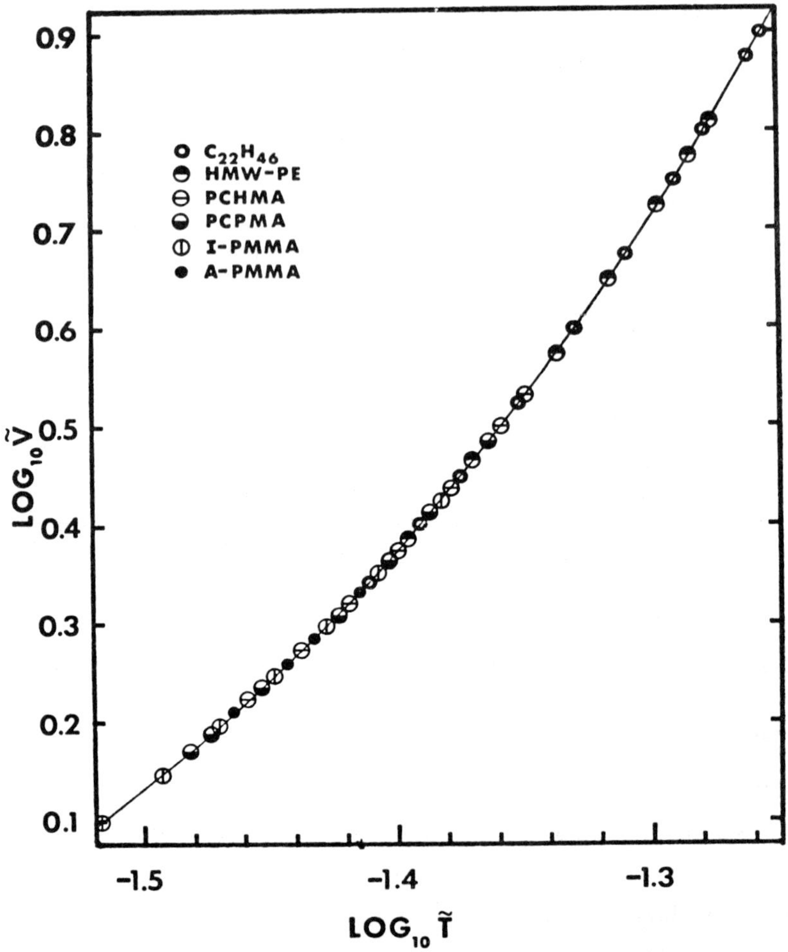

FIGURE 1. Atmospheric pressure isobar for representative polymer melts and a *n*-paraffin liquid. Line: Equations 1 and 4. (From Simha & Wilson.[6] By permission of *Macromolecules*.)

ourselves further with this question but revert to it in the discussion of thermal properties in the glassy state. Our procedure will be to adopt a value of $3c/s = 1$ in Equation 4. Physically this amounts to the replacement of the real (infinitely long) chain by an *s*-mer with effectively unrestricted bond rotations. The structural distinctions between different polymers then are reflected in the relation of the segment to the actual repeat unit. In a structurally simple chain, for example in polymethylene, more than 2 CH_2 units turn out to define the segment. In the highly substituted poly(cyclohexyl methacrylate) in contrast, a half (averaged) unit defines the segment.[5] The assignment of a universal value to the above flexibility ratio in Equation 4 has two consequences. It validates a formal principle of corresponding states and secondly it makes the temperature scaling parameter T^* ($\tilde{T} = T/T^*$) a comparative measure of the maximum segmental cohesion.[1,5]

A few examples will suffice for our purposes to illustrate the application of Equations 1–4. In FIGURE 1 a reduced isobar at atmospheric pressure is displayed, with the solid line representing the theory.[6] The reduced temperature range has been enlarged by the inclusion of a C_{22} paraffin. In FIGURE 2 a series of reduced isotherms for polymers of styrene and *o*-methyl styrene is exhibited.[7] The maximum pressure is 2 kbar and the temperatures extend to 90 and 70 degrees respectively above the glass temperature T_g. Finally we show in FIGURE 3 a reduced plot of the internal energy as a function of the applied pressure.[5] Similar and detailed results for poly(vinyl acetate) at a series of temperatures have been described recently.[8] Having demonstrated the position of the theory in respect to the equation of state, one anticipates a similar kind of agreement for the compressional entropy.[5,8]

The Liquid-Glass Transition

The preceding discussion serves as a prelude to the examination of the intersections of liquid and glassy PVT surfaces. The analysis will center around the behavior of the hole fraction, introduced in Equations 1–4 as a structural parameter. As will be shown in the next section, we have gone farther in formulating a *PVT* surface for a properly defined glass than was hitherto possible. However, the aim of predicting a priori the *existence* of a transition, remains elusive. Such a theoretical prediction must of course arise from kinetic arguments.

In "fast" *PVT* experimentation two general types of glasses and hence inter-

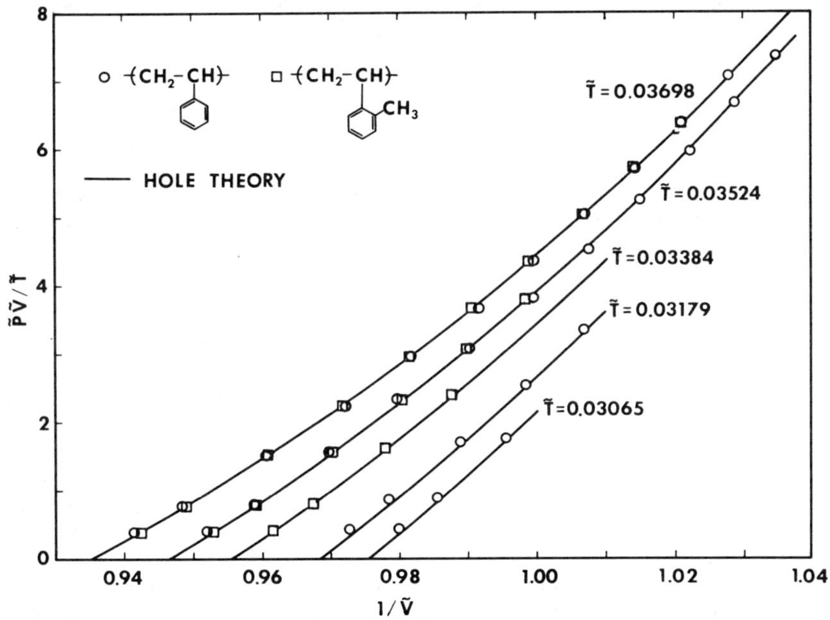

FIGURE 2. Reduced isotherms for styrene polymer melts. Lines: Equations 1 and 4. (From Quach & Simha.[7] By permission of the *Journal of Applied Physics*.)

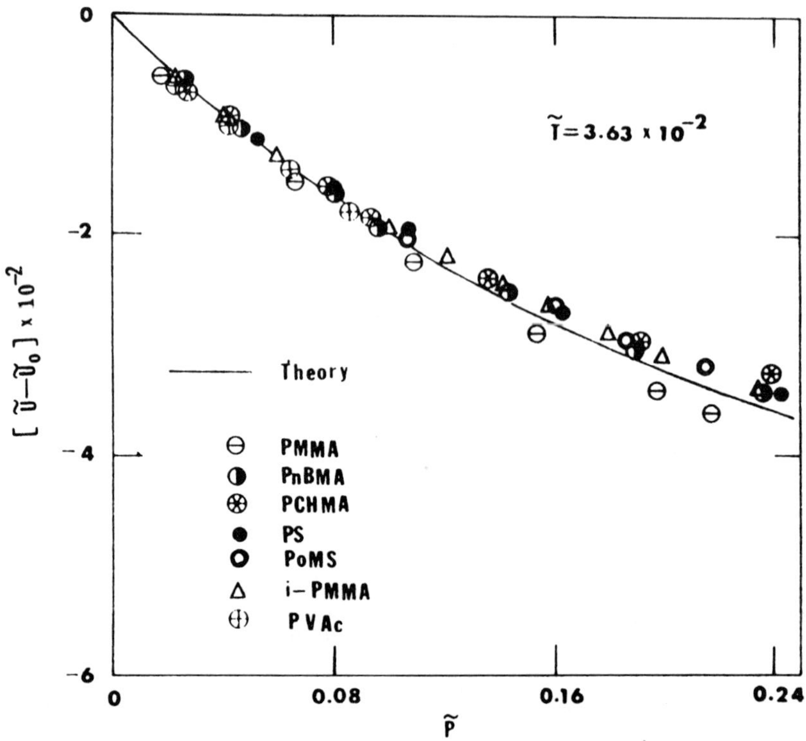

FIGURE 3. Reduced internal energy as a function of reduced pressure at fixed reduced temperature. Line: Equation 2. (From Olabisi & Simha.[5] By permission of *Macromolecules*.)

section lines can be distinguished as a consequence of their nonequilibrium character. Any characteristic quantity Q such as the volume may be regarded as a function of two sets of variables, i.e.,

$$Q = Q(P, T; P' \text{ or } T', r).$$

Besides the usual variables P and T, there is a set of "historical" quantities, namely a formation pressure or temperature and a time scaling factor r, such as a cooling rate. A constant formation history is generated, for example, by cooling at constant r and P' into the glassy range.[7,9–11] The intersection of the PVT surface of this glass with the liquid surface then yields a $T_g^{\dagger}$–P line, or a series of such lines for different formation histories. In the more usual procedure the liquid is subjected to different pressures and an examination of a series of isobars intersecting with liquid isobars then yields a T_g–P line. The two sets of lines may intersect but in general will not coincide. In the first instance we can think of a "single physical substance"[11,14] and ask meaningful quasi-thermodynamic questions, whereas in the second case we are dealing with different substances. We note that as an alternative, a constant formation system may be generated by pressurizing at a constant rate r and a formation temperature T'. One may then inquire into the relations between different transition lines. We will deal with this in the frame of the theory, that is, in terms of the hole parameter $h = 1 - y$.

Consider the following equation:

$$dT_g/dP = (\partial T/\partial P)_h + (\partial T/\partial h)_p \, dh/dP. \quad (5)$$

The first derivative on the right hand side defines a line along which the structural parameter h remains constant. The relation between the three variables T, P, and h is governed by the equilibrium equation of the state, i.e., Equations 1 and 4. On the other hand we have, in terms of the changes in thermal expansion (α) and compressibility (κ), the equation[11,13,14]:

$$dT_g^{\dagger}/dP = \Delta\kappa/\Delta\alpha. \quad (6)$$

By considering the volume V as a function of T, P, and h, the right hand side can be transformed with the result[15]:

$$dT_g^{\dagger}/dP = (\partial T/\partial P)_h F_P/F_T. \quad (7)$$

Here F_P and F_T represent the so-called freezing fractions[6,16] defined as follows:

$$F_{X_i} = 1 - (\partial h/\partial X_i)_{X_{k,g}} / (\partial h/\partial X_i)_{X_{k,l}} \quad i \neq k \quad (8)$$

where X_i and X_k stand for pressure or temperature and the subscripts g and l refer to the glass and liquid. The F_{X_i} measure the extent of freeze-in of the ordering parameter h at the transition and may vary between 1 and 0. The derivatives for the melt are obtained from Equations 1 and 4. We defer a further consideration of the F_{X_i} to the next section, except to mention that *both* F_P and F_T have been evaluated at the transition temperature for two systems, namely selenium[12] and poly(vinyl acetate.[16] Although the numerical values are quite different, the former being practically completely frozen in, within less than 7% $F_P \simeq F_T$ for both. Thus, we should have

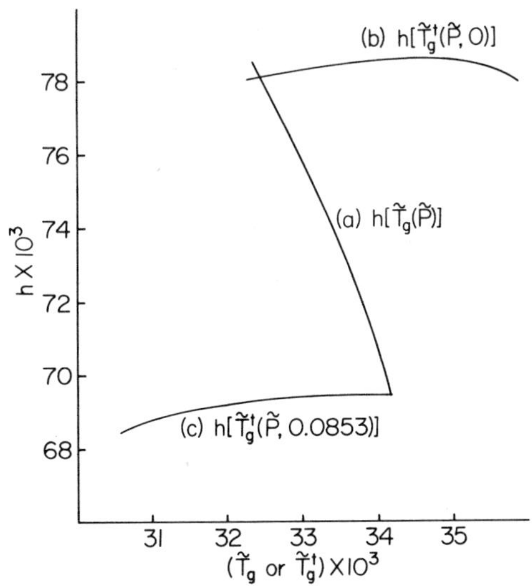

FIGURE 4. Behavior of hole fraction h along transition lines of variable and two constant formation glasses of poly(vinyl acetate). (From McKinney & Simha.[16] By permission of *Macromolecules*.)

$$dT_g^\dagger/dP = \Delta\kappa/\Delta\alpha \simeq (\partial T/\partial P)_h, \tag{7'}$$

and hence a generalized Ehrenfest-type relation[11]

$$dT_g/dP \simeq \Delta\kappa/\Delta\alpha + (\partial T/\partial h)_P \, dh/dP. \tag{8}$$

Since the last term is negative, there results: $dT_g/dP \leq \Delta\kappa/\Delta\alpha$, in accord with observation. The near constancy of h along the $T_g^\dagger$–P line and the validity of Equations 7′ and 8 have been the object of several investigations.[10,12,16] We illustrate by means of poly(vinyl acetate) where two constant formation glasses are available, generated at $P' = 1$ and 800 bar, respectively.[11] FIGURE 4 contrasts the pronounced variation of h along the T_g–P line, to be anticipated, with the near constancy along the two $T_g^\dagger$–P lines. This result enables us to predict or at least estimate the pressure coefficient of $T_g^\dagger$ without a knowledge of the compressibility and expansivity changes occurring at the transition. Moreover, it becomes possible to predict the densification coefficient $(\partial V/\partial P')_{P,T}$.[15] Detailed numerical examinations of Equation 8 for polymer glasses[8,10,16] indicate that the relationship between the transition lines of the constant and variables formation glasses is regulated by the behavior of the h function, which plays the role of an ordering parameter.

The Glassy State

Our objects of investigation are constant formation glasses. The basic assumption here is that the behavior of the h function is the crucial issue, everything else remaining as in the equilibrium melt. It is pertinent to note the fundamental differences between this and the approaches of other authors invoking hole models. First, of course, they arrive at different expressions than are shown in Equations 1–4. Secondly, they do not examine the experimental data of the melt to the extent necessary. Finally they assume without any proof that their hole parameters freeze at the transition and proceed to derive analytical relationships. While h has been shown to be constant along the $T_g^\dagger$–P lines, this does not necessarily imply constancy in the glassy state. Consider then the standard relations involving the Helmholtz free energy F:

$$-P = -P_1 - P_2 = (\partial F/\partial V)_{T,h} + (\partial F/\partial h)_{V,T}(\partial h/\partial V)_T, \tag{9}$$

$$-S = -S_1 - S_2 = (\partial F/\partial T)_{V,h} + (\partial F/\partial h)_{V,T}(\partial h/\partial T)_V, \tag{10}$$

and a corresponding relation for $U = F + TS$. The subscript 1 denotes the value of the function at thermodynamic equilibrium which is characterized by the vanishing of the second derivative on the right hand side of Equations 9 and 10. This is the condition expressed by Equation 4. However, the first term only survives also if h represents indeed a frozen ordering parameter and the last derivatives in Equations 9 and 10 vanish. This term may then be regarded as a quasi-lattice contribution. This, of course, does not render the equations of state of the melt and the frozen glass identical. If we accept Equation 1, y is an explicit function of V and T in the case of the melt, whereas in the frozen glass y is a constant equal to its value at the transition. Formally, the expressions 1–3 become identical with those of the cell theory.[4] To proceed and be consistent with our basic hypothesis, which treats the different behavior of the hole function h as the distinguishing feature of liquid and glass, we retain the mathematical form of the configurational partition function and hence of F and its derivatives, Equations 9 and 10. It remains then to reevaluate the derivatives of h. If this is to be accomplished on theoretical grounds, an additional postulate must be introduced as a replacement of the previous minimization of F. Alternatively this dependence may be derived from the experimental equation of state. This requires the numerical solution of the partial differential equation, Equation 9. The accuracy and physical adequacy of this procedure can then be tested by comparing the resulting thermodynamic functions with experiment. Such a program has been executed recently[8] for the poly(vinyl acetate) glasses studied by McKinney and

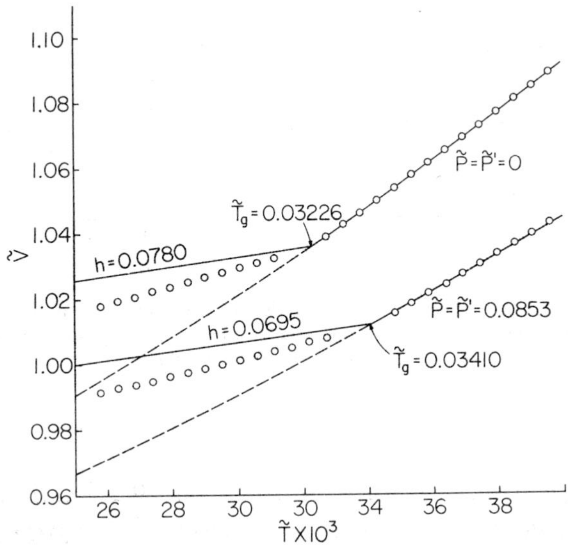

FIGURE 5. Isobars for melt, two glasses, and undercooled melt (dashed line) of poly (vinyl acetate). Points experimental. (From McKinney & Simha.[16] By permission of *Macromolecules*.)

Goldstein.[11] The numerical labor is somewhat involved, but on the other hand, it is desirable to study glasses with a range of molecular structures and glass temperatures. Hence it is gratifying to find that the results do not differ very significantly from those derived by a simplified procedure.[5,6,10,16] It rests entirely on Equation 1–3. That is, the equation of state is utilized to obtain y from Equation 1 and the result then substituted into Equations 2 and 3.

The next two figures serve as illustrations. In FIGURE 5 isobars with $P = P'$ are displayed for three sets. For the melts we have a satisfactory coincidence between experimental and theoretical curves, with the latter extrapolated into the glassy region. Also shown are the lattice contributions, h = constant, and finally the measured volumes. Clearly, h does not represent a frozen ordering parameter in the sense of Davies and Jones,[17] in this instance down to some sixty degrees below the normal glass temperature. The temperature dependence of h continues

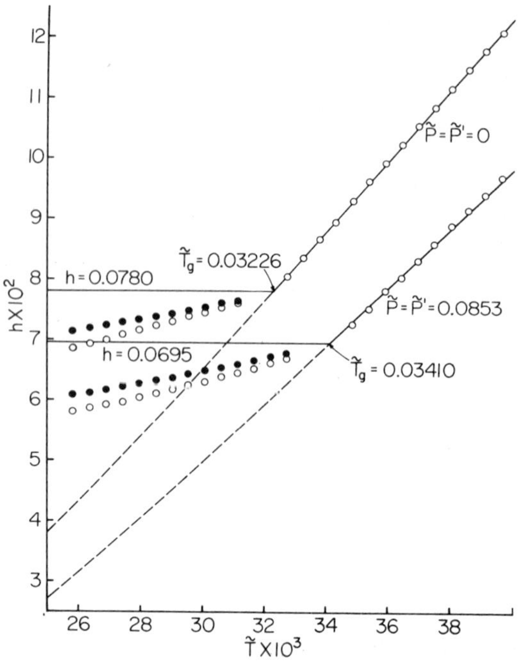

FIGURE 6. Temperature dependence of hole fraction above and below transition in poly(vinyl acetate). Open circles, simplified procedure, see text; full circles, Equation 9. (From McKinney & Simha.[8] By permission of *Macromolecules*.)

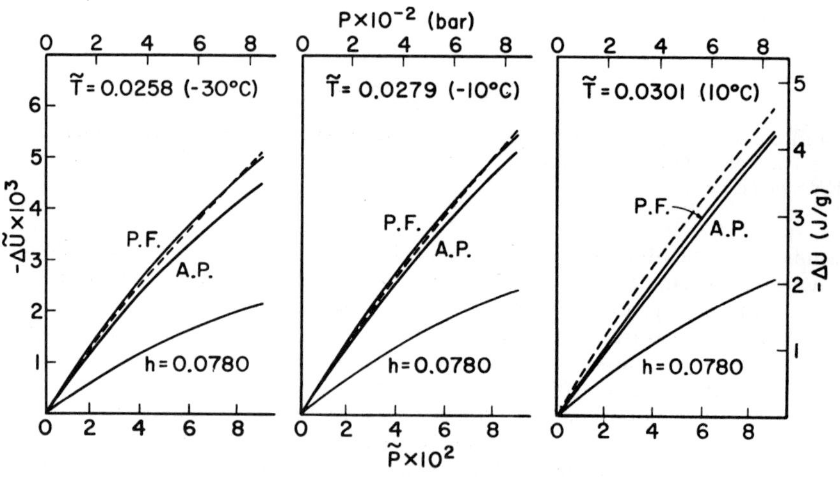

FIGURE 7. Internal energy as a function of pressure for constant formation (P' = 1 bar) glass. Dashed lines: experimental; lower lines: for h = const; P.F.: from Equations 9 and 10; A.P.: simplified procedure, see text. (From McKinney & Simha.[8] By permission of *Macromolecules*.)

to make a significant contribution to the thermal expansivity. This is explicitly seen in FIGURE 6, which shows the behavior of h in the melt and the two glasses, computed by means of Equation 9 or by the simpler procedure and Equation 1. With h so determined one can calculate thermodynamic functions by means of Equations 2 and 3, or by Equation 10 and a corresponding relation for U, without any further adjustment admissible. In FIGURE 7 the change ΔU in internal energy is plotted as a function of pressure for the poly(vinyl acetate) glass formed under atmospheric pressure. Three experimental isotherms are exhibited and three procedures illustrated. The adoption of a fixed value for the free volume fraction h is seen to be untenable. The two other solid curves represent the results of the simple adjustment procedure (A.P.) and of solving the complete Equation 9 (P.F.) respectively. A significant improvement appears, but the differences between the consistent and the simplified method of computation are comparatively minor. The same conclusion obtains in regard to the entropy. The differences become large however for the internal pressure $(\partial U/\partial V)_T$.[8] It is fair to say then that the liquid theory provides a quantitative description of the PVT surface in the glassy state when the temperature and pressure dependence of the free volume fraction is evaluated from experiment.

We remark finally that constructions like that shown in FIGURE 6 have yielded the freezing fractions F_T for a number of polymers. Quite generally F_T at atmospheric pressure correlates inversely with the reduced glass temperature.[6] Only in two systems with a very low $\tilde{T}_g$ has a value of F_T as high as 0.9 been found, namely poly(dimethyl siloxane)[6] and selenium.[12] The equation of state for a particular selenium glass is actually well described by assuming a constant value of $h = 0.17$ in Equation 1.

On the basis of the equation-of-state results obtained so far, the temperature and pressure dependence of h automatically introduces several ordering parameters in the majority of cases.[10] Just as this dependence changes in the transition from the melt to the glass, it will change in the course of the familiar subglass relaxations encountered in low and high molecular weight systems and revealed by a variety of dynamic and quasi-static methods. This has been explicitly demonstrated for some polymers.[5,6,19] One may inquire whether and where on the temperature scale a practical freeze-in of the free volume fraction h can be discerned. It can be shown that this occurs for organic polymers in the region below about 50–70 K, depending on the system.[20] A theory, based on this assumption and introducing appropriate quantum corrections, gives a proper account of the experimental thermal expansivity at atmospheric pressure. This is shown in FIGURE 8, which summarizes data for a variety of polymers. We note the following points: First, the actual temperatures do not extend below about 15 K and hence none of the low temperature anomalies, which are a subject of this conference, are visible. Secondly, the principle of corresponding states expressed by the graph, arises from the assumption $\tilde{\theta}$ = constant = 0.005, where $\tilde{\theta}$ represents the reduced quantum temperature at absolute zero. Thirdly, the systematic departures from the theoretical curve at a reduced temperature of about 0.004 are indicative of relaxation processes. For systems not undergoing such phenomena, the theory indeed remains adequate to higher temperatures than shown here.[21]

The discussion has so far dealt with the equation of state and the pressure dependence of the configurational internal energy and entropy, all quantities where an unequivocal confrontation between experiment and theory is possible. We note now some additional predictions of the latter.[8]

The notion has been advanced on various occasions that contributions to the

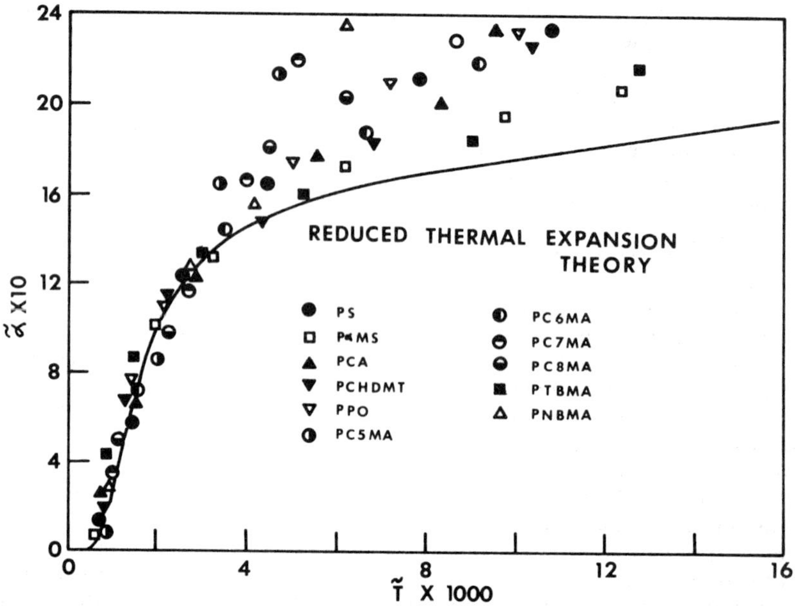

FIGURE 8. Reduced thermal expansivity of organic polymers at low temperatures. Line: theory, see text. (From Simha *et al.*[20] By permission of the *Journal of Applied Physics*.)

thermodynamic functions other then lattice-type ones are effectively frozen not too far below the glass transition region. This is contradicted by the results discussed, and this contradiction can be illustrated again in terms of the relative magnitudes of lattice and hole contributions to the configurational entropy. We write

$$S(\text{hole}) = S(h) - S(0),$$

where the last term is computed by means of the cell theory. At some 60 degrees below the T_g of poly(vinyl acetate) an appreciable fraction of the total computed configurational entropy is due to hole structure as is seen in TABLE 1, with the smaller contribution for the densified species.

Next we turn to the heat capacities and derived entropy data by making use of recent measurements of Weeks[22] at atmospheric pressure and computations[8]

TABLE 1

ENTROPY RELATIONS FOR POLY(VINYL ACETATE) AT −30°C AND ATMOSPHERIC PRESSURE

	V	$h \times 10^2$	$-\tilde{S}(h)$ + const	$\tilde{S}$(hole)	$\tilde{S}$(hole) / $-\tilde{S}(h)$ + const
Liquid	0.9953	4.22	0.477	0.0817	0.17
Glass ($P' = 0$)	1.0181	7.15	0.431	0.111	0.26
Glass ($P' = 800$)	1.0110	6.25	0.444	0.103	0.23

based on the equation of state results for poly(vinyl acetate) described above. The information is summarized in TABLE 2. We note first that the computed theoretical C_p, which represents the contribution of the external degrees of freedom, amounts to 19% of the total in the melt and only 8% in the glass. A somewhat smaller value, 12%, is found for liquid polystyrene and poly(methyl methacrylate).[8] Next we observe that less than one half of the total change of C_p at the transition can be ascribed to the configurational terms computed. The ratio is even further reduced in C_v. This however should not be ascribed to purely numerical inadequacies of the theory. Such do not appear in the pressure dependence of the thermodynamic functions. Moreover consider the standard relation

$$C_p - C_v = TV\alpha^2/\kappa,$$

which expresses the fact that the difference between the two heat capacities is practically configurational in origin. The experimental and computed values of this difference, as derived from the equation of state, are in good agreement for

TABLE 2

HEAT CAPACITY DATA FOR POLY(VINYL ACETATE) AT $T_g = 304$ K*

	Liquid		Glass ($P' = 0$)
$C_p(T = T_g)$ (exptl)	1.77		1.27
C_p(theor)/C_P(exptl)	0.19		0.08
$(C_p - C_v)(T = T_g)$(exptl)	0.261		0.069
(theor)	0.250		0.055
ΔC_p (exptl)		0.500	
(theor)		0.234	
ΔC_v (exptl)		0.310	
(theor)		0.039	
$S_g - S_l(T = 273)$(exptl)		0.055	
(theor)		0.023	

*All units in J/(g K).

both liquid and glass. Next it is of interest to estimate the entropy difference between the glass and the hypothetical melt below T_g. From the calorimetric data[22] there follow the results in the last two lines of TABLE 2. Again, the computed difference is only 42% of the experimental value.

Finally, we refer to observations of the enthalpy difference between a normal and a depressurized glass. The theory predicts the latter to have the lower value. Experimentally[23] the reverse is found for formation pressures exceeding about 800 bar, with practically no difference at smaller pressures.

The results described are suggestive of an incompleteness in the theory. Such an incompleteness, however, is not apparent in pressure studies, at least below 2 kbar. Recall the basic assumption, which ascribes the difference between the *PVT* surfaces of liquid and glass solely to a different dependence of the hole function h on the variables of state and otherwise maintains the partition function, developed for the equilibrium liquid. We see that more is required to account for the relation between the entropy surfaces. Phenomenologically, one may raise the question whether different temperatures $T_g^\dagger$ may be defined by the intersections of different thermodynamic surfaces.

Reverting to the theory, we recall the assignment of a fixed number $3c$ of external degrees of freedom or "soft" modes per chain. The scaling temperature T^* is inversely and the reduced temperature $\tilde{T}$ is directly related to c. If some of these modes freeze out over the transition range, the reduced temperature will be lower for a given T than we have assumed. It is pertinent to note in this connection that the temperature coefficient of C_p is usually larger in the glass than in the liquid. That is, the curvature of the entropy isobar is more pronounced in the glass.

Referring to the entropy, Equation 10, it appears that an additional term, arising from the temperature dependence of a second parameter, must be introduced. Even if the formal expression 9 is maintained, that is, this parameter does not sensitively vary with volume, the pressure will also be affected by this modification. This then is one of the problems requiring experimental *and* theoretical attention. A second question concerns the hole function $h(V, T)$. So far, it has been extracted from experimental PVT surfaces. Can a theory be devised that accounts for the partial freeze-in observed? This partial effect is particularly pronounced in high T_g polymers. These also retain the largest values of h at T_g. To illustrate: For poly(dimethyl siloxane) with a T_g of 150 K, $h(T_g) \simeq 1\%$. In poly(α-methylstyrene), $T_g = 455$ K, and $h(T_g) \simeq 10\%$.[6] Correspondingly, in the former, hole clustering will be minimal and actually a number average cluster size of 1.06 is computed. In the second polymer, this number has increased to 2.5.[5] Thus, a partial freeze-in of molecular motion near small holes, while keeping large clusters thermally alive,[24] will result in additional contributions to the thermal expansivity and other configurational functions.

References

1. Simha, R. & T. Somcynsky. 1969. Macromolecules **2:** 342–350.
2. For example, Simha, R. 1975. Rheol. Acta **14:** 12–18.
3. Lennard-Jones, J. E. & A. F. Devonshire. 1938. Proc. R. Soc. (London) **A165:** 1–11.
4. Pirgogine, I. 1957. The Molecular Theory of Solutions. North Holland Publishing Co.. Amsterdam.
5. Olabisi, O. & R. Simha. 1975. Macromolecules **8:** 211–218.
6. Simha, R. & P. S. Wilson. 1973. Macromolecules **6:** 908–914.
7. Quach, A. & R. Simha. 1971. J. Appl. Phys. **42:** 4592–4606.
8. McKinney, J. E. & R. Simha. 1976. Macromolecules **9:** 430–441.
9. Quach, A. & R. Simha. 1971. Macromolecules **4:** 268–270.
10. Quach, A. & R. Simha. 1972. J. Phys. Chem. **76:** 416–421.
11. McKinney, J. E. & M. Goldstein. 1974. J. Res. Nat. Bur. Stand., Sect. A, **78:** 331–353.
12. Berg, J. I. & R. Simha. 1976. J. Non-Cryst. Sol. In press.
13. Passaglia, E. & G. M. Martin. 1964. J. Res. Nat. Bur. Stand., Sect. A, **68:** 273–276.
14. Goldstein, M. 1973. J. Phys. Chem. **77:** 667–673.
15. McKinney, J. E. & R. Simha. J. Res. Nat. Bur. Stand., Sect. A. Submitted for publication.
16. McKinney, J. E. & R. Simha. 1974. Macromolecules **7:** 894–901.
17. An excellent review of Ehrenfest relations and their physical basis is presented in: Rehage, G. & W. Borchard. 1973. *In* Physics of Glassy Polymers. R. N. Haward, Ed.: 54–107. Applied Science Publishers, Ltd. London.
18. Moynihan, C. T. & U. E. Schnaus. 1971. J. Amer. Ceram. Soc. **54:** 136–140.
19. Quach, A., P. S. Wilson & R. Simha. 1974. J. Macromol. Sci. **B9**(3): 533–550.
20. Simha, R., J. M. Roe & V. S. Nanda. 1972. J. Appl. Phys. **43:**4312–4317.
21. Midha, Y. R. & V. S. Nanda. 1975. J. Appl. Phys. **46:** 3710–3711.
22. Weeks, J. J. 1975. Private communication.
23. For example: Price C., R. C. Williams & R. C. Ayerst. 1972. Amorphous Materials. R. W. Douglas & B. Ellis, Eds.: 117–124. Wiley-Interscience. New York, N.Y.
24. Somcynsky, T. & R. Simha. 1971. J. Appl. Phys. **42:** 4545–4548.

STRUCTURAL RELAXATION IN VITREOUS MATERIALS*

C. T. Moynihan, P. B. Macedo, C. J. Montrose, P. K. Gupta, M. A. DeBolt, J. F. Dill, B. E. Dom, P. W. Drake, A. J. Easteal, P. B. Elterman, R. P. Moeller, H. Sasabe, and J. A. Wilder

Vitreous State Laboratory
Catholic University of America
Washington, DC 20064

Introduction

When a liquid is subjected to a sudden change in temperature T or pressure P, its properties (volume V, enthalpy H, index of refraction n, shear viscosity η, etc.) exhibit an instantaneous, solidlike change. This is followed by a slower, liquidlike structural relaxation to new equilibrium values at the new temperature or pressure. It is generally presumed that this structural relaxation involves some change of the average molecular configuration of the liquid. The time scale for the structural relaxation increases rapidly with decreasing temperature and increasing pressure and in the so-called glass transition region—which should be thought of as an area in the T–P plane—reaches magnitudes (seconds to days) readily perceptible to human investigators. Above the glass transition region, (i.e., at temperatures above and pressures below) the structure rearranges promptly in response to changes in T or P and measured properties (H, V, n, etc.) are said to be those of the equilibrium liquid. Below the glass transition region (i.e., at temperatures below and pressures above), the structural rearrangement is kinetically arrested, measured changes in properties (H, V, n, etc.) in response to changes in T and P do not contain contributions from the structural rearrangement, and the material is referred to as a glass. As a consequence, there is in general a difference between the second derivatives of Gibbs free energy—namely, heat capacity C_p, the thermal expansion coefficient α, and isothermal compressibility, κ—for equilibrium liquid and glass.

In FIGURES 1 and 2 the time dependence of liquid properties due to the structural relaxation is shown schematically for the the isobaric response of enthalpy to temperature changes. In FIGURE 1 the system is initially at equilibrium at temperature T_0; the temperature is stepped at time t_1 by an amount ΔT. Immediately the system exhibits the solidlike enthalpy change ΔH_g from the initial equilibrium value H_{e0} at T_0; this is followed by a further change with time by an amount ΔH_r due to the structural relaxation to the equilibrium value H_{e1} at the new temperature. The equilibrium liquid and glass heat capacities, C_{pe} and C_{pg}, are then defined in terms of this experiment by

$$C_{pg} = \lim_{\substack{\Delta T \to 0 \\ (t - t_1) = 0}} [(H - H_{e0})/\Delta T] = \lim_{\Delta T \to 0} \Delta H_g/\Delta T,$$

$$C_{pe} = \lim_{\substack{\Delta T \to 0 \\ (t - t_1) \to \infty}} [(H - H_{e0})/\Delta T] = \lim_{\Delta T \to 0} [(\Delta H_g + \Delta H_r)/\Delta T],$$

*This research was supported by contracts from the Office of Naval Research and the Air Force Office of Scientific Research.

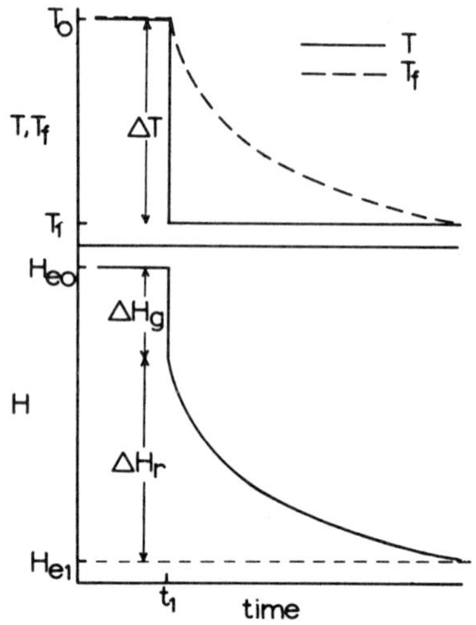

FIGURE 1. Isothermal evolution of enthalpy and fictive temperature following a single temperature step.

where the limitation to small ΔT is introduced to take into account that C_{pg} and C_{pe} may in general be temperature dependent.

FIGURE 2 shows the response of the enthalpy when the liquid is cooled isobarically through the glass transition region at a constant rate

$$q = \mathrm{d}T/\mathrm{d}t,$$

and subsequently reheated through the same temperature interval at a rate of the same magnitude. Rate heating or cooling may be thought of as a series of differential temperature steps, dT, each of which is followed by an isothermal hold of duration dt = dT/q. During the initial part of the rate cool the temperature is sufficiently high that the time required for the structural relaxation is short compared to the experimental time scale established by the cooling rate, so that the H-T curve follows that for the equilibrium liquid. At lower temperatures the time required for structural relaxation becomes longer, so that following a temperature step dT the time dT/q is not sufficient for the liquid to equilibrate and the experi-

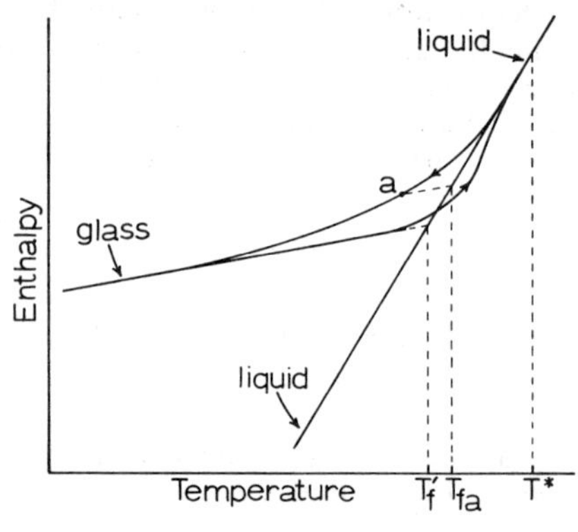

FIGURE 2. Evolution of enthalpy during cooling and subsequent heating at a constant rate.

mental H-T curve departs from the equilibrium liquid curve. Finally, well below the glass transition region the structural relaxation times become so long that no further changes take place in the configurational state of the system on further cooling, and the H-T curve corresponds to that for the glass.

Irrespective of the direction of temperature change, the direction of the structural relaxation process is always toward equilibrium, that is, at any given point on either the heating or cooling H-T curve, the structural relaxation acts in such a fashion as to eventually bring the experimental H-T curve into coincidence with the equilibrium liquid H-T curve. Consequently on reheating the H-T curve evolves along a different path from that for the prior cool, as shown in FIGURE 2. Typically on reheating at a rate comparable to the cooling rate, the H-T curve "overshoots" the equilibrium liquid curve and then at higher temperatures, where the structural relaxation is rapid, rejoins it from below.

The heat capacity, C_p, is the slope of the H-T curves of FIGURE 2. Consequently during cooling through the transition region C_p drops monotonically from the value C_{pe} associated with the equilibrium liquid to the value C_{pg} associated with the glass. On reheating C_p typically departs from the C_{pg} value rather sharply, passes through a maximum, and then decreases at high temperatures to C_{pe}.

In the present paper we report some recent results of an ongoing program of study at the Vitreous State Laboratory of the structural relaxation in and slightly above the glass transition region. We have carried out experiments exemplified by FIGURES 1 and 2, as well as other studies accomplished by a novel and markedly different technique—digital correlation spectroscopy.

Our primary aim at the present has been to develop and test a phenomenological treatment of the kinetics of the structural relaxation capable of describing the time evolution of liquid properties in response to any arbitrary T-P-t program. Secondarily, by comparing the kinetic parameters for different properties of the same liquid, we hope to gain some insight into the microscopic nature of the structural relaxation. Additional detail on the material presented below, particularly with regard to historical background and experimental techniques, has been presented in a series of recent papers from this laboratory.[1-9]

KINETICS OF THE STRUCTURAL RELAXATION

In this section we outline briefly the phenomenological description of the kinetics of the structural relaxation for the general nonlinear case in which the system is far removed from equilibrium. We will confine our discussion to the case in which the system is removed from structural equilibrium by rapid isobaric temperature changes, since this is the case corresponding to our experiments. An analogous treatment of structural relaxation following rapid isothermal pressure changes is straightforward.

Fictive Temperature

It is convenient to characterize the configurational or structural state of a system at temperature T as measured in terms of a macroscopic property by a fictive temperature T_f. In terms of FIGURE 1 for the property enthalpy, T_f is defined by

$$\frac{T_f - T_1}{\Delta T} = \frac{H - H_{e1}}{\Delta Hr}, \tag{1}$$

for temperature changes ΔT small enough that C_{pe} and C_{pg} may be taken as constant. Hence, as shown in FIGURE 1, T_f changes from T_0 to T_1 in parallel with the evolution of the enthalpy from $(H_{e1} - \Delta H_r)$ to H_{e1}.

A more general definition of T_f, applicable to the characterization of the structural state during any arbitrary T-t program, is, again in terms of the property enthalpy,

$$H(T) = H_e(T_f) - \int_T^{T_f} C_{pg}\, dT', \tag{2}$$

where $H_e(T_f)$ is the equilibrium value of the enthalpy at temperature T_f. As shown in FIGURE 2, T_f via Equation 2 is determined by the temperature of intersection with the equilibrium liquid H-T curve of a line drawn through the (H, T) point of interest parallel to the glass H-T curve, e.g., the fictive temperature at point a on the cooling curve is T_{fa}. In terms of Equations 1 and 2, T_f is thus the relaxational part of the enthalpy expressed in temperature units, while differentiation of Equation 2 shows that the isobaric temperature coefficient of T_f at temperature T

$$\frac{dT_f}{dT} = \frac{(C_p - C_{pg})\mid_T}{(C_{pe} - C_{pg})\mid_{T_f}} \tag{3}$$

is the relaxational part of the heat capacity normalized to zero for the glass and to unity for the equilibrium liquid. The equilibrium state at temperature T thus corresponds to the condition $T_f(T) = T$. Note also from FIGURE 2 that on rate cooling through the transition region the glass at low temperatures eventually reaches a constant value designated T_f'.

T_f may be defined analogously in terms of other macroscopic properties (V, n, η, etc.). It is important to note that T_f as used here is strictly a measure of the relaxational part of the macroscopic property, so that values of T_f assessed from different macroscopic properties for the same nonequilibrium glass are not necessarily identical.

Isothermal Relaxation in Response to a Single Temperature Step

The time evolution of T_f following a single isobaric temperature step from equilibrium at time t_1 as shown in FIGURE 1 may be described by a relaxation function, $\phi(t - t_1, t)$ defined by

$$T_f(t) = T_0 + \Delta T[1 - \phi(t - t_1, t)], \tag{4}$$

so that (cf. Equation 1)

$$\lim_{t - t_1 \to 0} \phi(t - t_1, t) = 1,$$

$$\lim_{t - t_1 \to \infty} \phi(t - t_1, t) = 0.$$

Experimentally $\phi(t - t_1, t)$ is found to be both *nonexponential* and *nonlinear*.

It is nonexponential in the sense that for very small departures from equilibrium ($\Delta T \to 0$) $\partial \ln \phi(t, t - t_1)/\partial t$ is not constant. In such cases, however, an equilibrium relaxation function, $\phi_e(t - t_1)$, may be represented as an integral of weighted exponential terms:

$$\lim_{\Delta T \to 0} \phi(t - t_1, t) \equiv \phi_e(t - t_1)$$

$$= \int_{-\infty}^{\infty} g\left(\ln \frac{\tau_e}{\tau_e'}\right) \exp[-(t - t_1)/\tau_e] \, d \ln \frac{\tau_e}{\tau_e'} \qquad (5)$$

where τ_e and τ_e' are temperature-dependent relaxation times, τ_e' being a reference time. The function $g(\ln \tau_e/\tau_e')$ is the relaxation time probability density function subject to the normalization condition

$$\int_{-\infty}^{\infty} g\left(\ln \frac{\tau_e}{\tau_e'}\right) d \ln \frac{\tau_e}{\tau_e'} = 1.$$

In common parlance $g(\ln \tau_e/\tau_e')$ represents the spectrum of relaxation times.

An empirical expression for the equilibrium relaxation function of Equation 5 that has been found to give an excellent fit to a wide variety of relaxation processes in vitreous systems and which we will assume throughout the remainder of this paper is of the form

$$\phi_e(t - t_1) = \exp\{-[(t - t_1)/\tau_{0e}]^{\beta}\}, \qquad (6)$$

where τ_{0e} is a characteristic relaxation time. A given value of $\beta(0 < \beta \leq 1)$ uniquely specifies the probability density function $g(\ln \tau_e/\tau_e')$.[10] The spectrum of relaxation times corresponding to Equation 6 broadens with decreasing β and is asymmetric on a logarithmic relaxation time scale, being skewed toward shorter times, although not as asymmetric as the Davidson-Cole density function.[11]

For substantial departures from equilibrium the relaxation function exhibits marked nonlinearity in the sense that $\phi(t - t_1, t)$ depends both on temperature T and on structure, i.e., on T_f. Narayanaswamy and Gardon[12,13] have shown that this may be dealt with phenomenologically by allowing the relaxation time in expressions such as Equation 6 to depend explicitly on T and T_f, so that for the nonlinear case far from equilibrium Equation 6 becomes

$$\phi(t - t_1, t) = \exp\left[-\left(\int_{t_1}^{t} dt'/\tau_0\right)^{\beta}\right], \qquad (7)$$

with the relaxation time given by

$$\tau_0 = A \exp\left(\frac{x \Delta h^*}{RT} + \frac{(1 - x)\Delta h^*}{RT_f}\right), \qquad (8)$$

where A, $x(0 \leq x \leq 1)$, and Δh^* are constants, and R is the ideal gas constant. Note that τ_0 of Equations 7 and 8 and τ_{0e} of Equation 6 become identical in the limit very close to equilibrium where $\Delta T \to 0$ and $T_f \to T$. That is, Δh^*, the activation enthalpy for the relaxation process, expresses the temperature dependence of the relaxation time for the linear regime close to equilibrium:

$$\Delta h^* = R \lim_{T_f \to T} \left(\frac{\partial \ln \tau_0}{\partial(1/T)}\right) \equiv R\left(\frac{\partial \ln \tau_{0e}}{\partial(1/T)}\right) \qquad (9)$$

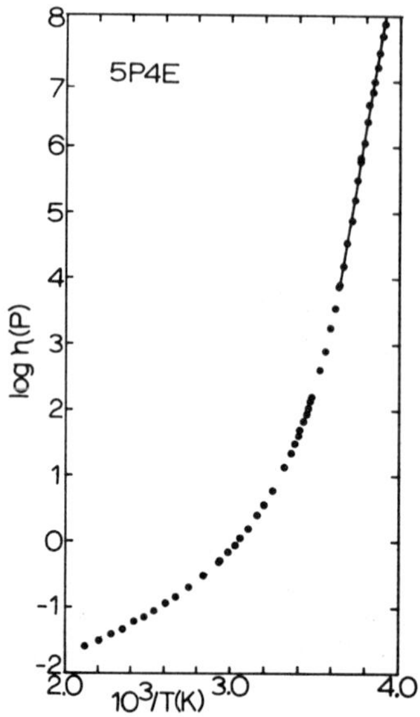

FIGURE 3. Arrhenius plot of shear viscosity of 5-phenyl-4-ether at 1 atm. The solid line is a least squares fit of the data above $10^4 P$ to the Arrhenius equation $\eta = B\exp(\Delta h^*/RT)$ with $B = 6.8 \times 10^{-53}$ P and $\Delta h^* = 70{,}322$ cal/mole.

The assumption that Δh^* is both constant and the same for each relaxation time in the spectrum implied by Equations 6 or 7 signifies respectively Arrhenius behavior and "thermorheological simplicity" or a "temperature independent spectrum of relaxation times." The former assumption may be justified in part on the basis that, as will be shown below, Δh^* for the structural relaxation is generally quite close to the activation enthalpy for the shear viscosity η. In the high viscosity regime, which includes the glass transition region, most liquids—and this includes all liquids considered in our studies to date—exhibit an Arrhenius temperature dependence.[14-16] This is illustrated in FIGURE 3 with viscosity data obtained by us with capillary and rotating cylinder viscometers for the lubricant 5-phenyl-4-ether [5P4E, $C_6H_5(OC_6H_4)_3OC_6H_5$].

FIGURE 4. Evolution of the fictive temperature calculated from refractive index n for vitreous B_2O_3 following a single temperature step at time $t_1 = 0$ from $T_0 = 539.2$ K to $T_1 = 536.4$ K. Solid curve is calculated from Equations 4, 7 & 8 using $A = 5.1 \times 10^{-34}$ s, $\Delta h^* = 92$ kcal/mole, $\beta = 0.83$, and $x = 0.50$.

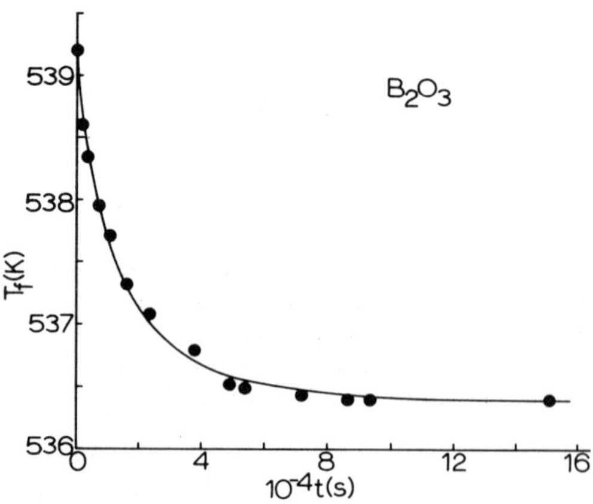

In FIGURE 4 is shown the evolution of the fictive temperature calculated from refractive index n for vitreous B_2O_3 following a single temperature step at time $t_1 = 0$ from $T_0 = 539.2$ K to $T_1 = 536.4$ K.[17] In these experiments the index n was monitored during heat treatment at T_1 by periodically quenching the sample, which arrests the structural relaxation, and measuring n at room temperature, after which the sample was reintroduced into the furnace at T_1 for additional heat treatment. The solid curve in FIGURE 4 is a fit of the data to Equations 4, 7, and 8 using the parameters given in the figure caption. The A and β parameters were adjusted to give the best fit, while the Δh^* and x parameters were set equal respectively to the shear viscosity activation enthalpy[14] and the mean x value (0.50) found by Narayanaswamy[13] for a variety of network glasses.

A similar experiment has been carried out for As_2Se_3 in which the evolution of enthalpy was monitored. A number of As_2Se_3 samples were annealed to equilibrium at temperature $T_0 = 441.2$ K, quenched to room temperature, which arrests

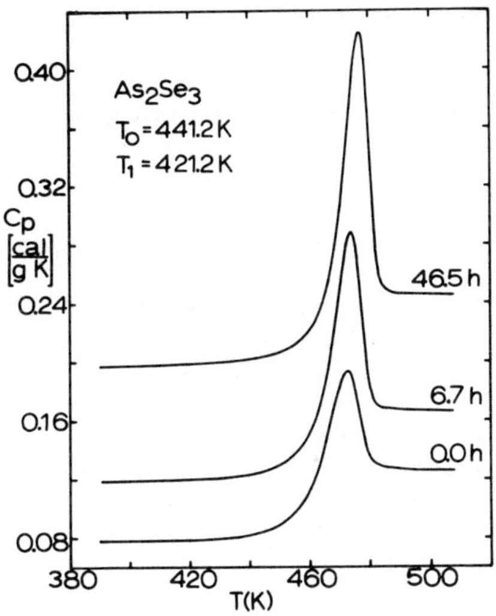

FIGURE 5. Heat capacities of As_2Se_3 glass measured by DSC during heating at 10 K/min for three samples annealed for different times at temperature T_1 following a step change from temperature T_0. The C_p scale is correct for the bottom plot; for clarity the middle and topmost plots have been displaced upward by 0.04 and 0.12 cal/g K, respectively.

the structural relaxation, reintroduced into the furnace at temperature $T_1 = 421.2$ K, annealed at T_1 for various times t, and again quenched to room temperature. The heat capacities were then measured on a differential scanning calorimeter (DSC) in the glass transition region. Typical C_p scans are shown in FIGURE 5 for different annealing times. The increase with annealing time in the area under the heat capacity maximum corresponds to the sample regaining during heating the increasing amounts of enthalpy lost during the correspondingly longer anneals at temperature T_1. The fictive temperatures of the As_2Se_3 glasses following the anneal at T_1 were calculated from the C_p data by integrating Equation 3 from a temperature $T^*(= T_f^*)$ in the equilibrium liquid region (cf. FIGURE 2) to a temperature well below the glass transition region.

In FIGURE 6 these fictive temperatures are plotted versus the logarithm of annealing time. The solid line is the evolution of T_f calculated from Equations 4, 7, and 8. The A, Δh^*, β, and x parameters are given in the caption to FIGURE 12 and

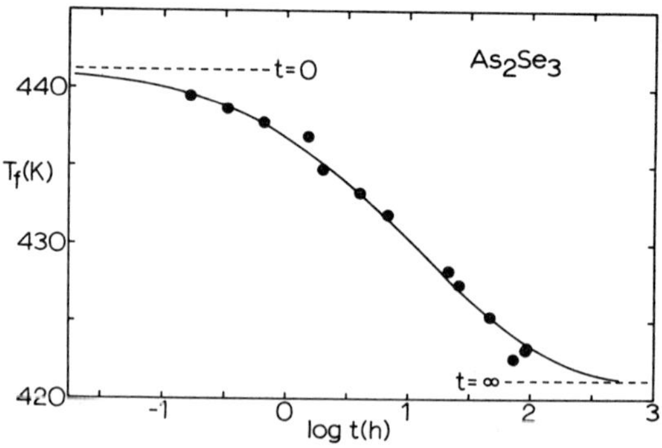

FIGURE 6. Evolution of the fictive temperature calculated from enthalpy H for vitreous As_2Se_3 following a single temperature step at time $t_1 = 0$ from $T_0 = 441.2$ K to $T_1 = 421.2$ K. Solid curve is calculated from Equations 4, 7, and 8 using the parameters given in the caption to FIGURE 12.

were obtained independently from an analysis of entire C_p versus T curves during rate heating, as will be explained in a subsequent section.

Isothermal Relaxation in Response to More Than One Temperature Step

Suppose a liquid initially at equilibrium at temperature T_0 is subjected to a number of temperature steps: ΔT_1 at time t_1, ΔT_2 at time $t_2, \ldots, \Delta T_m$ at time t_m. Provided that the relaxation function is linear—or has been linearized by a procedure such as the Narayanaswamy method[12,13] described in the preceding section—the evolution of T_f for $t \geq t_m$ may be expressed as the superposition of the responses (given by Equation 4) of the system to the various temperature changes at their respective times.

$$T_f(t) = T_0 + \Delta T_1[1 - \phi(t - t_1, t)] + \Delta T_2[1 - \phi(t - t_2, t)] + \cdots + \Delta T_m[1 - \phi(t - t_m, t)$$

$$= T_0 + \sum_{j=1}^{m} \Delta T_j[1 - \phi(t - t_j, t)]. \qquad \textbf{(10)}$$

In evaluating the integrals in the relaxation functions (Equation 7) one must take into account the effect of changes in both T_f and T on the relaxation times (Equation 8).

Situations of the above sort have been investigated in the so-called "crossover" structural relaxation experiment.[13,17–19] Two temperature steps are involved in this experiment. (Recently Corsaro[20] has reported and analyzed by a method identical to that described here crossovers involving two pressure steps.) The temperature is stepped at time t_1 by an amount $\Delta T_1 (= T_1 - T_0)$ and the glass allowed to relax partly to equilibrium at temperature T_1. At time t_2 the temperature is stepped a second time by $\Delta T_2 (= T_2 - T_1)$ to a temperature T_2, which lies between T_0 and T_1, and the evolution of some property and hence of T_f is monitored for times

$t \geq t_2$. Using the relaxation function of Equation 7 in Equation 10 the fictive temperature for $t \geq t_2$ is given by

$$T_f(t) = T_0 + \Delta T_1 \left\{ 1 - \exp\left[-\left(\int_{t_1}^{t_2} \frac{dt'}{\tau_0} + \int_{t_2}^{t} \frac{dt'}{\tau_0} \right)^{\beta} \right] \right\} + \Delta T_2 \left\{ 1 - \exp\left[-\left(\int_{t_2}^{t} \frac{dt'}{\tau_0} \right)^{\beta} \right] \right\} \quad (11)$$

The first integral in the second term on the right hand side does not need to be evaluated explicitly, since, for a given value of β, it may be determined via Equation 11 from the measured fictive temperature at time t_2:

$$\int_{t_1}^{t_2} \frac{dt'}{\tau_0} = \left[-\ln\left(\frac{T_1 - T_f(t_2)}{T_1 - T_0} \right) \right]^{1/\beta}. \quad (12)$$

Results of a crossover experiment of this sort for B_2O_3[17] are shown in FIGURE 7, where T_f was calculated from the index of refraction n. The solid curve is a fit of the data to Equations 8 and 11 using kinetic parameters A, Δh^*, β, and x given in the figure caption and in agreement within experimental error with those used to fit the B_2O_3 data of FIGURE 4. The behavior exhibited in FIGURE 7, i.e., that T_f first moves away from the equilibrium position ($T_f = T_2$) and then eventually reverses its direction of change and approaches equilibrium at long times, is due to two factors in Equation 11. The first is that ΔT_1 and ΔT_2 are of opposite sign so that the second and third terms on the right side of Equation 11 act respectively to decrease and increase T_f, but at different rates. The second is that the relaxation is nonexponential and requires a spectrum of relaxation times for its description, i.e., $\beta \neq 1$. That is, if we set β equal to 1 in Equation 11 and substitute from Equation

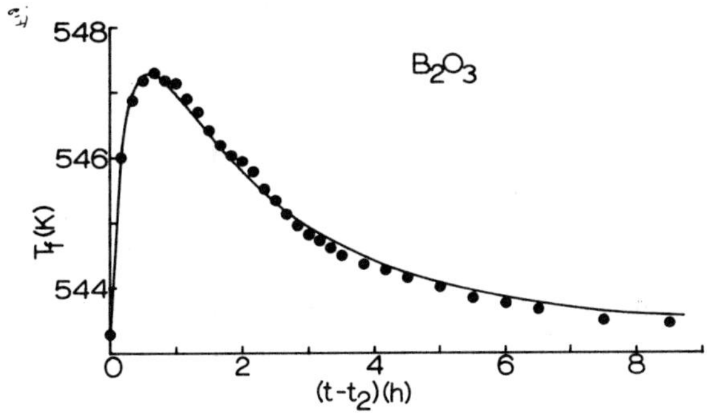

FIGURE 7. Evolution of the fictive temperature calculated from refractive index n for vitreous B_2O_3 following two temperature steps, ΔT_1 at time t_1 from equilibrium at $T_0 = 583.2$ K to $T_1 = 498.7$ K and ΔT_2 at time t_2 from T_1 to $T_2 = 543.4$ K. Solid curve is calculated from Equations 8 and 11 using $A = 5.6 \times 10^{-34}$s, $\Delta h^* = 92$ kcal/mole, $\beta = 0.82$, and $x = 0.50$.

12 we obtain

$$T_f(t) = T_f(t_2) + [T_2 - T_f(t_2)]\left[1 - \exp\left(-\int_{t_2}^{t} \frac{dt'}{\tau_0}\right)\right],$$

which would predict that $T_f(t)$ varies smoothly from $T_f(t_2)$ to T_2 with no reversals in its direction of evolution with time. Hence behavior of the sort exhibited in FIGURE 7 is a direct manifestation of the nonexponential character of the structural relaxation, irrespective of whether the relaxation is linear or nonlinear. This sort of behavior is often referred to as the "memory effect" in glass. That is, the B_2O_3 sample of FIGURE 7 "remembers" that at time t_2 as a result of its previous thermal history it does not possess a structure corresponding to the equilibrium structure at any temperature. Hence its properties evolve in a different fashion than that of FIGURE 4, where at the start of the experiment the structure corresponded to the equilibrium structure at temperature T_0.

Previous physical rationalizations[13,17-19] of the memory effect exhibited in FIGURE 7 suggested that it was due to the existence of two or more independent relaxation mechanisms in the glass. From the present treatment we see that to account for it one need assume only the validity of the superposition principle and a nonexponential macroscopic relaxation function. No assumptions are needed about the microscopic nature of the process, a fact also pointed out by Douglas.[21]

Relaxation During Continuous Heating or Cooling

If we think of continuous heating or cooling at rate q as a series of differential temperature steps, dT, followed by isothermal holds, $dt = dT/q$, Equation 10 may be extended to the case of a continuous change in temperature by replacing the summation by an integral. Using the relaxation function of Equation 7 this gives

$$T_f(T) = T_0 + \int_{T_0}^{T} dT'\left\{1 - \exp\left[-\left(\int_{T'}^{T} dT''/q\tau_0\right)^{\beta}\right]\right\} \qquad (13)$$

The integration of Equation 13 is carried out over the actual temperature-time path followed by the system and must commence at a temperature T_0 at which the system is in equilibrium.

To evaluate the ability of Equation 13 to describe the structural relaxation during continuous heating or cooling we have carried out number of experiments by DSC in which we cooled a liquid through the glass transition region at a number of different cooling rates and subsequently measured the heat capacity while reheating through the transition region at a fixed rate. Typical data of this sort are shown in FIGURE 8 for 5-phenyl-4-ether. For this experiment the temperature T_0 in Equation 13 is a temperature above the glass transition region at which for the heating and cooling rates of interest the equilibrium liquid heat capacity C_{pe} is observed; the corresponding temperature-time path starts at T_0, follows the liquid during cooling to below the transition region at a given constant rate, and finally follows the glass during reheating at a (possibly different) constant rate.

In FIGURES 9 and 10 are shown the evolutions of T_f and dT_f/dT (calculated from the C_p data using Equations 2 & 3) during rate heating at 5 K/min of 5P4E

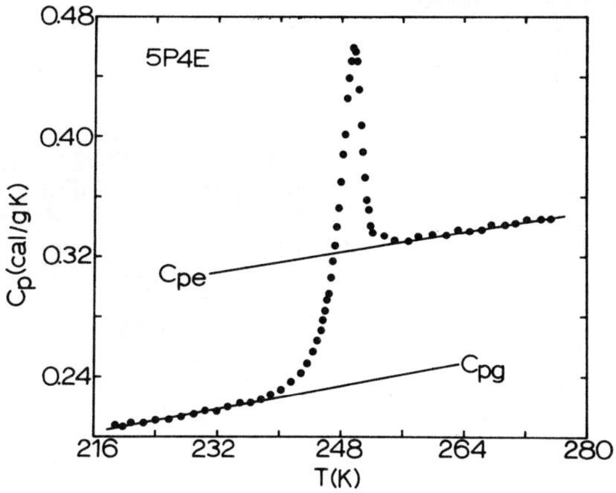

FIGURE 8. Heat capacity of 5-phenyl-4-ether measured by DSC at a heating rate of 5 K/min following a rate cool through the transition region at −1.25 K/min. C_{pg}(cal/g K) = −0.005 + 9.68 × 10^{-4} T(K). C_{pe}(cal/g K) = 0.111 + 8.58 × 10^{-4} T(K).

following rate cools at three different rates. It will be noted from FIGURE 9 that an increase in cooling rate leads to a corresponding increase in the limiting glass fictive temperature, T_f' (corresponding to the level low temperature region of the $T_f - T$ plots of FIGURE 9), attained at the end of the rate cool. The reason for this is immediately apparent from the occurrence of the product $q\tau_0$ in Equation 13. Increasing the magnitude of the cooling rate $|q|$ by a given factor is equivalent to increasing the relaxation time τ_0 by the same factor. Since τ_0 decreases with increasing temperature, this tends to move the region of relaxational effects up in temperature. In fact, it is easily shown[1,3] (if not intuitively obvious from Equations 8 and 13) that the relation between isobaric cooling rate q and T_f' is approximately

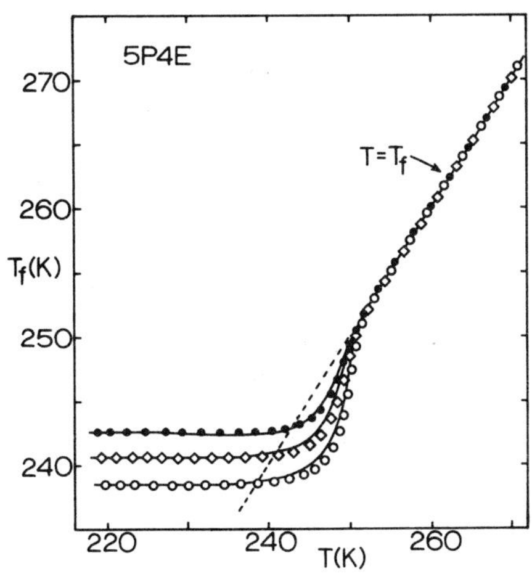

FIGURE 9. Fictive temperature calculated from enthalpy H versus temperature for 5-phenyl-4-ether during heating at 5 K/min following rate cools through the transition region at (•) −5 K/min, (◇) −1.25 K/min, and (○) −0.31 K/min. Solid lines are calculated from Equations 8 and 13 using the parameters $A = 1.21 \times 10^{-67}$ s, $\Delta h^* = 77$ kcal/mole, $\beta = 0.70$, $x = 0.40$.

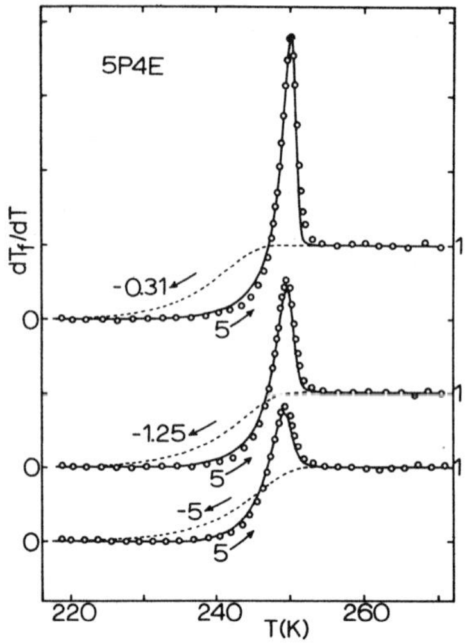

FIGURE 10. dT_f/dT calculated from enthalpy H versus T during rate heating and cooling of 5-phenyl-4-ether. Points are experimental data for heating at 5 K/min following rate cools at (bottom to top) −5, −1.25, and −0.31 K/min. Dashed lines are calculated cooling curves and solid lines are calculated heating curves using Equations 8 and 13 and parameters given in the caption for FIGURE 9.

equivalent to that between τ_{0e} and T (cf. Equation 9):

$$\partial \ln |q| / \partial(1/T'_f) \approx -\Delta h^*/R. \qquad \textbf{(14)}$$

As predicted from Equation 14 for constant Δh^*, the Arrhenius plot of ln $|q|$ versus $(1/T'_f)$ for 5P4E in FIGURE 11 is linear.

Fits of the 5P4E enthalpy relaxation data to Equations 8 and 13 using the procedure described in Reference 4 are shown in FIGURES 9–11; the kinetic parameters are given in the caption to FIGURE 9. The A and Δh^* parameters are fixed by imposing the condition that the calculated solid line in FIGURE 11 match the experimental ln $|q|$ versus $(1/T'_f)$ plot. The β and x parameters are fixed by matching the calculated and experimental dT_f/dT versus T plots of FIGURE 10; the height and position of the maxima in the calculated dT_f/T curves are quite sensitive to small variations in these parameters.

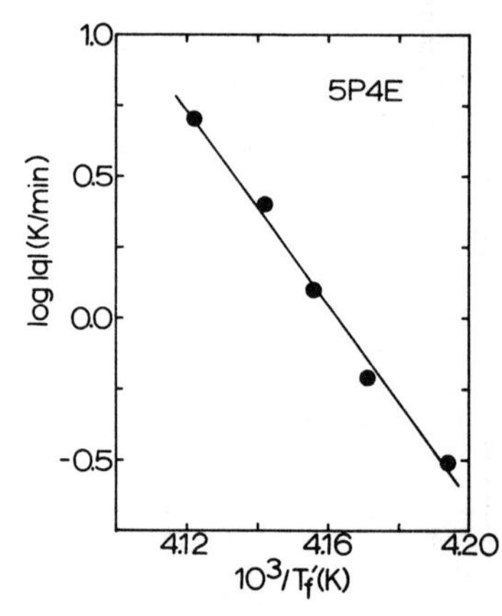

FIGURE 11. Arrhenius plot of cooling rate $|q|$ versus limiting glass fictive temperature T'_f for 5-phenyl-4-ether. Solid line is calculated from Equations 8 and 13 using parameters given in caption for FIGURE 9.

A similar set of experiments (measurement of C_p during rate heating following rate cooling at a variety of rates) has been carried out for As_2Se_3 glass. Experimental dT_f/dT versus T heating curves are shown in FIGURE 12, along with the cooling and heating curves obtained by fitting this data to Equations 8 and 13. The best fit parameters are given in the caption to FIGURE 12. These parameters have also been used to calculate the solid line in FIGURE 6, showing that kinetic parameters assessed from rate heating data give an excellent description of the (much simpler) structural relaxation during isothermal annealing following a single temperature step.

It is of interest to note that the experimental T_f versus T curves during rate heating of FIGURE 9 cross the equilibrium liquid line ($T_f = T$) with a positive slope. Since the condition of equilibrium is $T_f = T$, the system at this point during rate heating appears to be moving away from equilibrium. This behavior is analogous to that observed in crossover experiments (cf. FIGURE 7) and is attributable to the same phenomenological cause, namely, the need for a spectrum of

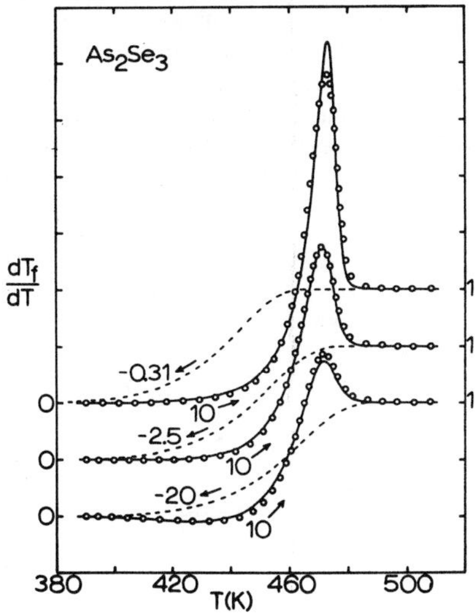

FIGURE 12. dT_f/dT calculated from enthalpy versus T during rate heating and cooling of As_2Se_3 glass. Points are experimental data for heating at 10 K/min following rate cools at (bottom to top) −20, −2.5, and −0.31 K/min. Dashed lines are calculated cooling curves and solid lines are calculated heating curves using Equations 8 and 13 and the parameters $A = 7.6 \times 10^{-38}$ s, $\Delta h^* = 81.8$ kcal/mole, $\beta = 0.67$, and $x = 0.49$.

relaxation times in describing the structural relaxation. Experimenters in the past have, for the most part, failed to remark on this rather direct manifestation of the memory effect readily apparent in rate heating curves, DTA traces, and so forth in the transition region.

STRUCTURAL RELAXATION BY DIGITAL CORRELATION SPECTROSCOPY

The theoretical background and experimental details for structural relaxation studies by digital correlation spectroscopy have been covered exhaustively in previous publications,[6-8,22] so that in the present paper we will confine ourselves to a brief qualitative description of theory and experiment.

Thermally driven density (and, hence, index of refraction) fluctuations in a liquid grow and decay by the same mechanism that gives rise to the structural relaxation. Since these density fluctuations cause light scattering from the liquid, experimental information on the time dependence of the intensity of scattered light contains information on the kinetics of the structural relaxation.

In the digital correlation experiment a laser of optical wavelength Λ is focused into the liquid. The light scattered through some angle Θ is collected by a photomultiplier whose output is fed to a digital autocorrelator. The autocorrelator monitors and stores the photomultiplier output in terms of $n(t)$, the number of photopulses received in the time period t to $(t + \theta)$, where θ is a bin size, and computes a singly clipped autocorrelation function

$$G(t) = \langle n_m(t')\, n(t' + t) \rangle .$$

$G(t)$ is the time average of the product $n_m(t')n(t' + t)$, where $n_m(t') = 0$ if $n(t') \leq m$, $n_m(t') = 1$ if $n(t') > m$, and m is a preset clipping level.

The experimental time-scale of the digital autocorrelator is roughly 10^{-6} to 10 s, so that in turn it may be used to study structural relaxation occurring on this time scale, i.e., structural relaxation at the upper end and somewhat above the glass transition region. For a time scale t in this range for typical liquids the condition holds that the thermal diffusion time constant $C_p\rho/\lambda k^2 \ll t$, where ρ is density, λ thermal conductivity, and $k[= 4\pi \sin(\Theta/2)/\Lambda]$ the wave vector of the density fluctuation. This means that at and slightly above the glass transition region density fluctuations grow and decay isothermally.

The measured autocorrelation function $G(t)$ is given by

$$G(t) = a + b\, \phi_e(t)^2, \qquad (15)$$

where $\phi_e(t)$ is the equilibrium isothermal relaxation function for longitudinal strain in response to changes in longitudinal stress. The constants a and b are determined by experimental factors such as the total duration and the geometry of the experiment; they may be evaluated directly from the measured $G(t)$ by imposing the conditions $\phi_e(0) = 1$ and $\phi_e(\infty) = 0$.

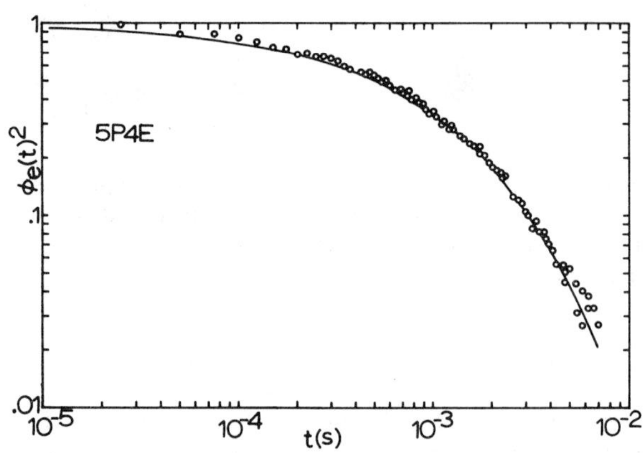

FIGURE 13. Square of equilibrium longitudinal strain relaxation function $\phi_e(t)$ versus time t for 5-phenyl-4-ether measured by digital correlation spectroscopy at -10.7°C and atmospheric pressure. Solid line is calculated from Equation 6 using $\tau_{oe} = 2.5 \times 10^{-3}$ s and $\beta = 0.65$.

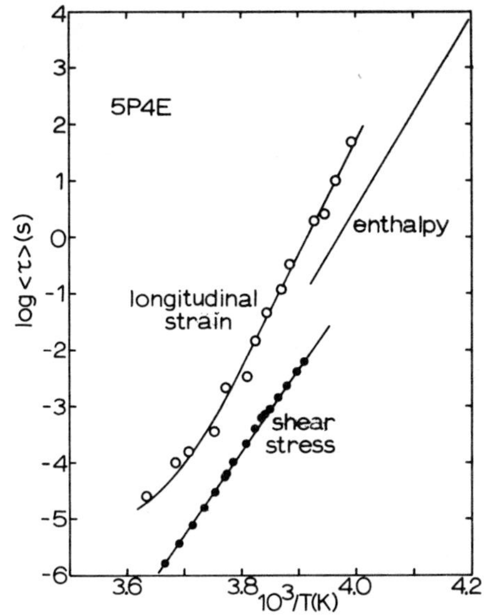

FIGURE 14. Temperature dependence of mean isothermal, isobaric equilibrium relaxation times for shear stress, enthalpy, and longitudinal strain for 5-phenyl-4-ether.

In FIGURE 13 is shown a typical plot of $\phi_e(t)^2$ versus t obtained by digital correlation spectroscopy for 5-phenyl-4-ether and covering some three orders of magnitude in time. The relaxation function is well-described by Equation 6 with $\beta = 0.65$; the same value of β accounts for similar data for 5P4E over the entire temperature range in which the structural relaxation is accessible to correlator studies (cf. FIGURE 14).

COMPARISON OF STRUCTURAL RELAXATION TIMES FOR DIFFERENT PROPERTIES

In this section we compare the time scales and detailed kinetics of the structural relaxation in the glass transition region of a given material when monitored in terms of different properties. We must begin with two caveats. The first is that the relaxation time (more properly, retardation time) characterizing the evolution of a strain in response to an applied stress is in general different from the relaxation time characterizing the evolution of stress in response to an applied strain.[23] We shall in general confine ourselves to comparing strain relaxation times in response to applied stresses, where "strain" is used here to denote not only the usual mechanical shear, dilatational (volume) and longitudinal strains, but also properties such as enthalpy and index of refraction, while "stress" donotes both mechanical shear, compressional (pressure), and longitudinal stresses and temperature changes. The one exception to this is that we will list the mean shear stress relaxation time in response to applied shear strains, since the glass transition region is frequently characterized in terms of viscosity and since it is readily calculated from

$$\langle \tau \rangle = \eta / G_\infty, \tag{16}$$

where G_∞ is the solidlike (i.e., short time, high frequency) shear modulus. The second caveat is that relaxation times are in general different for different constraints on the state variables not monitored directly in the relaxation experiment, e.g., the volume relaxation time in response to pressure changes is different for isothermal and for adiabatic conditions.[17,22,24] We shall compare relaxation times for isothermal isobaric conditions.

In FIGURE 14 the mean isothermal, isobaric equilibrium shear stress, enthalpy, and longitudinal strain relaxation times are compared on an Arrhenius plot for 5P4E. The shear stress times were calculated via Equation 16 using the data of FIGURE 3 and G_∞ values determined by Brillouin light scattering as a function of temperature:

$$G_\infty(\text{dyne/cm}^2) = 9.26 \times 10^9 - 1.68 \times 10^8\, T(^\circ\text{C}).$$

The equilibrium enthalpy and longitudinal strain relaxation functions are of the form of Equation 6 for which the mean relaxation time is given by[10]

$$\langle\tau\rangle = \tau_{0e}\,\Gamma(1/\beta)/\beta.$$

For enthalpy τ_{0e} was calculated over the glass transition region from Equation 8 for the condition $T = T_f$ and the parameters given in the caption to FIGURE 9. For longitudinal strain the τ_{0e} were obtained from digital correlation spectroscopy measurements (cf. FIGURE 13). In TABLE 1 values of $\langle\tau\rangle$ at a given temperature in the transition region and other structural relaxational parameters are compared for different properties for four glass-formers: 5P4E, B_2O_3, As_2Se_3, and an alkali silicate glass.

From FIGURE 14 and TABLE 1 we may draw several conclusions. The first is that the shear stress relaxation time—which recall is not strictly comparable with the other "strain" relaxation times—is typically shorter than these strain times by factors ranging from 2 to 300. Second, the activation enthalpies Δh^* for the different properties of a given material are all of comparable value. For B_2O_3 and the alkali silicate glass the various Δh^* values are probably the same within experimental error, but for 5P4E and As_2Se_3 the relaxational data are of good enough quality to suggest that the small differences in the measured Δh^* values for the different properties are probably real. (That the Δh^* values for the different materials in TABLE 1 are all of comparable magnitude is of no particular significance; much higher (147 kcal/mole for BSC glass[1,3]) and much lower (32 kcal/mole for glycerol[6]) Δh^* values have been observed in or near the transition region.)

The third conclusion is that the time scales (the $\langle\tau\rangle$ values) and the spectra of relaxation times (the β parameters) for the strain relaxations appear in general to be somewhat different for different properties of the same material. This is not unexpected either on the basis of qualitative speculations about the nature of the structural relaxation or on the basis of the order parameter model for the thermodynamics of the structural relaxation.

Consider first the microscopic nature of the structural relaxation. It is fair to say that for the most part the details of this are not known. Nonetheless, many workers have speculated that it involves a cooperative, inherently nonexponential rearrangement of the average configuration of the liquid. It follows that those macroscopic properties that are more affected by the early stages of this process will appear to relax faster than those that are more affected by the later stages. For example, the enthalpy changes occurring during the approach to equilibrium of a network glass following a change in temperature could be considered to arise from the breaking of some of the network bonds, while the volume changes are due to rearrangement of the structure into less densely packed configurations. One cannot say a priori, however, which of these two processes should on the average occur earlier in time. That is, bond breaking might be a necessary precursor to volume-changing rearrangements of the structure, so that one would expect H to relax faster than V. On the other hand, configurational rearrangements leading to large volume changes might occur early in time, stressing the network and leading to subsequent bond breaking, so that one would expect V to relax faster than H. A posteriori, however, information on the relative rates of relaxation of, say, H and V may provide important clues to the detailed mechanism of the structural relaxation. Bearing in mind that relaxation of longitudinal strain involves changes in both volume and shear strain in response to applied pressure and shear stress, we can see that data for the three network glasses of TABLE 1 suggest that the rate of volume relaxation in these materials is slightly faster (B_2O_3) to considerably faster (As_2Se_3 and the alkali silicate glass) than the rate of enthalpy relaxation. We must hedge a bit, however, in view of the fact that there is evidence to indicate that for a given property, e.g., H, the kinetics of the isothermal, isobaric return to equilibrium following a change in T may be different from those following a change in P.[30] Consequently, only the data for As_2Se_3 in TABLE 1 in which both H and V changes in response to T changes were measured is completely clearcut in indicating different kinetics for H and V relaxation.

TABLE 1

MEAN ISOTHERMAL, ISOBARIC EQUILIBRIUM RELAXATION TIMES IN THE GLASS TRANSITION REGION AND STRUCTURAL RELAXATION KINETIC PARAMETERS FOR VARIOUS MATERIALS

System	Relaxing Property	In Response to Changes in	T(K)	$<\tau>$ (s)	Δh^* (kcal/mole)	β	x	Reference
5P4E	H	T	250	3.2	77	0.70	0.40	—
	long. strain	long. stress	250	5.1×10^1	92	0.65	—	—
	shear stress	shear strain	250	1.6×10^{-1}	70	—	—	—
B_2O_3	H	T	536.4	9.7×10^3	90	0.65	0.40	4
	n	T	536.4	1.7×10^4	92	0.83	0.5	—
	V	P	536.4	6.7×10^3	83	0.60	—	22
	shear stress	shear strain	536.4	1.1×10^3	92	—	—	14, 25
As_2Se_3	H	T	450	5.4×10^2	81.8	0.67	0.49	—
	V	T	450	1.0×10^2	81.8	0.80	0.25	—
	shear stress	shear strain	450	4.5×10^1	68	—	—	26, 27
$0.125\ Na_2O$	H	T	727	2.1×10^2	98	0.66	0.70	5
$-0.125\ K_2O$	long. strain	long. stress	727	3.0×10^1	91	0.57	—	8
$-0.75\ SiO_2$	shear stress	shear strain	727	7.8	92	—	—	28, 29

The order parameter model[9,31–35] for the thermodynamics of the structural relaxation assumes that the state of a vitreous system needs to be specified in terms of N order parameters, Z_1, Z_2, $\ldots Z_N$, in addition to T and P, so that the Gibbs free energy is of the form

$$G = G(T, P, \vec{Z}),$$

where $\vec{Z}$ stands for the entire set of N order parameters. The microscopic significance of order parameters in liquids and glasses cannot be unambiguously specified at present, although they might correspond to such things as the number of flexed bonds and the number of "holes" in polymers, the number of broken bonds and the number of "holes" in network glasses, and so forth. For the equilibrium liquid at each T and P the order parameters are each subject to the constraint

$$\frac{\partial G}{\partial Z_i} = 0 \qquad \text{for } i = 1, 2, \ldots N.$$

Hence at equilibrium the order parameters depend only on T and P:

$$\vec{Z}_e = \vec{Z}_e(T, P),$$

as does the equilibrium liquid free energy

$$G_e = G_e[T, P, \vec{Z}_e(T, P)] = G_e(T, P).$$

It is presumed that the evolution of the order parameters in response to rapid changes in T and P is kinetically impeded. Thus, at any point (T_0, P_0) on the equilibrium liquid free energy surface one may generate a glass free energy surface by subjecting the liquid to instantaneous changes in T and/or P, freezing in the order parameters at their equilibrium values at (T_0, P_0):

$$G_g = G_g(T, P, \vec{Z}_0)$$

where $\vec{Z}_0 = \vec{Z}_e(T_0, P_0)$. The equilibrium liquid is never thermodynamically unstable with respect to the glass, so that the condition must apply

$$G_g(T, P, \vec{Z}_0) \geq G_e(T, P) \qquad \text{for } (T, P) \neq (T_0, P_0). \tag{17}$$

From this stability condition it may be shown[9,32,33] that at the point (T_0, P_0) of glass formation the following conditions hold

$$V_g = V_e$$

$$S_g = S_e$$

$$\Delta C_p \geq 0$$

$$\Delta\kappa \geq 0$$

and

$$\Pi \equiv \Delta C_p \Delta\kappa / TV(\Delta\alpha)^2 \geq 1, \tag{18}$$

where

$$\Delta C_p = C_{pe} - C_{pg} = \partial^2 G / \partial T^2 - \partial^2 G_g / \partial T^2,$$

$$\Delta\alpha = \alpha_e - \alpha_g = \partial^2 G_e / \partial T \partial P - \partial^2 G_g / \partial T \partial P,$$

$$\Delta\kappa = \kappa_e - \kappa_g = \partial^2 G_e / \partial P^2 - \partial^2 G_g / \partial P^2.$$

Equation 18 has been termed the Prigogine-Defay condition. The equality in Equation 18 applies in the case of a single order parameter ($N = 1$) or in the case of two or more order parameters ($N > 1$) that satisfy the condition for all i and k

$$(\partial V/\partial Z_i)/(\partial H/\partial Z_i) = (\partial V/\partial Z_k)/(\partial H/\partial Z_k). \tag{19}$$

The inequality in Equation 18 applies in the case of two or more order parameters that do not satisfy this condition.

A compilation of the experimental thermodynamic data needed for the cal-

TABLE 2

THERMODYNAMIC PARAMETERS AND PRIGOGINE–DEFAY RATIOS IN THE GLASS TRANSITION REGION AT ATMOSPHERIC PRESSURE FOR THREE GLASS-FORMERS*

	B_2O_3	40 mole% $Ca(NO_3)_2$ – 60 mole% KNO_3	Poly (vinyl acetate)
T(K)	550	340	303.8
$10^3 V(m^3/kg)$	0.558	0.459, <u>0.456</u>	0.84309
$10^{-2}\ C_{pe}$(J/kg K)	19.1, <u>19.3</u>	15.4, <u>14.9</u>	18.0
$10^{-2}\ C_{pg}$(J/kg K)	13.5, <u>13.0</u>	9.7, <u>9.5</u>	13.0
$10^{-2}\ \Delta C_p$(J/kg K)	6.3	5.4	<u>5.0</u>, 5.1
$10^4\ \alpha_e(K^{-1})$	4.0	3.64, <u>3.5</u>	7.117
$10^4\ \alpha_g(K^{-1})$	0.58, <u>0.5</u>	1.2	2.795
$10^4\ \Delta\alpha(K^{-1})$	3.5	2.3	4.322
$10^{11}\ \kappa_e(m^2/N)$	38, <u>40</u>	13.2	49.81
$10^{11}\ \kappa_g(m^2/N)$	7.9, <u>12</u>	6.3, <u>6.3</u>	28.96
$10^{11}\ \Delta\kappa(m^2/N)$	28	6.9	20.85
Π	4.7	4.5	2.2

*Where more than one value of a parameter is listed, the one used to determine ΔC_p, $\Delta\alpha$, $\Delta\kappa$, and Π is underlined.

culation of the Prigogine-Defay ratio Π has been made recently[9] for three glass-formers for which the data were considered to be of unusual reliability and is reproduced in TABLE 2. The data suggest that in general $\Pi > 1$, so that the state of glass-forming systems may be expected to require a many order parameter description not subject to the constraint of Equation 19. For isothermal, isobaric relaxation in a system not greatly removed from equilibrium evolution of properties such as H or V is related to the evolution of the order parameters by

$$\frac{dV}{dt} = \sum_{i=1}^{N} \left(\frac{\partial V}{\partial Z_i}\right) \frac{dZ_i}{dt},$$

$$\frac{dH}{dt} = \sum_{i=1}^{N} \left(\frac{\partial H}{\partial Z_i}\right) \frac{dZ_i}{dt}.$$

For a system for which $\Pi = 1$, so that Equation 19 is satisfied, it follows from Equations 1, 4, and 5 and the analogous equations for volume relaxation that

$$\phi_{eH}(t) = \phi_{eV}(t),$$

that is, the equilibrium relaxation functions are the same for volume and enthalpy. Conversely, one expects that if $\Pi > 1$, so that Equation 19 is not satisfied,

$$\phi_{eH}(t) \neq \phi_{eV}(t).$$

Hence the indications from FIGURE 14 and TABLE 1 that volume and enthalpy relax at different rates are consistent with the predictions of the order parameter model of the structural relaxation in systems for which $\Pi > 1$, a condition that seems to be fairly generally satisfied.

Conclusions

We have shown here that the nonlinear structural relaxation in glass in response to a wide variety of temperature-time programs can be accounted for phenomenologically in terms of a small number of kinetic parameters. The kinetic parameters used in our analyses (A, Δh^*, x, and β) are the minimum number required to give an adequate account of the structural relaxation in the sense that they reflect four fundamental aspects of the phenomena that are immediately apparent in the experimental data. That is, A determines the temperature at which the structural relaxation is observable on a given experimental time scale, Δh^* determines how that temperature changes with a change in time scale, β accounts for the nonexponential character of the relaxation (the memory effect), and x accounts for the nonlinear character. Relaxation in systems other than those studied here may of course require a slightly different detailed phenomenological treatment, e.g., a different spectrum of relaxation times from that implied by Equation 6 or a different temperature dependence of the equilibrium relaxation times (perhaps a Vogel-Tamann-Fulcher equation type of dependence) from the Arrhenius dependence of Equation 9. However, we expect that the general method of accounting for the nonlinearity by making the relaxation times depend on both temperature and average structure and of dealing with complicated temperature histories by means of the superposition principle should remain valid.

Currently available data indicate the structural relaxation kinetics are different for different macroscopic properties of the same material. We have shown both by qualitative arguments and by a consideration of the order parameter model for the thermodynamics of the structural relaxation that this is in general expected. More important, we have tried to indicate that a comparison of the kinetics for different properties can serve as an important a posteriori check on the correctness of detailed microscopic models that may be proposed for the structural relaxation. Clearly more experimental studies of this sort are needed and hopefully will be carried out in the future.

Summary

A phenomenological treatment of the kinetics of the structural relaxation in liquids in the glass transition region in response to isobaric temperature changes was described. The important features of the treatment are the ability to account for the nonlinear character of the relaxation by allowing the relaxation times to depend both on temperature and on structure and the use of the superposition principle to deal with thermal histories that involve a number of temperature changes or a continuous change in temperature with time. Analysis of experimental data on the evolution of macroscopic properties for a number of different thermal histories was presented for a number of different glass formers. The technique of study of the kinetics of longitudinal strain relaxation by digital correlation spectroscopy was described briefly and typical results presented. Present results indicate that the kinetics of the structural relaxation are different for different macroscopic properties of the same material. It was shown that this behavior is expected both on the basis of qualitative speculations on the microscopic nature of the structural relaxation and on the basis of the order parameter model of the thermodynamics of the structural relaxation.

REFERENCES

1. MOYNIHAN, C. T., A. J. EASTEAL, J. WILDER & J. TUCKER. 1974. J. Phys. Chem. **78:** 2673.
2. MOYNIHAN, C. T., P. MACEDO, N. SAAD, M. DEBOLT, B. DOM, A. EASTEAL & J. WILDER. 1975. Fiz. Khim. Stek. **1:** 420.
3. MOYNIHAN, C. T., A. J. EASTEAL, M. A. DEBOLT, & J. TUCKER. 1976. J. Amer. Ceram. Soc. **59:** 12.
4. DEBOLT, M. A., A. J. EASTEAL, P. B. MACEDO & C. T. MOYNIHAN. 1976. J. Amer. Ceram. Soc. **59:** 16.
5. MOYNIHAN, C. T., A. J. EASTEAL, D. C. TRAN, J. A. WILDER & E. P. DONOVAN. 1976. J. Amer. Ceram. Soc. **59:** 137.
6. DEMOULIN, C., C. J. MONTROSE & N. OSTROWSKY. 1974. Phys. Rev. A **9:** 1740.
7. MACEDO, P. B. & C. J. MONTROSE. 1974. Proceedings 10th International Congress on Glass, No. 11, Kyoto, Japan: 68–72.
8. LAI, C. C., P. B. MACEDO & C. J. MONTROSE. 1975. J. Amer. Ceram. Soc. **58:** 120.
9. GUPTA, P. K. & C. T. MOYNIHAN. 1976. J. Chem. Phys. In press.
10. MOYNIHAN, C. T., L. P. BOESCH & N. L. LABERGE. 1973. Phys. Chem. Glasses **14:** 122.
11. DAVIDSON, D. & R. COLE. 1951. J. Chem. Phys. **19:** 1484.
12. GARDON, R. & O. S. NARAYANASWAMY. 1970. J. Amer. Ceram. Soc. **53:** 380.
13. NARAYANASWAMY, O. S. 1971. J. Amer. Ceram. Soc. **54:** 491.
14. MACEDO, P. B. & A. NAPOLITANO. 1968. J. Chem. Phys. **49:** 1887.
15. TWEER, H., N. LABERGE & P. B. MACEDO. 1971. J. Amer. Ceram. Soc. **54:** 121.
16. LAUGHLIN, W. T. & D. R. ULHMANN. 1972. J. Phys. Chem. **76:** 2317.
17. BOESCH, L., A. NAPOLITANO & P. B. MACEDO. 1970. J. Amer. Ceram. Soc. **53:** 148.
18. MACEDO, P. B. & A. NAPOLITANO. 1967. J. Res. Nat. Bur. Stand. **71A:** 231.
19. NAPOLITANO, A. & P. B. MACEDO. 1968. J. Res. Nat. Bur. Stand. **72A:** 425.
20. CORSARO, R. D. 1976. J. Amer. Ceram. Soc. **59:** 115.
21. DOUGLAS, R. W. 1972. *In* Amorphous Materials. R. W. Douglas & B. Ellis, Eds.: 3–22. Wiley-Interscience. New York, N.Y.
22. BUCARO, J. A., H. D. DARDY & R. D. CORSARO. 1975. J. Appl. Phys. **46:** 741.
23. MCCRUM, N. G., B. E. READ & G. WILLIAMS. 1967. Anelastic and Dielectric Effects in Polymeric Solids. Wiley. New York, N.Y.
24. BAUER, H-J. 1965. *In* Physical Acoustics, Vol. IIA, W. P. Mason, Ed.: 47–131. Academic Press. New York, N.Y.
25. CAPPS, W., P. B. MACEDO, B. O'MEARA & T. A. LITOVITZ. 1966. J. Chem. Phys. **45:** 3431.
26. SUZUKI, S., T. KOBAYASHI, H. OHNO & S. KAMIYA. 1973. Zairyo **22:** 134.
27. CHERNOV, A. P., S. A. DEMBOVSKII & S. F. CHISTOV. 1968. Izv. Akad. Nauk SSSR, Neorg. Mater. **4:** 1449.
28. POOLE, J. P. 1949. J. Amer. Ceram. Soc. **32:** 230.
29. DAY, D. E. 1972. *In* Amorphous Materials. R. W. Douglas & B. Ellis, Eds.: 39–47. Wiley-Interscience. New York, N.Y.
30. WEITZ, A. & B. WUNDERLICH. 1974. J. Polym. Sci. Polym. Phys. Ed. **12:** 2473.
31. DAVIES, R. O. & G. O. JONES. 1953. Proc. R. Soc. (Lond.) **A217:** 26.
32. DAVIES, R. O. & G. O. JONES. 1953. Adv. Phys. **2:** 370.
33. GOLDSTEIN, M. 1963. J. Chem. Phys. **39:** 3369.
34. GOLDSTEIN, M. 1973. J. Phys. Chem. **77:** 667.
35. GOLDSTEIN, M. 1975. J. Appl. Phys. **46:** 4153.

METASTABLE STATES IN THE LENNARD-JONES FLUID

Harold J. Raveché

National Bureau of Standards
Washington, DC 20234

Metastable states associated with the fluid–solid transition[1] in the classical Lennard-Jones system are simulated by means of the Monte Carlo algorithm in statistical mechanics. The simulations are concerned with both the thermal and structural properties of undercooled or overcompressed monatomic fluids.

The Lennard-Jones potential energy function is

$$U(r) = 4\epsilon[(\sigma/r)^{12} - (\sigma/r)^{6}],$$

where r is the internuclear distance and ϵ and σ are energy and length parameters, respectively. Using N_A for the Avogadro constant and k_B for the Boltzmann constant, the following units will be employed: volume, σ^3; pressure, ϵ/σ^3; energy, $N_A\epsilon$; and temperature, ϵ/k_B. For reference, the critical point density and temperature of argon is $\rho = 0.31$ and $T = 1.26$, and the triple point value for argon is $\rho = 0.84$, $T = 0.70$.

We investigate thermodynamic states in the range $T = 0.80$–2.74 and $\rho = 1.1$–1.3. For argon the pressures for these states would be well into the kilobar region.

Simulations are performed for 256 and 108 particle systems. The computations proceed as follows[2]: The atomic coordinates of a disordered fluid array, obtained from an equilibrated run at liquid densities,[1] are scaled to a high density at a temperature for which the lowest energy state is that of the crystalline (face-centered cubic, fcc) solid. That is, a random array is prepared at a density and temperature for which the equilibrium state is crystalline; see the schematic of an isotherm shown in FIGURE 1. Therefore the initial array is similar to a real fluid which has been undercooled or overcompressed. We then investigate whether the pressure and energy converge to a particular value and whether the convergence, on a microscopic level, is noticeably labile.

Results for 256 particles at $\rho = 1.105$ and $T = 0.80$, which is less than one-half the freezing temperature[1] are shown in FIGURE 2a. The solid curve with solid circles is the cumulative average (i.e., the average over all previous configurations) for the pressure and the dashed curve is the average over the most recent 10^5 configurations. The average root mean square displacement of a particle from its initial position in the disordered array is shown by the solid curve with open circles. The results illustrate that convergence is approached only after 10^7 configurations have been generated. For reference, the equilibrated pressure of a run begun from fcc coordinates is 9.03 and this should be compared to 8.93, the value in FIGURE 2a. The internal energy for both the initially random and initially fcc-ordered arrays converged to same value, namely, −7.17.

The behavior of the rms as a function of the number of configurations is a qualitative measure of diffusion. Although the sequence of configurations in a Monte Carlo simulation is produced by a random process, each configuration of atoms differs from the preceding one by at most a small displacement of a single atom. In this sense, the progress of the simulation can be qualitatively interpreted

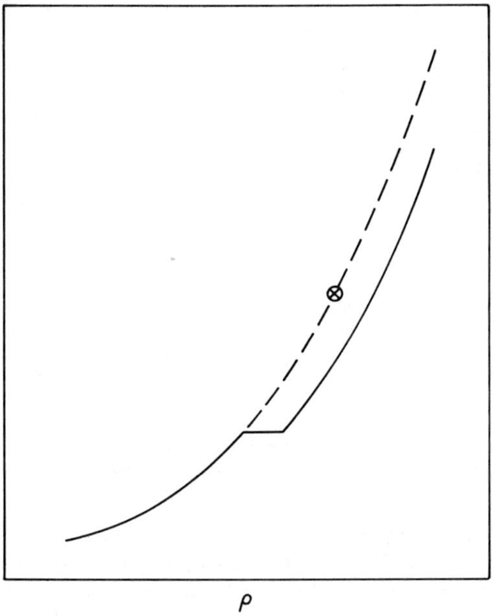

FIGURE 1. Schematic plot of an isotherm for fluid—solid transition. The circled crisscross indicates density of metastable state.

as progression in real time. Considering this, the rms in FIGURE 2 indicates that as the system equilibrates, the position of the atoms are not particularly labile. This is suggestive of limited diffusive motion.

The pair correlation function, $g(r)$, for this run at 2.0×10^7 configurations is shown by the solid curve in FIGURE 2b. The correlation function for the run begun

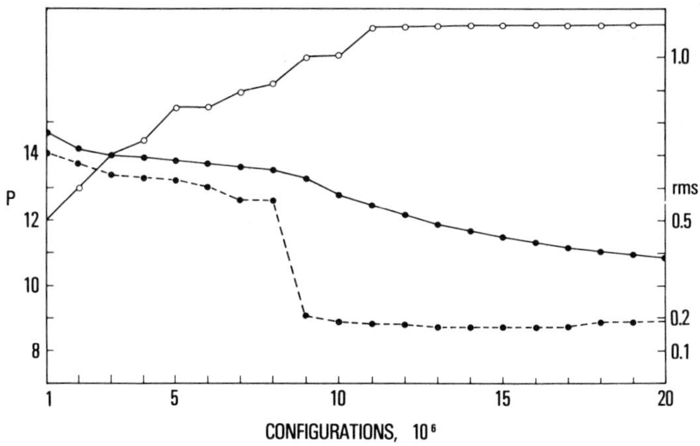

FIGURE 2a. Simulation at $T = 0.80$ and $\rho = 1.105$ begun from random array. Open circles denote the average root mean square displacement of an atom from its initial position. Solid circles on solid curve denote cumulative average of pressure and the solid circles on the dashed curve denote averages over the most recent 10^5 configurations.

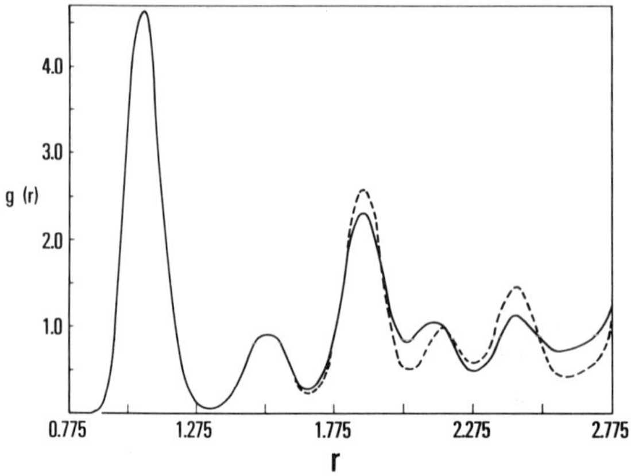

FIGURE 2b. Pair correlation function, solid curve denotes result at 2.0×10^7 configurations and dashed curve is result of simulation begun from fcc array.

from the fcc array is given by the dashed curve. Both curves are identical to radial distances comparable to the second nearest-neighbor distance and they are quite similar in form for larger internuclear separations. The local structure which is initially present in the random array, that is, at 2.0×10^6 configurations, is shown in FIGURE 2c. Evidently the local order changed substantially as the simulation converged.

The results can be interpreted as homogeneous nucleation. The formation of a perfect lattice in these simulations is greatly hindered by the periodic boundary conditions which are used to avoid surface effects. Strains in the crystal are to be expected unless the crystal nucleates with its principle axes parallel to the axes of the reference coordinate system.

Similar computations for the 256 particle system were performed on the $T = 2.74$ isotherm at $\rho = 1.30$ which is approximately 20% beyond the freezing

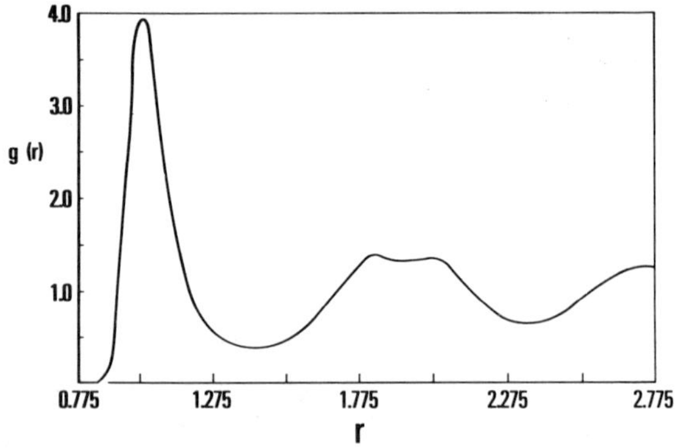

FIGURE 2c. Pair correlation function for simulation begun from random array at 2.0×10^6 configurations.

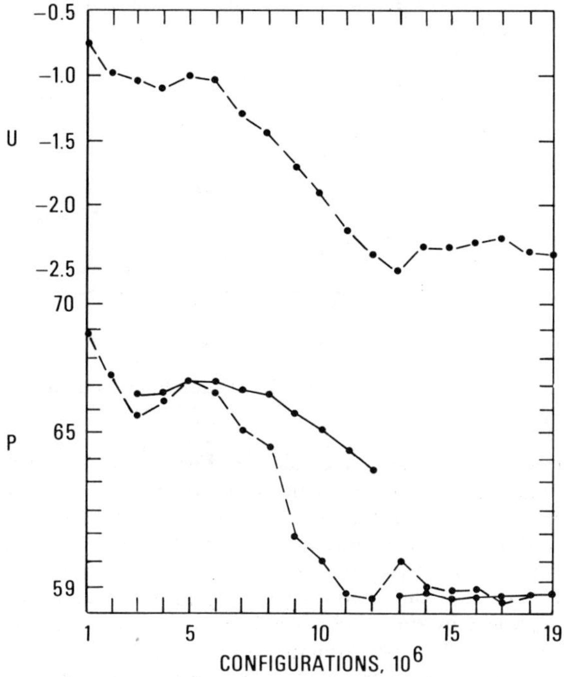

FIGURE 3a. Pressure and energy for $T = 2.74$ and $\rho = 1.30$. The solid curve indicates the cumulative average and the dashed, the averages over the most recent 10^5 configurations. The break in the solid curve indicates that the coordinates and these points were used to begin a new simulation.

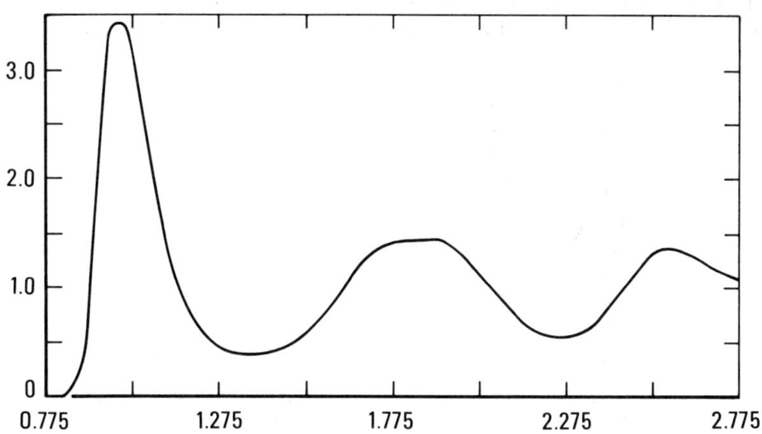

FIGURE 3b. Pair correlation function at 1.9×10^7.

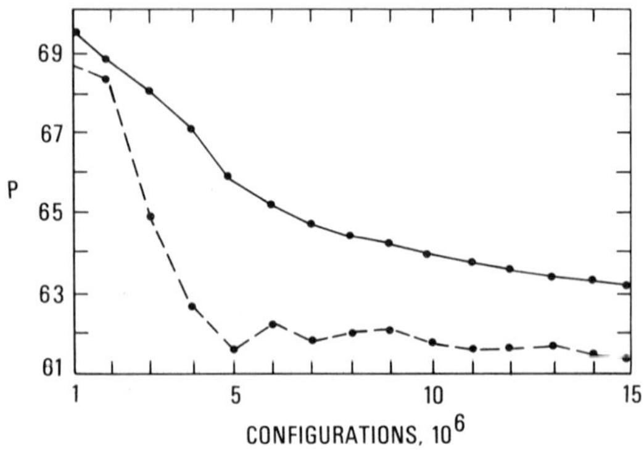

FIGURE 4a. Simulation at $T = 1.30$ and $\rho = 1.30$ begun from random number generator.

density.[1] The pressure and energy are shown in FIGURE 3a. The breaks in the solid curve indicate that the coordinates at those points were used to begin a new simulation. The pressure and energy after convergence are 59 and -2.4, respectively, compared to 53 and -3.3 for a simulation of the fcc array. The molecular order, however, suggests features that are different from those in FIGURE 2b. The pair correlation at 1.9×10^7 is shown in FIGURE 3b and the curve shows no evidence of the fcc ordering shown by the solid curve in FIGURE 2b. Visual inspection of the atomic coordinates at 1.9×10^7 configurations by means of stereoscopic pairs of photographs indicates an amorphous structure with little evidence of crystallinity. During the same sequence of 1.4×10^7 to 1.9×10^7 configurations, the molecular order ceased to be labile. The pair correlation function did not change by more than $\pm 1\%$ beyond 1.4×10^7 configurations. The correlation function did change, however, from the initial array to 1.4×10^7 configurations. The maxima and minima became more pronounced indicating that the amorphous structure became locally more close-packed as the simulation converged.

The amorphous structure at convergence is suggestive of the formation of a glassy state. In FIGURE 3b there is no evidence of the subdued second nearest-

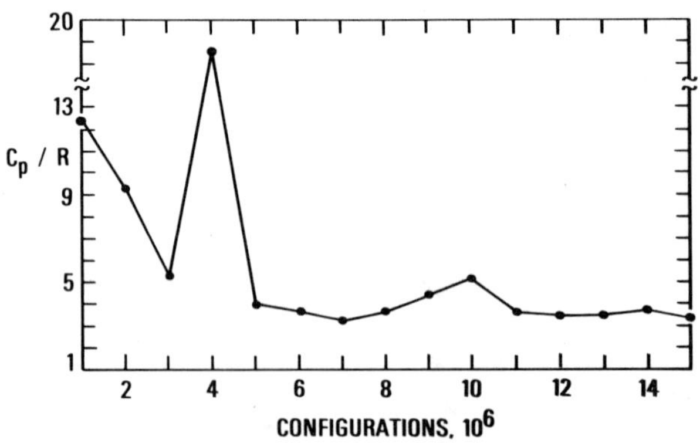

FIGURE 4b. Constant pressure heat capacity in units of the gas constant.

neighbor peak at $r \sim 1.45$ present in the solid curve of FIGURE 2b. In previous studies[3] we have observed that the existence of fcc lattice structure results in a subdued peak in this range of internuclear separation. The pair correlation function shown in FIGURE 3b exhibits some of the features found in studies of the random close-packed arrays of hard spheres.[4] In particular, the broad second maximum can be interpreted as two separate peaks centered at approximately $r = 1.75$ and $r = 1.95$. Bernal[5] attributes the first of these to the presence of tetrahedra which share a common base, and the second to the collineation of three particles.

The relation between the structure of a random close-packed system and that of an ideal glass has been discussed in detail by Turnbull.[6] It is sufficient to remark here that the structure of the glass state in macroscopic systems is still an important unresolved problem.

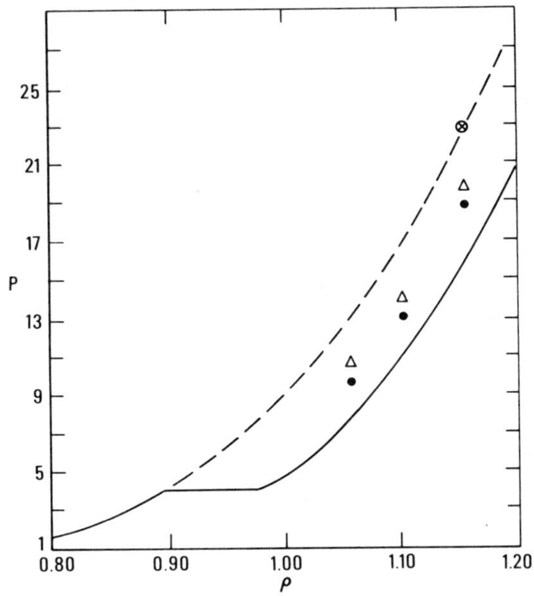

FIGURE 5. Results on the $T = 1.17$ isotherm for 108 (△) and 256 (●) particle systems. The circled crisscross denotes the original density of the random arrays. The density was successively decreased and the coordinates of each preceding state were used to begin a new simulation.

The reproducibility of the calculations has been checked by repeating a simulation with initial coordinates obtained from a random number generator. The results for $\rho = 1.30$ and $T = 2.74$ are shown in FIGURE 4a. These results should be compared to those in FIGURE 3a which correspond to a simulation begun from the coordinates of an equilibrated run at liquid-like densities.[1] Comparison shows that the simulations are reproducible to within 4% and we conjecture that the differences would be smaller if the simulation shown in FIGURE 4a had been continued to the same number of configurations as that in FIGURE 3a.

It is also possible to calculate the constant pressure heat capacity for the Lennard-Jones system. The results are shown in FIGURE 4b. For reference, we note that the heat capacity of the crystalline solid was estimated to be 3.4 which is close to the result for the glassy state shown in FIGURE 4b.

We have investigated size effects by performing simulations on 108 particle systems. There is one noticeable difference between 108 and 256 particle systems: the convergence is not as complete in the smaller system. That is, the converged values of the pressure and energy in the smaller system are higher than those in the larger system at the same density and temperature. This is shown in FIGURE 5 where we have plotted results for both the 108 (denoted by triangles) and 256 (solid circles) particle systems on the $T = 1.17$ isotherm.[1] The circled crisscross denotes the density at which both systems were initially prepared.

In summary we have shown that nucleation from a fluid to a crystalline array is possible in small three dimensional systems with periodic boundary conditions. The results of these and other simulations[2] indicate that there is an amount of overcompression or undercooling which must be exceeded to observe the characteristic decrease in pressure and internal energy. That is unless the overcompression is of a certain magnitude, the thermodynamic properties of the initially random array appears to fluctuate about values that are typical of a smooth continuation of the equilibrium phase into the metastable region. For isotherms we have investigated, the lower limit of compression appears to be 15%–20%. For a given density the calculations suggest that even a large amount of undercooling is required, as much as 50% or more. However, these results must be investigated further for their size dependence.

In addition we have found evidence for the existence of an amorphous close-packed array which has some of the characteristics of a model proposed[6] for the glass in a macroscopic system. If the existence of this state can be confirmed in further studies, it may prove useful in the study of the molecular structure of the glass state. Since we have shown that nucleation is possible, this suggests that the amorphous solid state may be a well-defined state between the fluid and crystalline phases.

References

1. STREETT, W. B., H. J. RAVECHÉ & R. D. MOUNTAIN. 1974. J. Chem. Phys. **61:** 1960.
2. RAVECHÉ, H. J. & W. B. STREETT. To be published.
3. RAVECHÉ, H. J., R. D. MOUNTAIN & W. B. STREETT. 1974. J. Chem. Phys. **61:** 1970.
4. FINNEY, J. L. 1970. Proc. R. Soc. Lond. A **319:** 479.
5. BERNAL, J. D. 1964. Proc. R. Soc. Lond. A **280:** 299.
6. TURNBULL, D. 1969. Contemp. Phys. **10:** 473.

REMARKS ON POLYMER VISCOSITY

A. A. Miller

1070 Hickory Road
Schenectady, New York 12309

The theme of these remarks is that in some respects the behavior of polymer liquids is *simpler* than that of "simple" (i.e., low-molecular-weight) liquids. Some of these results were presented in the Polymer Division of the ACS National Meeting in September 1974, and are reported in *Polymer Preprints* of that meeting.[1]

Considering Newtonian liquid viscosity as a function of p, v, and T, the following exact relationship can be derived by partial differentiation:

$$(\mathrm{d}T/\mathrm{d}p)_\eta = \frac{(\mathrm{d}v/\mathrm{d}p)_T}{(\mathrm{d}v/\mathrm{d}T)_\eta - (\mathrm{d}v/\mathrm{d}T)_p}$$

where $(\mathrm{d}T/\mathrm{d}p)_\eta$ and $(\mathrm{d}v/\mathrm{d}T)_\eta$ are constant viscosity terms, $(\mathrm{d}v/\mathrm{d}p)_T$ and $(\mathrm{d}v/\mathrm{d}T)_p$ are the compressibility and thermal expansibility, respectively. From literature data on several polymeric liquids it had been shown previously[2] that at constant (i.e., atmospheric) pressure, the denominator of the right-hand term is constant, K, for a given liquid over a broad temperature range down to T_g, the glass transition temperature. Considering this transition as an iso-mobility state, $(\mathrm{d}v/\mathrm{d}T)_\eta = \mathrm{d}v_g/\mathrm{d}T$ for the glass formed at elevated temperatures and pressures, and $(\mathrm{d}T/\mathrm{d}p)_\eta = \mathrm{d}T_g/\mathrm{d}p$ for the pressure dependence of T_g. Also, it was suggested that K is a "universal" constant for vinyl-type polymer liquids.

TABLE 1 lists the thermal expansibilities in decreasing order for 12 vinyl-type polymer liquids. It is seen that while there is a large change in the $(\mathrm{d}v/\mathrm{d}T)_p$ values, K remains quite constant at a value of about $-17(\pm 1) \times 10^{-4}$ cc/g deg.

TABLE 1

EXPANSIBILITIES AND K VALUES*

	$10^4(\mathrm{d}v/\mathrm{d}T)_p$ cc/g deg	-10^4K† cc/g deg
n-Pentadecane	14.0	17.4
n-Octadecane	12.5	16.7
Polydimethylsiloxane		
(MW = 8800)	9.6	17.7
(MW = 30,500)	9.7	18.1
Polyisobutylene (MW = 440)	8.3	16.7
Natural Rubber	7.1	17.9
Polyisobutylene (MW = 40,000)	6.0	15.8
Poly(methyl acrylate)	5.6	18.1
Polystyrene	5.5	16.8
Poly(methyl methacrylate)	5.0	19.0
Poly(vinyl acetate)	4.9	16.0
Poly(vinyl chloride)	4.0	20.0, 15.9

*See Reference 1 for sources of data.
†$K = (\mathrm{d}v/\mathrm{d}T)_\eta - (\mathrm{d}v/\mathrm{d}T)_p$.

On the other hand, this value does not apply to "simple" liquids such as carbon tetrachloride, benzene, and *n*-pentane, where $-10^4 K = 10$, 20, and 32, respectively.

Preliminary evidence suggests that the temperature dependence of viscosities of vinyl-type polymers conform to the Vogel equation: $\log \eta \sim B/(T - T_0)$, over broader viscosity ranges than for simple liquids. For example, in the case of polystyrene (MW = 47,000 and 38,000), the viscosity data of Plazek,[3] together with those of Allen and Fox,[4] can be expressed by the Vogel equation to well within a 0.1 decade over 8 decades of viscosity (and down to within 10° of T_g) with B = 632° and T_0 = 50.2°C. However, for a number of low-molecular-weight liquids it has been shown that at least two sets of Vogel constants are required to express the viscosities over only about 5 decades.[5,6]

Davies and Matheson[6] have attributed the failure of the Vogel equation to the complexity of molecular motions (rotation of the whole molecule about one or two axes, internal rotations, etc.) involved in the viscous flow of these simple liquids. By contrast, in vinyl-type polymer liquids only one mode of motion may be predominant in viscous flow, namely, internal rotation around main-chain bonds. Furthermore, for a given vinyl-type polymer, all of the main-chain bonds (except, of course, the terminal bonds) are identical with respect to the rotational energy barriers.

References

1. Miller, A. A. 1974. Polym. Preprints **15(2):** 410
2. Miller, A. A. 1971. Macromolecules **4:** 757.
3. Plazek, D. J. 1965. J. Phys. Chem. **69:** 3480.
4. Allen, V. R. & T. G. Fox. 1964. J. Chem. Phys. **41:** 337.
5. Barlow, A. J., J. Lamb & A. J. Matheson. 1966. Proc. R. Soc. **A292:** 322.
6. Davies, D. B. & A. J. Matheson. 1966. J. Chem. Phys. **45:** 1000.

DYNAMIC ORDER PARAMETER FLUCTUATIONS IN A DISORDERED SYSTEM

J. W. Haus*

National Bureau of Standards
Washington, D.C. 20234

J. R. Cullen

Naval Surface Weapons Center
White Oak, Maryland 20910

A modified Ginzburg-Landau free energy functional is introduced which includes order parameter fluctuations, $m(r, t)$ and a static local random variable, $A'(r)$, whose cumulant properties are assumed to be known:

$$F = \int d^3r \left[[A_0 + A'(r)] \frac{m^2}{2} + \frac{B}{4} m^4 + \frac{(\nabla m)^2}{2} - \mu m \right]. \tag{1}$$

The free energy of the system being studied is obtained by performing a functional integral over all values of the order parameter and the random variable. However, in this note our interest will be centered upon the system's dynamic susceptibility calculated within a mean field approximation, insofar as the order parameter is concerned, and for a quenched state with respect to the random variable. The interpretation of a quenched state has been amply discussed by Morita.[1] The equilibrium susceptibility in the mean field theory was solved by Shapero, Cullen, and Callen[2] using a self-consistent perturbution theory. We have calculated the dynamic susceptibility for a nonconserved order parameter in the mean field approximation under the equation of motion:

$$-\gamma_0 \frac{\delta F}{\delta m(q, \omega)} = i\omega m(q, \omega). \tag{2}$$

Neglecting inhomogeneities in the nonlinear term writing $A_0 + 3B\overline{m}^2 = A$ and assuming that only the second cumulant of the random variable exists

$$< A_{q'} A_{-q'} > = 2\pi^2 g e^{-(q/qc)^2},$$

where g is a strength and q_c^{-1} is a characteristic length of correlations among the inhomogeneities, then the dynamic susceptibility may be calculated by a method similar to Shapero's. The solution may be analytically calculated at $q = 0, \omega = 0$ and the suceptibility has a cusp at a value

$$A = A_N = \frac{\sqrt{\pi}}{2} g q_c - \frac{\pi^2}{8} g^2 (1 + \sqrt{\pi} g/q_c)^{-1} \tag{3}$$

a behavior that was found by Shapero *et al.* When the relaxation time is calculated as defined by Suzuki and Igarashi,[3] the renormalized transport coefficient dominates the expression; the relaxation time may be written as

*NBS-NRC Postdoctoral Fellow.

$$\tau = \langle \chi(0) \rangle^{-1} \frac{\mathrm{d}\langle \chi(0) \rangle}{\mathrm{d}A}. \qquad (4)$$

This diverges at A_N even though the susceptibility at this point is finite. The conventional vanHove theory where the transport coefficient stays finite would dictate that a critical slowing down would not occur for this system. In the theory presented above the fluctuations are prevented from diverging because of microscopic inhomogeneities in the system, but the renormalized transport coefficient manifests the approach to the maximum correlation length. This note generalizes the numerical results of Šimanek and Hayward[4] on the dynamics of the two-dimensional Ginzburg-Landau theory.

References

1. Morita, T. 1964. J. Math. Phys. **5:** 1401.
2. Shapero, D., J. R. Cullen & E. Callen. 1974. Phys. Lett. **50A:** 303.
3. Suzuki, M. & G. Igarashi. 1973. Prog. Theor. Phys. **49:** 1070.
4. Šimanek E. & J. C. Hayward. 1975. Phys. Lett. **53A:** 55.

DISCUSSION

R. F. Boyer, *Moderator*

Midland Macromolecular Institute
Midland, Michigan

A. A. MILLER (*Schenectady, N.Y.*): Dr. Simha, Flory has also given an equation of state for polymer liquids. How do the values of his characteristic parameters v^*, p^*, T^* compare with your scaling parameters, particularly with regard to their independence of pressure and temperature?

Also, the v^* parameter appears to be a "hard-core" volume of the hypothetical liquid at 0°K. Can you ascribe any similar physical significance to the p^* and T^* parameters so that they might be determined by independent methods and thus test these equations of state?

SIMHA: The numerical values of the scaling parameters naturally vary with the form of the equation employed, less so for v^* than T^* and p^*. Adjustments with temperature and pressure, required for a fit of equilibrium isotherms and isobars to experimental data indicate a fault in the theory. The illustrations shown suggest but small discrepancies in respect to the derivatives. Detailed examination shows deviations in organic polymers of less than 10% in the worst instance for the thermal expansivities α, and of course, experimental data may also be at fault. For a perfect fit in $d\alpha/dT$, T^* must be allowed to vary maximally by about 8% over 100°, with similar fluctuations in p^* for the compressibilities up to 2 kbar, and maximally 2% in v^*. Few instances, I believe, have been reported of such extensive and detailed testing of theory in chain-molecular, or simple liquids, for that matter. Nor have I seen quantitative agreement between theory and experiment to the same degree.

The definitions of the scaling parameters follow naturally from the theoretical model. As v^* indicates the range of the repulsion, so does p^* represent a cohesive energy density (maximum interchain attraction per unit repulsive volume). T^* is defined by a balance between this maximum attraction and a characteristic thermal energy. However, a theoretical prediction of these parameters from molecular characteristics is practically feasible only for the simplest structures. Comparisons of equation of state and transport data in gases have been customarily used to check on the consistency of the potential functions, which determine the scaling parameters. In any case, since an inadequate theoretical equation of state would not be saved in a meaningful way by numerical adjustments of T^*, p^*, v^*, comparisons between experiment and theory are meaningful without an independent knowledge of these quantities. However, their physical reasonableness may be investigated by comparisons between different systems. In this manner we have noted a correlation between p^*, v^*, and T^* in organic polymers and *n*-paraffins. In comparing v^* values with values obtained otherwise, it must be recalled that the segment is not necessarily identical with the repeat unit. We have given the relation between the two for several polymers.

E. HELFAND (*Bell Laboratories, Murray Hill, N.J.*): Dr. Simha, the theory that you presented is a single order parameter theory. At the end you touched on the question of how you can meet some of the objections to single order parameter theories by making c temperature dependent. Unfortunately c is so little understood that this only partially contributes to the fundamental understanding of the mechanism. Are you really referring to the question of whether one has reached equilibrium in a glass with respect to the conformational distribution, i.e., the distribution between *trans* and gauche bonds? Have there been any measurements in glasses of the *trans*-gauche distribution?

SIMHA: As applied to the *PVT* surfaces, the theory operates with a single (not implying frozen) ordering parameter. While c can be specified a priori only in extreme cases or in the frame of a normal coordinate description, it may be regarded as a comparative measure of chain flexibility. For the range of *PVT* and related data available we conclude that c is at most a very slowly decreasing function of T in the melt (see reply to Dr. Miller). A correlation between c and an intermolecular, as contrasted with an intramolecular contribution, to the conformational equilibrium distribution, may be expected for simple structures. Both have recently been computed by my colleagues for the crystalline state. Such an approach might lead to an explicit calculation of a c function.

A significant temperature dependent freeze-in of external degrees of freedom over the transition range would result in a nonequilibrium distribution. A direct determination of $t - g$ ratios would be of interest for several reasons. I believe, however, that thermodynamic studies, as discussed in Dr. Goldstein's and in my paper, have a more direct bearing and will be more helpful.

E. A. DIMARZIO (*National Bureau of Standards, Washington, D. C.*): Dr. Simha, I agree with you in the sense that the apportioning of c into external and internal modes has to be interpreted physically as the question of the stiffness of the molecule, because if you have a perfectly stiff molecule you know everything is internal. There are no internal degrees of freedom. If it's perfectly flexible, a large fraction of the degrees of freedom are external. The physical interpretation of the apportioning of c has to reside in the flexibility. As you pointed out, Gibbs and DiMarzio do have a theory, very crude, with regard to flexibility that makes the c effectively dependent on temperature.

Now I have a separate question. Would you describe the various contributions to the temperature variation of volume above and below the glass temperature. There seem to be three separate (a priori possible) contributions. (1) temperature variation in lattice site size, (2) temperature variation in hole size, and (3) temperature variation in hole number. I would inquire how each contribution is accounted for in your theory. In particular, does the hole size have the same temperature variation as the lattice site size?

SIMHA: In the analysis of the relation between the liquid and glass, the *formal* dependence of the partition function on V, T, and h is retained. What changes is the functional dependence $h(V, T)$ (but see concluding comments in paper). Thus the lattice contribution to the thermodynamic functions (h = constant) retains the identical form (Equations 9 and 10 and subsequent discussion).

Above T_g, the thermal expansion is quantitatively described by a lattice plus a structural contribution. The latter arises from a temperature and pressure dependence of the hole fraction in accord with a minimization of the configurational free energy.

As for an additional contribution arising from a hole expansion, this would seem to be an ad hoc device in a quasi-lattice model, besides not being warranted by experiment. The hole size is to be defined by the segment. Its size as measured by the volume-scaling parameter, does appear to increase slightly with temperature (see reply to Dr. Miller) for reasons inherent in the model (assumption of uniform lattice accomodating intra- and inter-molecular distances, fixed ratio c/s) but the numerical effects are minor at best, until one gest to the *third* derivatives of the partition function. One can, of course, consider in a lattice model a hole size, which arises from a temperature-dependent degree of hole clustering. We are suggesting this as an important element in the observed survival of structural contributions in the glassy state down to very low temperatures. It arises from the different temperature dependence of the numbers of small and large clusters, existing particularly in high T_g systems with their relatively large values of h at T_g.

S. MOSS (*University of Houston, Houston, Tex.*): I wanted to ask a question that I'm sure has been raised a number of times and has been beaten down. It is a sort of a ghost, and I think that I know the answer, but it seems worthwhile to ask it anyway. To what extent can one take these curves of specific heat and treat the glass transition as a phase transition? I have argued with enough people about that and I think that I bring imperfect information to my argument. I would like to know, for instance, even though those specific heat curves of yours could be fit very well using your considerations and the parameters that you are dealing with, and it's obviously a kinetic thing, a relaxation phenomenon, yet this issue comes up again and again, namely, that the glass transition really can be treated as a proper phase transition if only one could find the right order parameter. I wonder if the people who talked this morning would comment on that?

MACEDO: First of all, there is no question that the kinetic aspects dominate the behavior, that if you cool the system at a lower rate, the glass transition moves to a lower temperature; if you cool it faster, it moves to higher temperatures. The temperature at which the glass transition occurs depends entirely on the time scale of your apparatus. If I do ultrasonic measurements, and I work at 100 MHz, glassy behavior may set in several hundred degrees higher than in the specific heat experiment. The problem is, of course, to decide whether the type of kinetic behavior that one observes in the glass transition issues from some sort of thermodynamic phase transition that would occur at lower temperatures.

It is possible that somewhere in this never-never land below T_g that you can't touch experimentally because you just can't wait long enough to make the measurement, there is a second or some higher order phase transition. Or perhaps there is an "infinite" order phase transition where things just change slowly.

MOSS: Those are certainly different things.

MACEDO: You can fit the data in some liquids in with two-, three-, ... state-type models, and in so doing you come up with an infinite order phase transition. B_2O_3, for example, fits extremely well with a three-state model; on the other hand, you can turn it around and describe the data in terms of the type of second order phase transition that Gibbs and DiMarzio talked about.

MOSS: I mean certainly within the framework of a Landau theory you could say, well, is it a phase transition? And then you become involved in changes of symmetry, for example. It seems to be an open question.

MACEDO: It is an open question and it is one that experimentally we can never find out.

A. LEADBETTER (*University of Exeter, Exeter, England*): I have a comment addressed to Dr. Macedo. I first would like to say that I was delighted to see his application of auto-correlation techniques to these relaxations. I think that this is a very marked advance in what one can do, and one ought to emphasize this has only recently become possible with the advent of photon correlation techniques. What I wanted to comment on is that Dr. Macedo suggested that one could do this with other techniques such as neutron scattering. Although in principle of course he is correct, this time scale cannot be achieved using neutron techniques. The situation is that in neutron scattering you don't measure this correlation time directly, but rather the energy broadening of the signal, which is a Lorentzian broadening for an exponential correlation function exactly as for conventional light scattering. The problem is that with the best present neutron techniques the longest time scale you can measure is 10^{-9} sec, and of course the relaxations here are interesting, you can observe them, but these are in fluid liquids; they are not in the viscous liquids relevant to glass-forming systems. With possible advances in techniques, possible in the next year or so by a so-called spin echo technique, which has been developed at Grenoble, one will hopefully be able to measure directly the correlation times rather than their Fourier transforms and with characteristic times perhaps two orders of magnitude longer than at present. So perhaps in a year or two one might be able to see down to 10^{-7} sec with neutrons, but I don't think there is much prospect at the moment of getting beyond that, so these relaxations are perhaps still important only in rather fluid liquids.

MACEDO: There is no question that what you say is absolutely correct. My comments concerning neutron scattering were intended as pedagogical and not to suggest that the technique is useful in viscous liquids except perhaps for looking at the analogs of what would be Raman lines in an optical experiment.

LEADBETTER: Yes, except that I would dispute that last statement. The molecules are not moving in isolation. There is certainly coupling even in a liquid, and you don't know what the breadth is in that coupling. This is perhaps a side issue. I don't dispute your main thesis at all. I think it is a worthwhile thing to do.

MACEDO: Let me just agree with you; I think both kinds of experiments should be done and compared because life is complicated enough.

S. WEINBERG (*Owens-Illinois Corporation, Toledo, O.*): Dr. Macedo, this morning you discussed the use of light-scattering techniques and the interpretation of light-scattering experiments. In addition, you discussed normal fluctuation theories, which one usually applies to fluids. I would like to raise the following point: although the interpretation of light-scattering experiments from fluids is very straightforward, it seems to me that it is more difficult to interpret the scattering from a glass (or a fluid in the glass transition region). I'm sure you know that if one tries to express the total light scattering intensity in terms of density fluctuations for the glass, and then relates the latter to the compressibility, one finds disagreement with the experiment. Could you comment?

MACEDO: First of all if you do a light-scattering experiment in a glass you have to realize that whenever you are doing light scattering you are measuring light scattering from everything that changes the index of refraction, so in a multicomponent system composition fluctuations are important as well as density fluctuations. Only the latter are related to the compressibility. Both composition and density fluctuations contribute to the central (Rayleigh) line and unless you can separate them on the basis of their halfwidths, all you measure is the total scattered intensity. Now sometimes this separation can be made. The characteristic line widths which are associated with composition fluctuations are typically a factor of 10^6 or so different from that associated with density fluctuations. So if you are doing a correlation experiment for which the "time scale window" in your correlator is say 10^{-4} to 10 sec, you can say I want to look at density fluctuation or I want to look at composition fluctuations. The time scales are entirely different, and generally for a given temperature, only one or the other time scale is measureable.

QUESTION: Which time scales?

MACEDO: Let's talk about the glass transition region, say a viscosity of 10^{10} poise. At 10^{10} poise, the time scale for density fluctuations is around one second. Between one millisecond and a hundred seconds you get the whole density relaxation function. If you want to look at composition fluctuations under the same conditions, you need about fifty hours.

WEINBERG: Well, I'm not talking about composition fluctuations. Maybe I can make my question a little clearer, and I'm sure there are experts in the room who could respond to this point. The fluctuation theory presupposes that in fact you know how to do the expansion of the entropy in terms of the appropriate number of independent thermodynamic variables. In other words you have a local equilibrium state. You can characterize the state of a little-fluctuated region in terms of a certain number of independent variables, and then do the entropy expansion. For a simple fluid, (or even in a multicomponent fluid) this is a simple procedure, but it seems to be a lot trickier when one is in the glass transition region, since here it is not clear how to characterize the local equilibrium state.

MACEDO: I think I understand the difficulty now. Let's consider the case of a single-component glass former, such as SiO_2 or B_2O_3. At temperatures well above T_g the simple fluctuation theory works well; that is, the scattered intensity (the sum of the Rayleigh and Brillouin intensities) is correctly given in terms of the equilibrium compressibility multiplied by the temperature, i.e., TK_{eq}. However, if one lowers the temperature such that the structural (density) relaxation time is say 10^{-3} seconds (a viscosity of about 10^7 poise) the structural rearrangement component of the density fluctuation can no longer propagate with the phonon modes (which show up in the Brillouin lines at about 10^{10} Hz frequency shift), but rather appear in the central line of the spectrum. The total intensity is still correctly given in terms of TK_{eq}. However, if the temperature is lowered to well below T_g one finds that the structural density fluctuations are "frozen in," that is, kinetically arrested, so that even hundreds of degrees below T_g, their magnitude is essentially the same as at T_g. If we designate the part of the compressibility associated with structural rearrangements as K_{st} and that governing the phonons as K_{ph}, then as a first approximation we would replace the factor TK_{eq} by $T_gK_{st} + TK_{ph}$. All we are saying here is that while the phonons are in equilibrium at the temperature T, the structural state of the material is roughly that which would be the equilibrium state at T_g. If you do this the measured and calculated intensities agree quite well. A few years ago we published several papers on this subject (MACEDO *et al.* 1973. J. Amer. Ceram. Soc. **56:** 506, 510, for example) which discuss the matter rather thoroughly.

C. A. ANGELL (*Purdue University*): Dr. Macedo, in view of the fact that the heat capacity is the reflection of the entropy fluctuations, and an entropy fluctuation requires reorganization of molecules in space and therefore takes time, is it correct that one should think of the heat capacity as having a frequency dependence that is in principle measurable through light scattering? I have in mind the possibility that there may be a distribution of heat capacity elements each characterized by its own relaxation time, and each linked with a corresponding element in the structural relaxation time distribution.

MACEDO: Well, the most simple answer to your question is, anything that's time dependent if you analyze it in the frequency domain will show up as frequency dependent, so if you have a heat measurement that oscillated in temperature width as a function of time you would find a frequency-dependent heat capacity. That can be measured with light, but the problem with a heat capacity is that when you do measure the entropy fluctuations you find that in the liquid there is only one entropy fluctuation present, one component whose line width is connected with the thermal conductivity of the liquid. Near the glass transition you find two pieces to that line. One piece is glasslike and has a thermal conductivity characteristic of glass; the other piece which is liquidlike is characterized by a *thermal* conductivity of the liquid and a magnitude proportionate to the specific heat difference $C_p - C_v$. That liquidlike piece unfortunately gets buried in the structural relaxation contribution to the spectrum and it is very hard to isolate.

L. C. E. STRUIK (*T.N.O., Delft, The Netherlands*): My remark concerns the practical value of the question whether there are one, two, or more internal parameters. I can illustrate this as follows: We have seen this morning that if you quench a material and then reheat it, the curve of volume or entropy versus time shows a maximum. However, after a single quench starting from an equilibrium state, specific volume will decrease continuously with time. On the other hand, if you heat the material from an equilibrium state, there will be a continuous increase in volume with time (KOVACS, A. J. 1964. Fortschr. Hochpolymer Forsch. **3**: 394). This proves that there is a wide distribution of relaxation times or internal parameters. But what's the value of this conclusion? You also can perform other experiments. You can quench a polymer and then measure the mechanical properties, i.e., how they develop during volume relaxation. You can measure the mechanical relaxation time, or its reciprocal, the molecular mobility M. Then you find that M decreases continuously with time after a quench from equilibrium and increases continuously after a heating from equilibrium. After a quench followed by heating, M first increased and then decreases with time. So molecular mobility M behaves in exactly the same way as specific volume v. If you plot the momentary value of the relaxation time versus the momentary value of volume, you find a single curve. This means that although there is a wide distribution in internal parameters, the actual behavior of the material can be described by a single macroscopic and measurable quantity.

My question is: what's the value of saying that there is a large number of internal parameters when it appears possible to describe the behavior of the material in terms of one macroscopic quantity?

MACEDO: I can think of several reasons for approaching the problem this way. At the fundamental or theoretical level our conception of what governs molecular processes in a liquid should not sweep the dynamical details under the rug by consolidating them into a single parameter. If it looks like the elementary molecular motions require many dynamical variables for their description (and it does) then what one should look for is the interplay of these various quantities in a given experiment. But I think there is another value of such an approach that is much more engineering oriented. We are trying very hard at Catholic University to understand what happens to the properties of a liquid no matter what you do to it, whether you come in under a wide variety of external changes, whether these be low-amplitude ultrasonic waves or a 1-msec 500,000-psi pressure pulse and a 200-degree temperature jump. And when we try to do that we find that we cannot express the relaxational behavior in terms of a single parameter. The various order parameters respond separately and differently to different types of imposed disturbances; the result is that you have to go to a much more complicated formula in which the various order parameters are accorded their distinct status. Our formulas are still largely empirical, but at least they are providing insight in how to handle very complicated thermal histories. We have been able to use them to calculate rather accurately the values of, for example, the volume, the entropy, and the shear viscosity as functions of time during and following a variety of imposed pressure and temperature changes.

THERMODYNAMICS OF THE GLASS TRANSITION: EMPIRICAL ASPECTS*

C. A. Angell and W. Sichina

Department of Chemistry
Purdue University
West Lafayette, Indiana 47907

Introduction

The glass transition, at which a viscous liquid settles into the glassy or structurally arrested state, in some respects appears to be a very obvious process, while in other respects it is both subtle and provocative. The process is obvious because the major phenomena observed, changes in heat capacity, expansion coeffiicient, and so forth, are no more than the consequences of the system under observation falling out of complete thermodynamic equilibrium at some point in the experiment. It is subtle and provocative because (i) the kinetics of the process whereby equilibrium is lost/recovered are in general not simple exponential (first order) processes even when the system is very close to equilibrium, (ii) the magnitude of the changes, rather than the fact that they occur, are not predictable without a very detailed partition function for the high density liquid state, which is not available even for very simple liquids, and (iii) the question of what phenomena would be encountered under longer and longer experiment time scales remains to be properly resolved.

The purpose of this paper is to provide some understanding of the magnitude of this problem by drawing attention to the great range and variety of thermodynamic changes by which the glass transition, i.e., the process of falling out of equilibrium, can be manifested. From the mass of data available, few consistent and general relationships can be salvaged. Those that can, however, are useful and may point the way to improved phenomenological description and ultimately to coherent theory for the phenomenon.

We will consider, in turn, thermodynamic manifestations of T_g, their magnitude, variety, and interrelation, and finally their relation to dissipative (relaxation) processes in the liquid state. In these considerations it will be taken as read that the changes in properties observed at the glass transition actually occur over a range of temperatures that is larger the higher the temperature of the phenomenon. Quantities such as ΔC_p characterizing the thermodynamic aspects of the transition will always be based on values measured outside (above and below) the transformation range.

THERMODYNAMIC CHANGES AT T_g

Heat Capacities

If equilibrium with respect to some degree of freedom is to be lost during a cooling process, then fluctuations in the total entropy associated with that degree

*This work was supported by Grant DMR-73-02632-A01 from the National Science Foundation.

of freedom must cease to contribute to the heat capacity according to Equation 1[1]:

$$\overline{\Delta S^2} = kC_p. \quad (1)$$

Thus, the glass transition with falling temperature must always be accompanied by a decrease of heat capacity. This change may, in some cases, be very small, but the inequality C_p(liquid) $-$ C_p(glass) $= \Delta C_p > 0$ cannot be violated.

The quantity ΔC_p is a very interesting and important quantity for understanding liquid state processes since it is the direct energy manifestation of changes in particle ordering which occur once the glassy structure has been "unlocked" by sufficient increase of temperature, (i.e., when $T > T_g$ for ordinary time scale experiments). Liquids with rapidly degraded structures will be characterized by large ΔC_p values, while those with temperature-resistant short-range orders will show relatively small ΔC_p values. Unfortunately, for the purposes of comparing and correlating behavior amongst different substances, there is no clear-cut basis for reducing the observed heat capacity changes (which are usually reported as "per mole" quantities) to some common basis. A "per-gram-atom" basis is useful for heavy atom systems (e.g., the chalcogenide glasses) where all bonds in the system are susceptible to thermal rupturing. In organic liquids, however, the temperature-inviolate mutual arrangement of groups of atoms of different sizes (e.g., $—CH_2—$, $C_6H_5—$, $—CH{=}CH—$, $—NH_2$, and so forth) renders a per-gram-atom basis unsuitable for comparisons. A "per-bead" basis, where a bead is defined as any tightly bound group of single atoms that serves as a quasi-independent unit in the structure, has been proposed for glasses in general and shown to be associated with an approximately constant contribution of 2.7 cal deg^{-1} to ΔC_p for the cases considered.[2] However, the decision on what constitutes a bead in a given glass is often problematical, if not arbitrary.

A less arbitrary, though also not completely satisfactory, manner of reducing the data to a common basis is to reduce the liquid state C_p by the fixed-structure (glassy) C_p at each temperature for which the comparison is to be made. We will adopt this latter basis in the present paper, defining $C_{p,r} = C_p(\text{liquid})/C_p(\text{glass})$ at T_g and $C_p(\text{liquid})/C_p(\infty)$ at other temperatures. Here $C_p(\infty)$ is the value of C_p appropriate to some fast experiment in which the structure does not change during the heat capacity measurement. Since very fast heat capacity measurements are not easily made, $C_p(\infty)$ is usually taken to be the same as C_p the value for the crystal at the same temperature.†

In FIGURE 1a complete molar C_p vs T plots are shown for two substances, GeO_2 and 2-methylpentane, which show very small and quite large $C_{p,r}$ values, respectively. These exemplify not only the extent of the differences in ΔC_p, but also the sort of differences in pre-T_g glass heat capacity functions, which may be encountered in practice. Glasses with heavy atom constituents or isotropic bonding usually approach their classical heat capacity values of 6 cal/g-atom before the glass transition occurs.

Also included in FIGURE 1a are plots for two molecular liquids *m*-fluorotoluene, and *m*-fluoroaniline, the constituent particles of which differ only in the replacement of a $—CH_3$ sidegroup by an $—NH_2$ sidegroup.[3] Attention was drawn to the latter by the unusually small boiling point-to-T_g ratio it exhibits. The great differ-

†This choice will somewhat underestimate the value at high temperatures where the liquid "instantaneous" structure will be considerably loosened with respect to the crystal structure (and to that of the liquid at T_g), but the difference will be of the nature of an anharmonicity correction, and should be small.

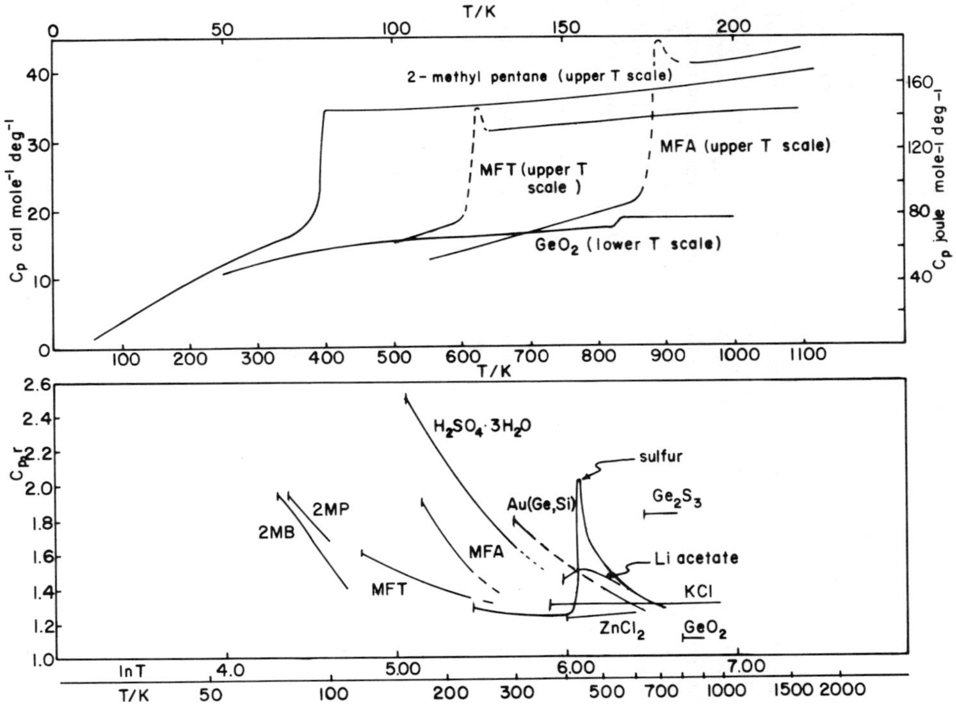

FIGURE 1. (a) A selection of heat capacity vs temperature functions for glass-forming liquids. (b) Reduced heat capacity $C_p[= C_p(\text{liquid})/C_p(\text{glass})]$ functions for glass-forming liquids at $T > T_g$. The sources of most data are referred to in the text. Data for Au(Si–Ge) are from Chen and Turnbull,[43] and for Ge_2S_3 from Schnaus *et al.*[44] (these data were included to demonstrate that large $C_{p,r}$ values are not limited to low-temperature liquids). The data for $ZnCl_2$ are from Angell,[22] for 2 MP (2-methylpentane) from Douslin and Huffman,[45] and for 2 MB (2-methylbutane) from Huffman *et al.*[46]

ence in thermal behavior is clearly a manifestation of the influence of hydrogen bonding (present in the fluoroaniline because of fluorine-enhanced —NH_2 donor strength) may have on liquid state properties. By contrast replacement of 50% of the *m*-fluorotoluene with *m*-methyl toluene (*m*-xylene, which is not itself glass-forming) produces only 5°C changes in T_g and no detectable change in ΔC_p at T_g.[3] It is believed that the study of series of molecular liquids, tailored like the above to exhibit specific differences in interaction potential at constant geometry, will be helpful in elucidating glass transition behavior.

In FIGURE 1b $C_{p,r}$ is shown as a function of temperature for a collection of liquids of different constituent particles and interaction types. $C_{p,r}$ usually decreases with increasing T though in a number of heavy atom cases a constant value is found. In unusual cases $C_{p,r}$ is increasing with T just above T_g. FIGURE 1 suggests that the structures of the inorganic tetrahedral network liquids GeO_2, BeF_2, and SiO_2 are particularly stable against temperature change, whereas the structures of hydrogen-bonded liquids in general, and occasional atomic and molecular liquids as well, degrade rapidly with changing temperature. In the case of hydrogen-bonded liquids the behavior can be understood in terms of the extra energetic degeneracy permitted by the broad minimum in the H-bond interaction potential.

These differences in structural stability would presumably be reflected in changes in the *X*-ray radial distribution functions for these liquids with changing temperature, though adequate data on this point are not, to the author's knowledge, available at the moment.

Data on sulfur,[4] the behavior of which is imitated by a number of (Ge + Te)-based alloys[5] show that in special cases, more than one type of disordering process can occur at the same time. The anomalous contributions, due to specific molecular equilibria [S_8(ring) → S_n(chain) in the sulfur case] or to a poorly understood geometrical or electronic effect (in the Ge-Te case), occur superimposed on "normal" liquid structure, disordering contributions in each case. Each disordering process has its own characteristic relaxation time, the times being definable by appropriate variable-scan-speed differential scanning calorimetry experiments.

The approximate $C_{p,r}$ shown for KCl is based not on laboratory experiments, (KCl being unvitrifiable), but on some computer simulation "experiments" currently being reported.[6-8] Although the computer experiment is conducted on a time scale some 11 orders of magnitude shorter than for normal heat capacity measurements, the value of $C_{p,r}$ for this very simple ionic substance is comparable with the values observed for its closest relatives among the laboratory glasses.

Expansion Coefficients

The expansivity $\alpha = (1/V)(\partial V/\partial T)_p$, will generally show more pronounced changes at T_g than the heat capacity because the glass expansivity is mainly determined by only the anharmonic component of the atomic motions, and thus is usually small. Comparison amongst different substances is facilitated by the fact that in the definition of α the temperature coefficient of the volume is reduced by the volume itself.

The behavior of α about T_g, like that of $C_{p,r}$, reflects changes in short-range order that occur when $T > T_g$. Thus, $\Delta\alpha$ can show all the variations associated with rate of short-range order breakdown seen for $C_{p,r}$, plus additional variations stemming from the fact that there are no inequalities governing the direction of expansivity changes at T_g. Thus $\Delta\alpha$ may be, and in some cases evidently is, negative depending on whether or not low-energy structures are also low-volume struc-

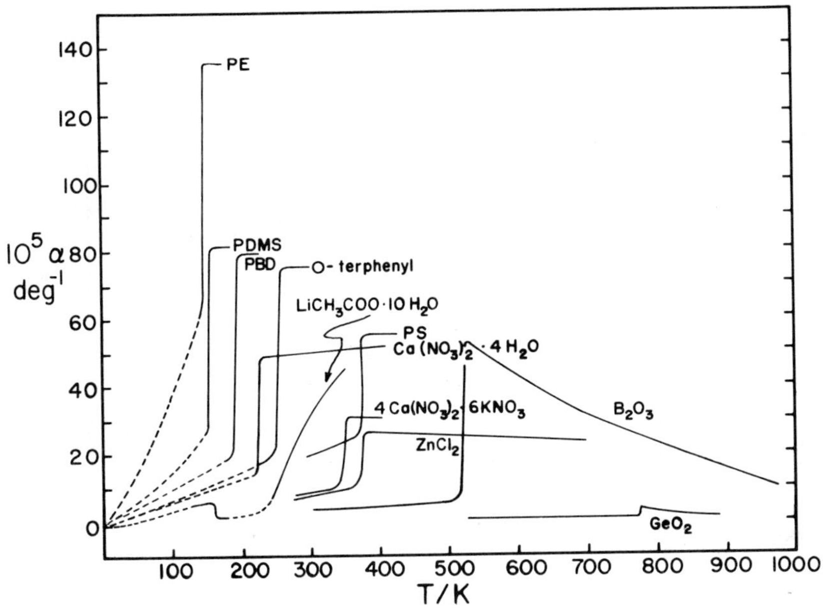

FIGURE 2. Expansion coefficients for a selection of glass-forming liquids through the glass transition region. Note negative $\Delta\alpha$ for the lithium acetate hydrate. For polymer liquids we have used the notation PE (polyethylene), PDMS (polydimethylsiloxane), PBD (polybutadiene), and PS (polystyrene). Data from References 9–11, 21, 36, 37, and also from Klemm[47] (for $ZnCl_2$), Goldstein and Nakoneczny[48] (for $ZnCl_2$), and Angell[49] [for $Ca(NO_3)_2 \cdot 4 H_2O$].

tures. Positive energy-volume correlations, hence positive values of $\Delta\alpha$, are the common finding. The opposite applies when open networks are the favored low-energy structure. The classical prototype glass, SiO_2, is such a case,[8] and recently some additional examples among aqueous salt solutions have been found.[9,10]

Some data for liquids of different structural types are collected in FIGURE 2. In FIGURE 2 no attempt has been made to provide accurate representations of the variation of α with temperature below T_g beyond noting that α must approach zero as $T \rightarrow 0$°K. With the exception of the aqueous glasses and B_2O_3, these data all tend to support the correlation suggested by Simha and Boyer[11]

$$T_g \Delta\alpha = \text{constant} = 0.112 \pm 0.2,$$

for which a free-volume theory rationale can be provided.[11] The occurrence of the contrary aqueous solution cases is important because it serves to illustrate that "free volume" interpretations of liquid flow properties, which have found wide acceptance, cannot be of general validity. Rather they apparently depend on a positive correlation of configurational volume with some other configurational property, either entropy or enthalpy, which governs the relaxational behavior (see below). It should be noted that substances showing an almost unobservable change in α at T_g may still exhibit a very pronounced change in C_p (the converse is not true).

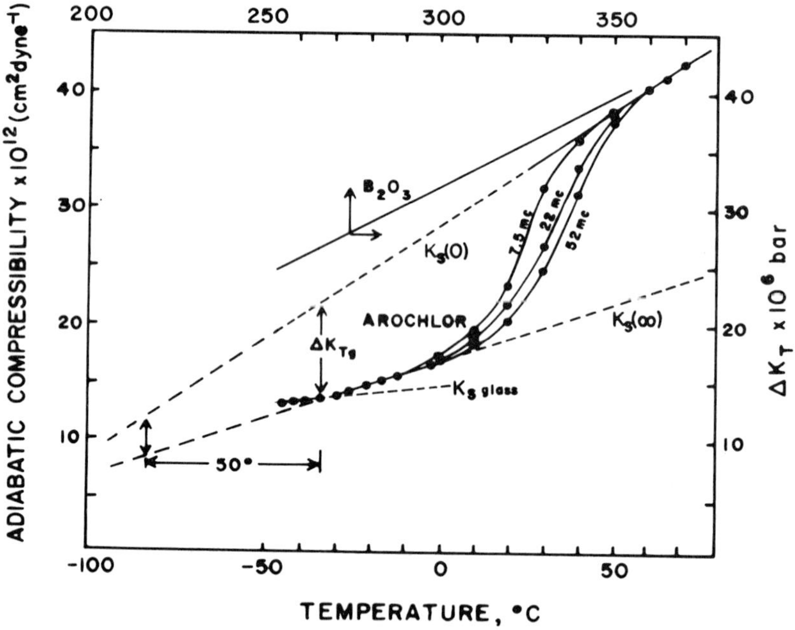

FIGURE 3. (i) Adiabatic compressibility K_s of arochlor from measurements made at different ultrasonic frequencies and (ii) the relaxing part of the isothermal compressibility of B_2O_3, $\Delta\kappa_T$ at temperatures above T_g. Note temperature dependence of $\Delta\kappa$ in each case.

Compressibility

The compressibility of a material, like its heat capacity, must decrease when equilibrium with respect to some degree of freedom is lost. This is again a consequence of the loss of a contribution to the mean square volume fluctuation, ΔV^2, which determines the compressibility through the relation[1]

$$\overline{\Delta V^2} = VkT\kappa_T. \tag{2}$$

The compressibility change at T_g is considerably more difficult to determine than the changes in expansivity or heat capacity, and few data are available. Those values that exist have mainly been obtained by ultrasonic absorption experiments, which are "fast" experiments compared with, e.g., differential scanning calorimetry. Thus, the change in (adiabatic) compressibility is only observed at a temperature well above the "normal" T_g and its value at T_g must be judged from experiments performed at different frequencies. The results of such experiments, an example of which[12] is given in FIGURE 3 show that the quantity $\Delta\kappa_S$ usually decreases with decreasing temperature, in contrast with the usual behavior of $\Delta\alpha$ and ΔC_p. That such decreases persist to T_g is shown by the results of a recent study of $\Delta\kappa_T$ for B_2O_3 in which pressure jump relaxation techniques were applied.[13] In the unusual B_2O_3 case, however, a reversal occurs as higher temperatures and $\Delta\kappa_T$, like $\Delta\alpha$, then decreases with increasing temperature.[14]

Relations Amongst Excess Thermodynamic Quantities

Davies and Jones[15,16] showed that if the position of equilibrium in a relaxing system is determined by a single ordering parameter, then the relationship

$$\frac{\Delta\kappa_T}{\Delta\alpha} = \frac{TV\Delta\alpha}{\Delta C_p} \tag{3}$$

must hold. Although this was the focus of a recent controversy,[17-19] it now seems clear that in the event that the position of equilibrium can only be properly described by use of more than one order parameter Equation 3 becomes an inequality

$$\frac{\Delta\kappa_T}{\Delta\alpha} > TV\frac{\Delta\alpha}{\Delta C_p}. \tag{4}$$

Since the available data support Equation 4 rather than 3, it is generally accepted that at least two,[14] and probably a spectrum of order parameters need to be specified to adequately describe the thermodynamic behavior of supercooled liquids near T_g. Equation 4 is often cast in the form

$$\frac{\Delta\kappa_T\Delta C_p}{TV(\Delta\alpha)^2} > 1 \tag{5}$$

Further relationships may be obtained by introducing the pressure dependence of the glass transition temperature, which is quite easily determined in the laboratory.

For a second-order thermodynamic transition, or for a nonequilibrium transition in a single-order parameter relaxing system, the relations

$$dT/dP = TV\,\Delta\alpha/\Delta C_p \tag{6}$$

and

$$dT/dP = \Delta\kappa_T/\Delta\alpha \tag{7}$$

may be derived.[15,16] Since the glass transition is neither a second-order transition nor a relaxation process characterized by a single ordering parameter, there is no immediate reason to expect either Equation 6 or 7 to describe the observed behavior of T_g with P. In practice, however, it is found that while Equation 7 never holds, Equation 6, which has been tested for a large number of cases, is generally successful.[20,21] Only two real failures have been recorded to date[22] (see below). Comparisons of calculated with experimental T_g vs P functions are shown in Figure 4. Note that when $\Delta\alpha$ is negative ($LiCH_3COO \cdot 10\,H_2O$ in Figure 2), T_g decreases with increasing pressure.

Equation 6 may be derived from the recognition that $\Delta S = 0$ along a line of second order transitions or from the assumption, for a nonequilibrium transition, that $\Delta S = 0$ at each pressure irrespective of the pressure at which the glass if formed, i.e., that $S_{ex}(P) =$ constant. Since the temperature at which the glass transition is observed in practice is determined by the temperature at which the average relaxation time for the structure reaches some characteristic value (determined by the particular experiment detecting T_g) the success of Equation 6 implies a simple relation between structural relaxation time and S_{ex}.

This matter and the related exception to Equation 6, will be discussed in a later section on relations between thermodynamic and relaxational properties. As emphasized by Goldstein[23,24] the failure of Equation 7, which follows from the

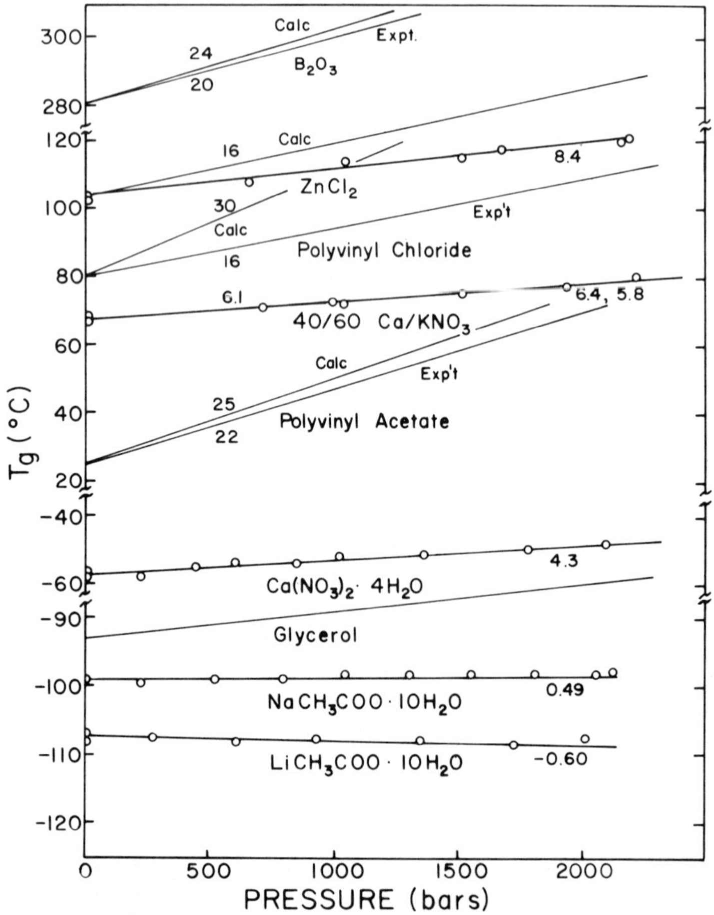

FIGURE 4. Plots of experimental T_g vs pressure functions for various liquids of interest. Calculated plots are based on Equation 6. Note pronounced discrepancies for cases of $ZnCl_2$ and polyvinyl chloride.

assumption that V_{ex} = const along the line of glass transitions, provides further evidence for the irrelevance of volume as a state-determining quantity for viscous liquids and glasses.

EXTRAPOLATIONS BELOW T_g

Since it is well recognized that the glass transition as studied in the laboratory is a kinetic phenomenon determined by the relation between the liquid structural relaxation time and the experimental time scale, it is reasonable to ask how the phenomenon would appear when studied on longer and longer time scales. The effect of different time scale experiments on the magnitude and sharpness of $\Delta\kappa_S$, for instance, has already been noted in FIGURE 3.

The necessity for some changes at very long times, or at temperature well below T_g, can be seen immediately. For instance, the decrease of $\Delta\kappa_S$ observed with increasing experiment time could not continue indefinitely since $\Delta\kappa_S$ cannot become negative.

That some lower limit should exist on the temperature range over which the glass transition will be manifested as a kinetic phenomenon, is also demonstrated by extrapolating the heat capacity versus temperature plots for liquids with large $C_{p,r}$ values and observing the way in which the difference in entropy between liquid and crystalline states (which was ΔS_F at the fusion point) changes with temperature. Data for $H_2SO_4 \cdot 3H_2O$ based on the very accurate calorimetric work of Kunzler and Giauque,[25] and for $Ca(NO_3)_2 \cdot 4H_2O$ using data from this laboratory,[26,27] are shown in Figure 5. These plots suggest that at a temperature only some 20° below the "normal" T_g, the difference in entropy between liquid and crystalline phases would vanish. Because the existence of amorphous phases with significantly lower total entropies than those of the stable crystalline phases at the same temperature is unacceptable as a general rule, these plots demonstrate that in extremely slow (equilibrium) experiments, the heat capacity of liquid $H_2SO_4 \cdot 3H_2O$ and $Ca(NO_3)_2 \cdot 4H_2O$ would have to decrease precipitously at, if not before, 130 or 200 K, respectively. The point of interest that is usually not recogized is just how sharply these considerations bound the possible forms that the *equilibrium* heat capacity can have in cases with large $C_{p,r}$ values (such on those exemplified in Figure 5). The most gradual possible decrease of ΔC_p below T_g that remains consistent with the requirement that S (liquid) > S (cryst) still amounts to a very sharp change in C_p, comparable with the high temperature end of a common lambda transition. It is tempting to see the sharply falling C_p vs T function at the low temperature end of the liquid sulfur reverse lambda transition (see FIGURE 1b) as a possible model for the form of the equilibrium glass transition.

Consideration of the FIGURE 5 cases, of which a great many parallel examples exist, thus supports rather strongly the original Gibbs–Dimarzio idea[28] that the glass transition observed in the laboratory is the kinetically limited reflection of an underlying equilibrium transition of approximately second-order character.

The possible existence of such vanishing-excess-entropy or "ideal" glass transitions T_0 at temperatures some tens of degrees below the experimental T_g has of course been a recognized consequence of the thermal data on glass-forming systems since Kauzmann[29] drew attention to the paradox in 1948. T_g/T_0 seems to be smaller the larger the value of $C_{p,r}$, which is consistent with the notion[30,31] that T_g occurs at some more or less constant value of the (suitably reduced) excess entropy. When $C_{p,r}$ is close to unity, a meaningful extrapolation to establish a calorimetric T_0 cannot, of course, be performed.

Because of its different thermodynamic relation to ΔC_p, the excess enthalpy does not extrapolate to zero until temperatures well below T_0. Thus, at T_0 ΔG_{ex} remains positive and the glass is still metastable with respect to the crystalline phase. It is interesting to observe, after Miller,[32] that the excess volume frequently extrapolates to zero at the same temperature as the excess enthalpy, e.g., for *o*-terphenyl $T_0(S_{ex} = 0)$ is 200 K whereas $V_{ex} = 0$ at 178°K and $H_{ex} = 0$ at 171 K. For polythene $T_0(S_{ex} = 0)$ is 160 K while $V_{ex} = 0$ at 56 K and $H_{ex} = 0$ at 50 K.‡

‡Miller has also pointed out that T_0 of Equation 13 consistently falls above T_0 (calc) for chain polymers with bulky side-chain groups, and suggests as a reason, that side-chain configuration randomization contributes to entropy of fusion but is not important in comparison with backbone degrees of freedom in determination of the viscosity temperature dependence.

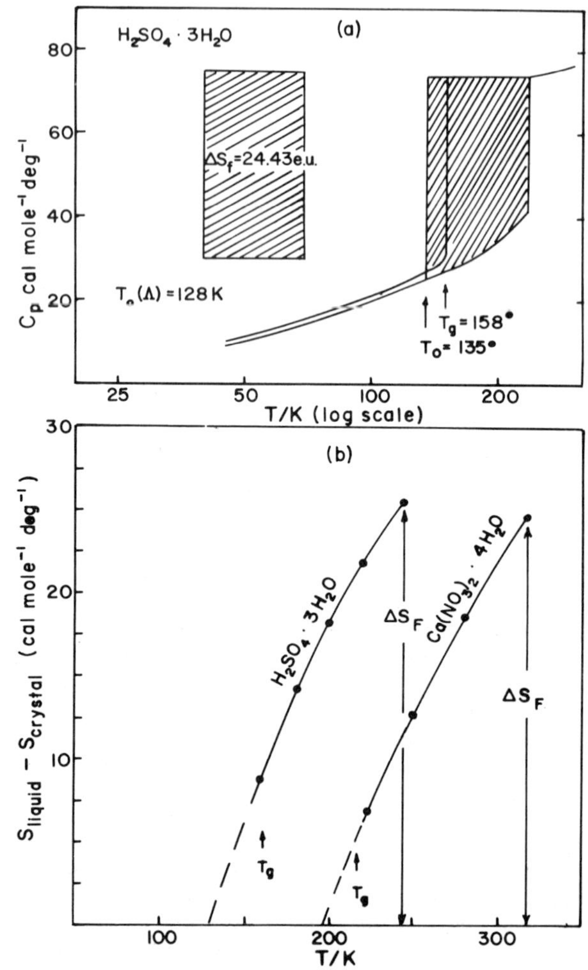

FIGURE 5. Graphical estimates of the limits on the temperature range below T_g over which the observed equilibrium liquid heat capacity could be maintained in "slow" (equilibrium) experiments. The condition $(S_{liquid} - S_{crystal})_T = 0$ would appear to define a temperature $T = T_0$ at which, if not before, rapid decreases in the equilibrium liquid heat capacity must occur.

A question arises concerning the value assumed by the Prigogine–Defay ratio, R (see Equation 5), at T_0. Qualitatively, R tends to decrease with decreasing temperature because the trends in both $\Delta\kappa$ and $\Delta\alpha$ usually decrease R while only the trend in ΔC_p tends to increase it. Where the data are available, as in the case of poly(vinyl acetate), it appears that R would remain well in excess of unity even at T_0.[33] Indeed a value of unity can in general only be expected for equilibrium second-order transitions when the low temperature phase has a unique structure (either by virtue of a unique geometry or a mobile equilibrium between different geometries) hence a unique free energy surface. This will not be the case in glass-forming systems.

Correlations of Thermodynamic Changes at T_g with Liquid Relaxational Properties

A quite empirical basis for viewing the excess entropy of a glass-forming liquid as its most important state-characterizing quantity seems to be emerging from the foregoing observations. Not only is it this quantity whose vanishing is narrowly averted by occurrence of the glass transition, but, in view of what is generally considered the success of Equation 6 in predicting the effect of pressure on T_g, it is the arrival of this quantity at a predetermined value that causes the glass transition to occur. This is equivalent to stating that the structural relaxation time for a glass-forming liquid near T_g is determined to good approximation by the magnitude of S_{ex} alone. In this section we will examine the empirical evidence for general relationship between S_{ex}, ΔC_p, and relaxation behavior in viscous liquids.

The above observation

$$\tau = f(S_{ex}) \tag{8}$$

implies a relationship between thermodynamic and nonequilibrium properties that is too simple to be easily accepted. In fact, it comes almost as a relief to find[22] a clear exception to Equation 6, and hence to Equation 8. As shown in FIGURE 4, $ZnCl_2$ and polyvinyl chloride exhibit smaller temperature dependence of T_g than predicted from Equation 6, which implies that the glass transition occurs at smaller S_{ex} values the higher the pressure. The reason for the failure in these cases is probably that S_{ex} varies rather slowly with temperature due to a relatively small value of ΔC_p per gram-atom (or $C_{p,r}$) and this makes it possible for the influence of other factors, e.g., pure temperature, to show up. Since T_g increases with increasing pressure, the observations would be qualitatively consistent with a relationship of the form

$$\tau = f(TS_{ex}) \tag{9}$$

which is actually the relationship embodied in the Adam–Gibbs theory for relaxational properties of viscous liquids.[34] These authors derive

$$\tau = \tau_0 \exp(-C/TS_{ex}) \tag{10}$$

where C is a constant.

Goldstein[33] has derived the relationship between dT_g/dP and changes in thermodynamic quantities to a expected if constancy of TS_{ex} rather than of S_{ex} itself determines the occurrence of T_g. He obtains

$$dT_g/dP = V_g T_g \Delta\alpha/(S_{ex} + \Delta C_p). \tag{11}$$

Numerically, the general rules found by Bestul and Chang[30,31] and Wunderlich[2] are that $S_{ex} = 0.7$ cal deg^{-1} bead^{-1} and $\Delta C_p = 2.7$ cal deg^{-1} bead^{-1}. Thus ~25% discrepancies between observed values of dT_g/dP and those calculated using Equation 6 should be the general rule, with considerably larger differences possible for cases where ΔC_p is unusually small. Poly(vinyl acetate) and B_2O_3 show deviations in the expected direction and of the expected magnitude, although experimental uncertainties in $\Delta\alpha$ are probably of comparable magnitude.§ It may be significant that the $Ca(NO_3)_2$—KNO_3 glass in which the calculated (6.1 deg

§For B_2O_3 the calculated dT_g/dP value used in FIGURE 5 is smaller than that quoted by O'Reilly[20] because of an improved value of $\Delta\alpha$ from studies by Macedo *et al.*[36] and Napolitano *et al.*[37]

kbar^{-1})[21] and experimental values (5.8 and 6.4 deg kbar^{-1})[22] are very similar, is a glass which has shown other evidence of relative "ideality".[38] For $ZnCl_2$, at least, $C_{p,r}$ at T_g is indeed unusually small.

Since the accurate measurement of dT_g/dP presents no major problems, the systematic testing of Equations 6 and 11 should be enlightening and deserves attention.

Equation 10, which could rationalize the general success of Equation 6, suggests that, for substances such as GeO_2 and SiO_2 in which $C_{p,r}$ is very small, the relaxational properties will show Arrhenius behavior. This is found to be the case. On the other hand where ΔC_p (or $C_{p,r}$) is large, S_{ex} should change rapidly with temperature and non-Arrhenius behavior should be encountered.

Quantitatively, if the simplest reasonably accurate approximation of the form of ΔC_p (see FIGURE 1), viz.,

$$\Delta C_p = \text{constant}/T \tag{11}$$

is introduced, we obtain

$$S_{ex} = \int_{T_0}^{T} \frac{\Delta C_p}{T}\, dT = \int_{T_0}^{T} \frac{\text{constant}}{T^2}\, dT = \Delta C_{p(T_0)} \frac{(T - T_0)}{T}, \tag{12}$$

hence, from Equation 10,

$$\tau = \tau_0 \exp B/(T - T_0), \tag{13}$$

where B is another constant. Equation 13 is the well-known empirical Vogel–Tammann–Fulcher equation, which provides an excellent description of the behavior of most viscous liquids over considerable temperature and viscosity ranges not too close to T_g. T_0, obtained by fitting of experimental data to Equation 13, should agree with the vanishing entropy temperature obtained from thermal data via FIGURE 5 type constructions. This is often, though by no means always, found to be the case.[39] For $H_2SO_4 \cdot 3H_2O$, T_0 values of 130 and 128 are found from viscosity (extrapolated value) and conductance measurements, respectively,[26] cf. 130°K in FIGURE 5. For $Ca(NO_3)_2 \cdot 4H_2O$, near its melting point, viscosity conductance, and trace-ion diffusion all yield T_0 values within 2° of the calorimetric value.[27] Unfortunately, these pleasing findings do not always apply to data on the same substances taken close to T_g. Near, but still above T_g, it is frequently found that relaxation times revert to an Arrhenius temperature dependence[40,41] in clear contradiction to Equations and 10 and 13 although the temperature dependence still contains a major contribution from changing liquid structure.[35] The origin of this low temperature Arrhenius regime, which is found for most but not all liquids, has yet to be properly explained. In relation to this problem we believe there is value in Dworkin's suggestion[50] that the T_0 obtained from the vanishing excess entropy analysis illustrated in FIGURE 5 be taken as an independently determined constant, T_0, of the transport equation (Equation 13) and that the deviations from Equation 13 then found for various substances near their T_g be analyzed in relation to molecular structure.

An overall correlation of the characteristics of mass transport with the magnitude of the heat capacity change is usefully made using reduced plots of the type shown in FIGURE 6. In FIGURE 6 the viscosity–temperature relations for several different substances, including weak and strong inorganic network liquids, ionic liquids, and two molecular liquids, are brought together by plotting viscosities on

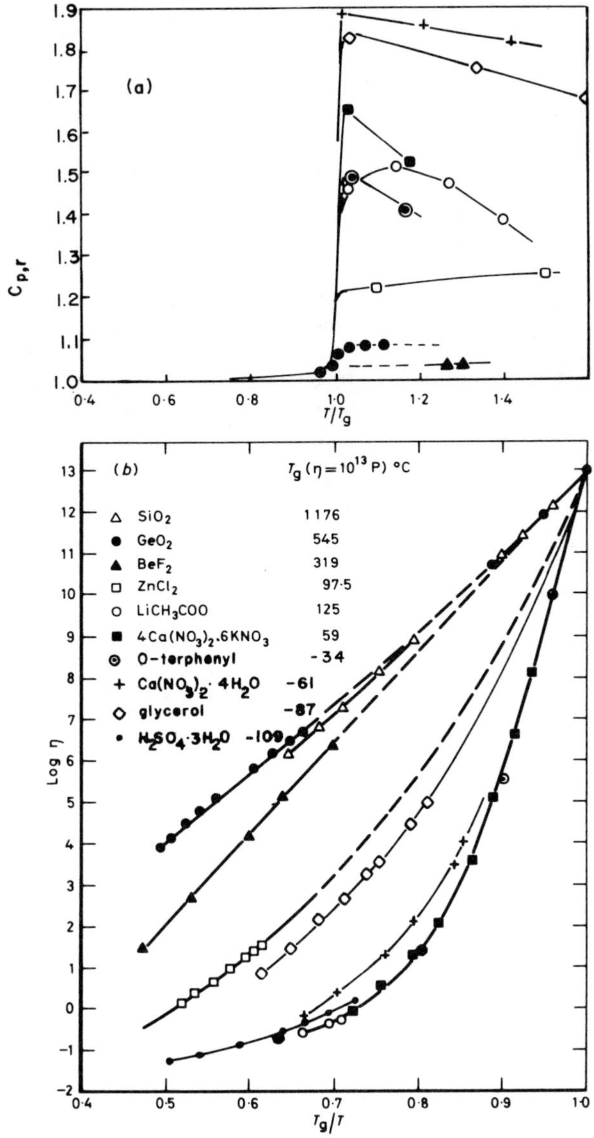

FIGURE 6 (a) Values of $C_{p,r}$ for simple inorganic glass-forming liquids, and some molecular and hydrated glasses, plotted vs reduced temperature T/T_g. (b) Viscosities of the same systems represented in part (a) plotted vs inverse reduced temperatures T_g/T in order to show the relation between viscous and thermodynamic properties. A maximum value of the limiting low-temperature slope seems to be reached when $E_{\text{act}} \approx 200RT_g$.

a reduced temperature scale, T_g/T, such that all liquids have a common point at a viscosity of 10^{13} poise.[36,37] This corresponds to the viscosity measured when the structural relaxation time is $\sim 10^4$ sec. A good qualitative correlation seems to exist between the magnitudes of $C_{p,r}$ for simple inorganic substances (SiO_2, GeO_2, BeF_2, $ZnCl_2$, and $4Ca(NO_3)_2 \cdot 6KNO_3$), the non-Arrhenius character of their transport properties, and the limiting low temperature slopes of the reduced Arrhenius plots (which are dimensionless quantities numerically equal to $E/2.303RT_g$, where E is the ordinary Arrhenius activation energy). This correlation, however, does not extend to the cases of $Ca(NO_3)_2 \cdot 4H_2O$ and glycerol, which have very large values of $C_{p,r}$ but fail to continue the series in FIGURE 6b. Unfortunately, suitable viscosity data are not available for $H_2SO_4 \cdot 3H_2O$, whose value of $C_{p,r}$ is exceptionally large (FIGURE 1b). Some values obtained by extrapolation of 30° to −50°C data in the composition range 0–16 mole% H_2SO_4,[51] are entered in FIGURE 6b to indicate (probably with good accuracy) that at least in the lower T_g/T range there is nothing extraordinary about the viscosity-reduced temperature relationship for this case. In general, there are insufficient data available for liquids of similar T_g values but of different constitution to elucidate these relationships satisfactorily at this point. There is some indication in FIGURE 6b that a limit to the low-temperature activation energy may be reached when $E \approx 200\,RT_g$.

The correlations between $C_{p,r}$ values and transport behavior for the simple inorganic liquids extend consistently to their disrupted-network binary solutions.[42] For instance, when alkali oxides are added to SiO_2 the behavior of $C_{p,r}$ changes to resemble that of $ZnCl_2$ in FIGURE 6b, and the viscosity becomes non-Arrhenius, also like that of $ZnCl_2$ in FIGURE 6b. Likewise, if the weaker $ZnCl_2$ network is disrupted by adding basic anions, then both $C_{p,r}$ and the viscosity behavior change in the direction of the ionic fused salts and molecular liquids shown in FIGURE 6.[42] The equivalent mixing experiments for strong hydrogen-bonded and non-hydrogen-bonded molecular liquids usually cannot be made because of immiscibility problems, but glycerol + monohydric alcohol mixtures may provide parallel cases, and therefore deserve examination.

CONCLUSIONS

A number of lines of empirical evidence support the notion that, except for strong-network liquids, the variation with temperature of the excess (or configurational) entropy of a liquid is the single most important factor determining the liquid behavior and, accordingly, the vitrification process.

ACKNOWLEDGMENT

We are indebted to Professor M. Goldstein for some very helpful discussions.

REFERENCES

1. LANDAU L. & E. M. LIFSCHITZ. 1958. Statistical Physics. Sect. **111:** 350. Pergammon Press, Ltd. London, Paris. Addison-Wesley Publishing Co., Inc. Reading, Mass.
2. WUNDERLICH, B. 1960. J. Phys. Chem. **64:** 1052–56.
3. ANGELL, C. A. & W. SICHINA. To be published.
4. WEST, E. D. 1959. J. Amer. Chem. Soc. **81:** 29–37.

5. De Neufville, J. P. 1972. J. Non-Cryst. Solids **8–10**: 85–105.
6. Woodcock, L. V., Proc. 1972 Summer Simulation Conference. IV. Physical Science.
7. Woodcock, L. V., P. A. Cheeseman & C. A. Angell. 1976. J. Chem. Phys. **65:** 1565.
8. Douglas, R. W., & J. O. Isard. 1951. J. Soc. Glass. Technol. **35:** 206–225.
9. Williams, E. & C. A. Angell. 1973. J. Polymer Sci. Polymer Lett. **11:** 383–387.
10. Williams, E., & C. A. Angell. Submitted to J. Phys. Chem.
11. Simha, R. & R. R. Boyer. 1962. J. Chem. Phys. **37:** 1003–1007.
12. Litovitz, T. A. & T. Lyon. 1950. J. Acoust. Soc. Amer. **30:** 856.
13. Corsaro, R. D. 1976. Phys. Chem. Glasses **17:** 13.
14. Leidecker, H. W., J. H. Simmons, T. A. Litovitz & P. B. Macedo. 1971. J. Chem. Phys. **55:** 2028–2031.
15. Davies, R. O. & G. O. Jones. 1953. Adv. Phys. **2:** 370–410.
16. Davies, R. O. & G. O. Jones. 1953. Proc. R. Soc. (London) A **217:** 26.
17. DiMarzio, E. A. 1974. J. Appl. Phys. **45:** 4143.
18. Goldstein, M. J. 1975. Appl. Phys. **46:** 4153–4156.
19. Gupta, P. K. & C. T. Moynihan. J. Chem. Phys. In press.
20. O'Reilly, J. M. 1962. J. Polymer Sci. **57:** 429–442.
21. Rao, K. J., D. B. Helphrey & C. A. Angell. 1973. Phys. Chem. Glasses **14:** 26–32.
22. Angell, C. A., E. Williams, K. J. Rao & J. C. Tucker. 1976. J. Phys. Chem. In Press.
23. Goldstein, M. 1963. J. Chem. Phys. **39:** 3369–3374.
24. Goldstein, M. 1973. J. Phys. Chem. **77:** 667–673.
25. Kunzler, J. E. & W. F. Giaque. 1952. J. Amer. Chem. Soc. **74:** 797–800.
26. Sare, E. J. 1971. Ph.D. Thesis, Purdue University (1971).
27. Angell, C. A. & J. C. Tucker. 1974. J. Phys. Chem. **78:** 278–280.
28. Gibbs, J. H. & E. A. DiMarzio. 1958. J. Chem. Phys. **28:** 373–83.
29. Kauzmann, W. 1948. Chem. Rev. **43:** 219–256.
30. Bestul, A. B. & S. S. Chang. 1964. J. Chem. Phys. **42:** 3731–33.
31. Chang, S. S., A. B. Bestul & J. A. Horman. 1966. VII International Congress on Glass, Brussels, 1965. Vol. **1:** 15. Gordon and Breach, New York.
32. Miller, A. A. 1970. Macromolecules **3:** 674.
33. Goldstein, M. Private communication.
34. Adam, G. & J. H. Gibbs. 1965. J. Chem. Phys. **43:** 139–46.
35. Howell, F. S., R. Bose, C. T. Moynihan & P. B. Macedo. 1974. J. Phys. Chem. **78:** 639–652.
36. Macedo, P. B., W. Capps & T. A. Litovitz. 1966. J. Chem. Phys. **44:** 3357–3364.
37. Napolitano, A., P. B. Macedo & E. G. Hawkins. 1965. J. Amer. Ceram. Soc. **48:** 613.
38. Angell, C. A. 1968. J. Amer. Ceram. Soc. **51:** 117–134.
39. Angell, C. A. & K. J. Rao. 1972. J. Chem. Phys. **57:** 470–481.
40. Laughlin, W. T. & D. R. Uhlmann. 1972. J. Phys. Chem. **76:** 2317–2325.
41. Bose, B., R. A. Weiler & P. B. Macedo. 1970. Phys. Chem. Glasses **11:** 117–123.
42. Angell, C. A. & J. C. Tucker. 1974. Physical Chemistry of Process Metallurgy: The Richardson Conference. M. M. Jeffes & R. J. Tait, Eds.: 207–214. Institute of Mining and Metallurgy. London.
43. Chen, H. S. & D. Turnbull. 1968. J. Chem. Phys. **48:** 2568–2571.
44. Schnaus, E. U., A. Marshall & C. T. Moynihan. 1970. J. Amer. Ceram. Soc. **54:** 1193–1198.
45. Douslin, D. R. & H. M. Huffman. 1946. J. Amer. Chem. Soc. **68:** 1704–1708.
46. Huffman, H. M., S. S. Todd & H. D. Oliver. 1949. J. Amer. Chem. Soc. **71**:584–592.
47. Klemm, W. 1926. Z. Anorg. Chem. **152**:235.
48. Goldstein, M. & M. Nakonecznyi. 1965. Phys. Chem. Glasses **6:** 126–132.
49. Angell, C. A. 1966. J. Phys. Chem. **70:** 3988–3997.
50. Dworkin, A. 1974. J. Chim. Phys. 929.
51. Vinal, G. W. & D. N. Craig. 1933. J. Res. Nat. Bur. Stand. **10:** 781–793.

STATISTICAL THERMODYNAMICS OF CONFIGURATIONAL PROPERTIES*

Martin Goldstein

Belfer Graduate School of Science
Yeshiva University
New York, New York 10033

Structure vs Structures

The question a student of glass structure asks is of the form: What is the structure of a glass of a particular composition, e.g., SiO_2 or a Au—Pd—Si alloy? He is usually aware that the properties of a glass, for example, its density, is somewhat dependent on its thermal history—how rapidly it was cooled through the glass transition range or whether it was annealed or not. But as a practical matter, the radial distribution function (the usual means of specifying structure) is not particularly sensitive to the thermal history, and the latter is therefore regarded as of only peripheral relevance to the problem of structure.

For the student of the statistical thermodynamics of the glass transition, however, the notion of *the* structure is too simplistic. His focus of interest is on all the structures possible. If there were only one structure of a glass, the thermodynamics would be a lot easier than it is, though it wouldn't be easy. It would presumably be a problem in the vibrational spectrum of a nonperiodic arrangement of atoms—an extremely difficult and as yet unsolved problem.

As a glass is warmed up above its transition temperature T_g and becomes a liquid, there are fairly rapid though not discontinuous changes in the second derivative properties specific heat C_p, thermal expansion coefficient α, and isothermal compressibility β. The values of these properties in the liquid are higher than in the glass. Accounting for their changes at T_g in molecular terms is the problem the statistical thermodynamicist is concerned with.

Now the fact that there are such changes near T_g is not itself a mystery. Their occurrence can be well accounted for without invoking a thermodynamic phase transition, although the behavior can be partly described using some of the mathematics of a second-order transition of the Ehrenfest type.[1] It is assumed that below T_g the substance is kinetically frozen into a single structure, with only vibrational degrees of freedom active, while above T_g, in the metastable supercooled liquid state, the kinetic restriction is removed by the higher temperature, and the substance is able to explore many structures over the time scale of an observation. And further, as temperature is raised, structures of higher energy and volume become accessible. Hence increases of ΔC_p, $\Delta\alpha$, and $\Delta\beta$ in C_p, α, and β are observed at T_g.

Molecular models of the glass transition based on these concepts have been constructed, from which predictions of the thermodynamic changes at T_g have been made. The models permit the calculation of the number of structures of a given energy and volume, and hence of the thermodynamic properties.

*This work was supported by the Air Force Office of Scientific Research under Grant 73-2540.

The Gibbs-DiMarzio Theory

The most successful theory we have so far is one proposed by Gibbs and DiMarzio.[2] It is a theory strictly applicable to polymeric molecules, which consist of long chains of carbon atoms chemically bonded to each other, with other atoms or groups of atoms attached to the chains. Single carbon-carbon bonds allow rotational freedom about the bond, but there is a wealth of evidence that the rotation is not free, but hindered. There are potential barriers that resist the rotation, but above the glass temperature T_g enough thermal energy is available so that they are crossed frequently. There are several minima in the potential as rotation about the full 2π of angle associated with a given C—C bond takes place. The statistical thermodynamics of such systems has been studied for many years by means of lattice models with considerable success in predicting the thermodynamics of polymers, in spite of certain approximations that must be introduced because of the so far intractable problem of excluded volume.[3]

Because each bond has a choice of several potential minima, and because there are many bonds in a chain, each chain has a large number of distinct configurations accessible to it. The chains are flexible—they can change configurational state with time—and thus they have a high entropy.

What Gibbs and DiMarzio based their theory on was the fact that not all the potential minima associated with rotation around a single C—C bond need have the same depth. It follows that as temperature is lowered the chains tend to assume those configurations for which each rotational coordinate occupies the lowest available minimum. This in turn means that the flexibility of the chain molecules—their ability to choose among many different configurations—is gradually lost with lowering temperature. And with this loss in flexibility (and entropy) there occurs a greater and greater difficulty in finding ways to pack the molecules together on a lattice. The packing difficulty, inversely related to the entropy, increases so severely as temperature is lowered that it becomes infinite, and the configurational entropy becomes zero, at a finite temperature rather than absolute zero.

This would imply a thermodynamic phase transition of the Ehrenfest type at the temperature T_2 where the entropy vanishes. Now in fact the glass transition we observe experimentally is clearly kinetic rather than thermodynamic, arising from rapidly increasing viscosity and relaxation times. However Gibbs and DiMarzio have argued that the packing difficulty must also reflect a difficulty of producing configurational change, and hence an increasing viscosity, so the kinetic and thermodynamic behavior are interrelated. Adam and Gibbs[4] have used this qualitative but plausible interrelation as the basis for an equation for liquid viscosity that works about as well as the well known WLF free volume equation.[5] A critical test of the relative merits of the two theories can be made by comparing their predictions of the pressure dependence of viscosity near T_g: the free volume theory fails badly, and the Gibbs-DiMarzio approach predicts it quite well.[6]

The Gibbs-DiMarzio theory asserts therefore that the kinetic behavior seen at T_g is in a sense of a reflection of a thermodynamic transition we would observe at a lower temperature T_2 if the metastable supercooled liquid could be studied at thermodynamic equilibrium below T_g. Unfortunately it cannot, because of the impossibly long time scale involved. That configurational entropy should vanish at T_2 is such a surprising prediction that no one would believe the Gibbs-DiMarzio theory if it weren't for the fact that there is experimental evidence that it is exactly what happens. At T_g the configurational entropy, estimated as the difference in entropy between liquid and crystal, is still finite. Below T_g, where its course cannot be followed experimentally, it can be estimated by extrapolation from above T_g.

Here it is falling so rapidly with lowering temperature that a relatively conservative extrapolation suggests it would vanish some 40°–60°K below T_g in most glasses, a point first made by Kauzmann, and confirmed by many studies since.[7,8]

The greatest strength of the Gibbs-DiMarzio theory in my view lies in its ability to suggest a molecular explanation for this so-called "Kauzmann Paradox."

Limitations of the Gibbs-DiMarzio Theory

The theory has several weaknesses. There is some uncertainty about the mathematical approximations necessary to get anywhere with this intractable cooperative problem and its excluded volume component. How would the most striking conclusion—the discontinuity in the temperature derivative of the configurational entropy at a finite temperature T_2—be altered if we could solve the problem rigorously? We do not know.

A second difficulty is that the model applies to chain molecules possessing the features of loss of flexibility with lowering temperature. But glasses can be formed from almost any liquid, not just organic high polymers. How is such a theory to be extended to network glasses without pushing the analogy with high polymers too far? How is it to be extended to glasses formed from simple rigid molecules such as *cis*-decalin and chlorobenzene-pyridine mixtures and the like? And most dramatically how can it be applied at all to the metal alloy glasses discovered after it was first proposed?

Attempts to develop other models applicable at least to network glasses have been made, in which the basic excitation of the lattice is assumed to be a broken primary bond in the structure. These however have not been able to provide a molecular basis for the cooperative character necessary to give rise to the entropy discontinuity, and it has had to be introduced in an ad hoc way.[8]

So we are left with the conclusion that the Gibbs-DiMarzio theory, with its limitations, is the best we have at the present time.

A Critical Examination of the Assumptions of Molecular Theories

The Gibbs-DiMarzio theory is based on two assumptions that no one expects to be strictly valid. I would like to describe an analysis I have performed using calorimetric data in an attempt to evaluate in a semiquantitative way how much of a contribution to the thermodynamics of glasses and of the transition arises from the limitations of these assumptions.

The first assumption is that the vibrational frequencies of the glassy lattice, and as a second order effect, their anharmonicities, are insensitive to the configurational state (as measured by the fictive temperature—the temperature at which the configurational state of the glass would be an equilibrium state of the liquid). That this might not be strictly true was considered by Angell and Rao.[8] These assumptions are needed to permit us to regard the configurational and vibrational partition functions as independent, and to assume the vibrational contributions to C_p, α, and β above T_g are equal to that of the glass below T_g. But we should not be surprised to find the higher energy, more open structures that are the equilibrium ones at a higher temperature in the liquid to have, on the average, lower vibrational frequencies and greater anharmonicities. If this were so, part of ΔC_p would include contributions from these changes. Are these effects large or small? How can we tell?

The second assumption has to do with the evidence that not all molecular mobility (other than vibrational) freezes out at T_g. There is extensive evidence from dielectric and mechanical relaxation and nuclear magnetic resonance that in almost all glasses there are molecular rearrangement processes that do not freeze out until much lower temperatures.[9,10] These motions, as shown by their activation energies, are hindered by potential barriers much lower than those that are associated with the main glass transition.

Motions of this type are commonly explained by the presence in the molecule of additional internal degrees of freedom other than those which are associated with the glass transition. Polymers for example often have molecular groups attached to the main chain, which are capable of internally hindered motions that could show up as additional glassy state relaxations even though the rotations about the C—C bonds of the main chain are kinetically frozen out below T_g.

These motions should make some contribution to C_p and α in the glass. No sudden changes in C_p are detected at the temperatures where mechanical or dielectric studies indicate these motions should freeze out, but R. Simha and associates have shown changes in thermal expansion coefficient of polymer glasses are observable at the expected temperatures.[11-13]

In addition to contributing to the glassy thermodynamic properties, these degrees of freedom could contribute to the configurational specific heat ΔC_p observed above T_g also. This could arise in a similar fashion to the way in which changes in vibrational frequencies that take place above T_g could contribute to ΔC_p: if the higher energy, more open structures that begin to be explored above T_g have more of the "looseness" that permits secondary relaxations to occur, there will be a contribution to ΔC_p from these degrees of freedom also.

Detection of Vibrational and Secondary Relaxational Contributions to ΔC_p

How can we detect such contributions, and distinguish those arising from changing vibrational frequencies and anharmonicities from those arising from changes in the numbers of molecular units capable of taking part in secondary relaxations?

It can be shown that if we compare the thermodynamic properties of two samples of glass produced in two different structural states (or fictive temperatures) by different thermal histories we can estimate the importance of these contributions to ΔC_p, and attempt to distinguish between them.[14]

First, if they make no significant contribution, and ΔC_p arises only from changes in the numbers of energetically equivalent structures explored by the liquid as temperature is changed, the entropy difference between the two samples of glass would remain constant as temperature is lowered down to 0°K.

If however there are appreciable changes in vibrational frequencies, so that the structures of higher energy (higher fictive temperature) have "softer" frequencies, the entropy difference between the two samples will fall with temperature. The fall-off would be expected to resemble a Debye specific heat curve, falling slowly at first, and then more rapidly at lower temperatures.

If there are differences in the anharmonicities of the vibrations, with the higher fictive temperature sample showing greater anharmonicity, there would be differences in C_v between the two samples, of a magnitude and sign not easy to determine, and differences in C_p due to the term $TV\alpha^2/\beta$, itself arising from anharmonicity.[15-17] This will contribute most at higher temperatures, so the entropy will fall off rapidly at first, and then more slowly at lower temperatures.

Finally, if there are changes in the number of molecular groups capable of engaging in secondary relaxations with temperature in the liquid state, with the higher fictive temperature sample having more such groups, there will also be a fall-off of the entropy difference with temperature, but like the effect of changes in anharmonicity the fall-off will be most rapid just below T_g, and then level off at lower temperatures, as these motions gradually freeze out.

We can thus anticipate a difficulty in distinguishing between the contributions of anharmonicity and of secondary relaxations.

Calorimetric Results

This experiment requires very accurate specific heat measurements, and such data has been obtained by only one group, that of S. S. Chang and associates at the National Bureau of Standards, and by them on only six substances.[18-22]

The first question to ask: is there an appreciable fall-off of the entropy difference between the two samples of glass at all, between T_g and the vicinity of 0°K? The results are shown in TABLE 1, in the third column, which gives the fraction of the entropy difference at T_g still present near 0°K. We find this fraction varies widely from substance to substance, ranging from 0.2 to 0.8, with an unweighted average about 0.5. So we conclude that about half the ΔC_p observed at T_g comes from these sources.

In FIGURE 1 I have plotted the fall-off of the entropy difference against temperature for the six substances. The curves show both rises at low temperature, consistent with a vibrational contribution to ΔC_p and high temperature rises consistent with contributions either from anharmonicity or from secondary relaxational degrees of freedom. In most cases (*o*-terphenyl is an exception) the contributions at higher temperature are more important. If the high temperature be-

TABLE 1

COMPARISON OF ENTROPIES OF GLASSES WITH DIFFERENT FICTIVE TEMPERATURES NEAR T_g AND NEAR 0°K

Substance	T_g, (°K)	ΔC_p (J/mole °K)	$S_Q - S_A$* (near T_g)	$S_q - S_A$ (0°K)	Configurational Fraction†
Diethyl phthalate	178	115	3.64	2.80	0.77
cis-1,4-Polyisoprene	200	30.5	0.97	0.77	0.79
o-Terphenyl	240	113	0.78	0.22	0.28
Selenium	300	14.4	0.51	0.35	0.68
Poly(ethyl methacrylate)	335	13.2	0.48	0.07	0.15
Poly(vinyl chloride)	350	18.4	0.19	0.11‡	0.58
Average					0.54

*S_Q = entropy of a rapidly quenched glass, a glass of higher fictive temperature than a slowly quenched or annealed glass of entropy S_A.

†The configurational fraction is the fraction of the entropy difference observed near T_g that remains at 0°K.

‡At 250°K; below 250°K the C_p of quenched and annealed glasses agreed within experimental error.

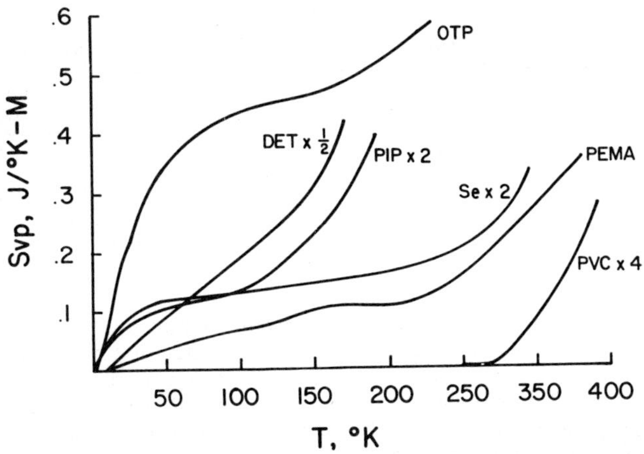

FIGURE 1. S_{vp}, the vanishing part of the entropy differences $S_Q - S_A$, plotted against temperature. For some of the substances $S_Q - S_A$ has been multiplied by a numerical factor for convenience in plotting. Vertical axis: S_{vp} in J/mole °K; horizontal axis: T in °K. OTP: *o*-terphenyl; DET × ½: diethylphthalate multiplied by ½; PIP: polyisoprene multiplied by 2; Se × 2: selenium multiplied by 2; PEMA: poly(ethyl methacrylate); PVC × 4: poly(vinyl chloride) multiplied by 4. (From Goldstein.[14] By permission of the *Journal of Chemical Physics*.)

havior could be shown to arise from the secondary relaxations, which freeze out kinetically, rather than from the anharmonicity, which doesn't, there would be an important consequence: it would imply that some of the residual entropy of the glass at 0°K may arise from these degrees of freedom. The usual assumption, that the residual entropy is associated with the configurational states that are kinetically frozen at T_g, would be called into question: the observed residual entropy would be at best an upper limit for this contribution. Further, the estimate that about 50% of ΔC_p arises from these degrees of freedom disregarded in the existing molecular theories of the glass transition would be at best a lower limit.

Anharmonicity or Secondary Relaxations?

It can be seen from FIGURE 1 that the entropy difference at higher temperatures shows a marked upward curvature in all six substances. This would seem to be inconsistent with an anharmonic contribution, which is usually assumed to be linear in temperature. However, Broadhurst and Mopsik[17] have given both theoretical arguments and experimental evidence that the contribution of anharmonicity in polymeric solids (and by extension, to other "soft" solids with similar intermolecular forces) shows a more marked temperature dependence: This is expressed in a temperature dependent Gruneisen constant γ, and results in upward curvature in plots of thermal expansion and specific heat against temperature.

In an attempt to shed light on this question, I have prepared TABLE 2 and FIGURE 2, which show entropy differences between the annealed glass and the crystal.[14] Chang obtained data on only three of the crystalline forms of the sub-

TABLE 2

COMPARISON OF GLASS AND CRYSTAL ENTROPIES NEAR T_g AND NEAR 0°K

	$S_A - S_C$* (near T_g)	$S_A - S_C$ (near 0°K)	Configurational Fraction.
Diethyl phthalate	22.25	20.17	0.91
o-Terphenyl	21.51	15.12	0.70
Selenium	6.34	3.59	0.57

*S_A is the entropy of an annealed glass; S_C, the entropy of the crystal.

stances for which glasses of different fictive temperatures were prepared: *o*-terphenyl, diethyl phthalate, and selenium. I have included his data in FIGURE 2 on the network glass As_2O_3, for which only one glass was studied, and for which in addition the absolute entropy of the glass was not determined. In all four substances there is a low temperature fall-off of the entropy difference consistent with vibrational frequency differences between glass and crystal. At higher temperatures there is no single pattern. In Selenium there is no high temperature rise at all, in *o*-terphenyl and As_2O_3 the high temperature rise is nearly linear, and in diethyl phthalate there is a marked upward curvature.

A rough estimate of the Gruneisen constants of polymer solids may be made from data by Warfield,[23] who determined Gruneisen constants on a number of crystalline and amorphous polymers by measuring the pressure dependence of the bulk modulus. The range of γ was 4–10, with no clear indication that the glassy polymers studied had a value of γ higher or lower than that of the crystalline polymers. In no case were crystalline and glassy forms of any one polymer compared, but if we can assume the Gruneisen constants for the two forms of a single substance can differ by as much as one or two units, we can make a crude estimate of the anharmonic contribution to the entropy difference between glass and crystal. Assuming representative values of the glassy compressibility, molar volume, and lattice specific heat C_v, and further assuming the Gruneisen constant

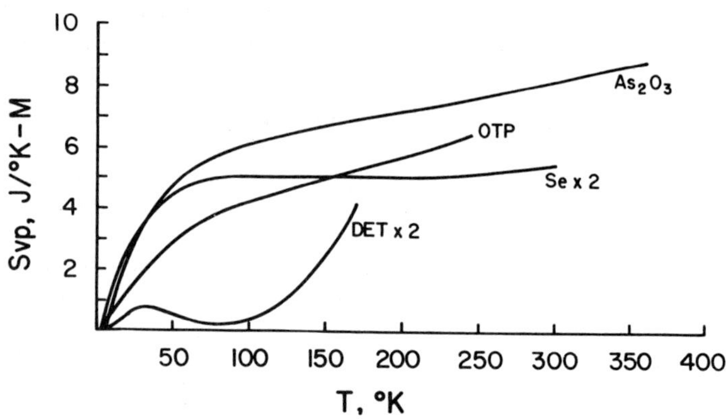

FIGURE 2. S_{vp}, the vanishing part of the entropy difference, $S_A - S_C$, between annealed glass and crystal. Vertical and horizontal axes and designation of curves as in FIGURE 1. The diethyl phthalate and selenium entropy differences have been multiplied by 2. (From Goldstein.[14] By permission of the *Journal of Chemical Physics*.)

$\gamma = V\alpha/\beta C_v$, we can calculate the contribution $TV\alpha^2/\beta$ to C_p of glass and crystalline phases. It makes a linear contribution to the entropy difference of about the order observed for *o*-terphenyl and As_2O_3.

On the other hand there are some facts that can be cited in support of a secondary relaxation interpretation. One is that while the excess thermal expansion observed in glassy polymers can also be accounted for by anharmonicity, Simha and associates noted that there are distinct changes in the slope of α vs T plots at the temperatures of secondary relaxations.[11,12]

Further, annealing experiments show that the strength of secondary relaxations diminish on annealing, a fact in qualitative accord with the possibility that they make a positive contribution to ΔC_p.[24]

It should be obvious that no clear answer to the question of the molecular origin of the fall-off of the entropy difference between glasses of different fictive temperatures with falling temperature is yet available. But it is also obvious that it is an important factor in the thermodynamics of the glass transition, and an answer is worth having.

The Kauzmann Paradox is a paradox because of the molecular interpretation we place on an extrapolation of ΔC_p below T_g. It appears that our molecular interpretation of ΔC_p accounts for only about half of it, and the significance of the extrapolation is made uncertain.

The Structural Significance of the Secondary Relaxational Processes

In our discussion above of the secondary relaxation processes we have given the generally accepted explanation of their origin: The molecules of which glasses are made are sufficiently complex to have internally hindered degrees of freedom that do not freeze out at T_g but at some lower temperature: such as side chains in polymer molecules.

To test this hypothesis G. P. Johari and I have done a study using dielectric relaxation on glasses made of molecules lacking such degrees of freedom: small, rigid, organic molecules such as pyridine, chlorobenzene and so forth.[24] According to the commonly accepted explanation these glasses should have shown a relaxation process only at the glass transition, and no further relaxational behavior below T_g. In fact we found a surprising and remarkably uniform pattern. Three-quarters of the systems we studied showed a secondary (β) relaxation (at about 0.75 T_g for a measuring frequency of 1 kHz), with a broad relaxation time spectrum, and low activation energies in the range 4–8 kcal (0.15 – 0.3 eV). It is interesting to note that about three-quarters of amorphous organic high polymers show a relaxation with characteristics so similar, that from the experimental dielectric data alone one cannot tell the polymers with their multitudinous internal degrees of freedom from the simple rigid molecules. We have found the same pattern in the few fused salt glasses we have studied, and in a group of alcohols which are not rigid molecules, and from which therefore more complicated behavior might have been expected.[25]

This remarkable uniformity of behavior, independent of the type of molecule or kinds of intermolecular forces present led us to conjecture that *the β-relaxation is a characteristic property of amorphous packing*.

There is evidence against this claim:

(1) About one quarter of our molecular and fused salt glasses, and about one quarter of amorphous polymers, do not show such a relaxation, a fact we can offer no convincing explanation for.

(2) Silicate glasses have not been shown to have such a relaxation. Most of them have a relaxation that used to be called "the singly-bonded oxygen" relaxation, in the right location in the temperature-frequency plane, which however has been shown recently to be present only if water is present as an impurity in the glass.[26]

(3) Metallic glasses, which can be studied by mechanical spectroscopy, have also not been shown to have such a relaxation. Chen and associates have failed to find one in a Pd—Au—Si alloy.[27] Eisenberg and Reich have found relaxations in a similar alloy whose presence or absence was highly sensitive to sample history.[28]

I still feel in spite of this contrary evidence that the most parsimonious conclusion is that the β-relaxation is somehow associated with amorphous packing as such rather than with the molecular nature of the glass former.

What feature of amorphous packing can give rise to the β-relaxation?

There is one significant feature distinguishing the random network theory from its rivals, the crystallite and amorphous cluster theories, that is relevant.[29] In the latter two there are two distinct kinds of environment for a molecule or molecular group in the structure: the highly organized, well-packed interior of a crystallite or amorphous cluster, and the more loosely packed material on surfaces and filling the interstices between the clusters—the "connective tissue."

The almost universal presence of the β-relaxation in glasses suggests that two distinct types of molecular environments are also almost universal, and is therefore evidence against the homogeneity implied by the random network model. My own preference is for the amorphous cluster theory, but this so far is an esthetic choice rather than a scientific one.

References

1. Goldstein, M. 1975. J. Appl. Phys. **46:** 4153. (This paper provides an entry into the extensive literature of this problem.)
2. Gibbs, J. H. 1960. *In* Modern Aspects of the Vitreous State. Vol. I, Chap. 7. Butterworths. London.
3. Flory, P. J. 1969. Statistical Mechanics of Chain Molecules. Wiley-Interscience. New York, N.Y.
4. Adam, G. & J. H. Gibbs. 1965. J. Chem. Phys. **43:** 139.
5. Williams, M. L., R. F. Landel & J. D. Ferry. 1955. J. Amer. Chem. Soc. **77:** 3701.
6. Goldstein, M. 1973. J. Phys. Chem. **77:** 667.
7. Kauzmann, W. 1948. Chem. Rev. **43:** 219.
8. Angell, C. A. & K. J. Rao. 1972. J. Chem. Phys. **57:** 470.
9. McCrum, N. G., B. E. Read & G. Williams. 1967. Anelastic and Dielectric Effects in Polymeric Solids. J. Wiley & Sons. New York, N.Y.
10. McCall, D. W. 1969. Nat. Bur. Stand. (U.S.) Spec. Pub. **301:** 475.
11. Simha, R., J. M. Roe & V. S. Nanda. 1972. J. Appl. Phys. **43:** 4312.
12. Wilson, P. S. & R. Simha. 1973. Macromolecules **6:** 902, 908.
13. McKinney, J. E. & R. Simha. 1974. Macromolecules **7:** 894.
14. Goldstein, M. 1976. J. Chem. Phys. **64:** 4767.
15. Keller, J. M. & D. C. Wallace. 1962. Phys. Rev. **126:** 1275.
16. Cowley, R. A. 1968. Rep. Prog. Phys. **31**(Pt. I): 123.
17. Broadhurst, M. G. & F. I. Mopsik. 1971. J. Chem. Phys. **54:** 4239.
18. Chang, S. S., J. A. Horman & A. B. Bestul. 1967. J. Res. Nat. Bur. Stand. (U.S.) **71A:** 293.
19. Chang, S. S. & A. B. Bestul. 1971. J. Res. Nat. Bur. Stand. **75A:** 113.
20. Chang, S. S. & A. B. Bestul. 1972. J. Chem. Phys. **56:** 503.

21. Chang, S. S. & A. B. Bestul. 1974. J. Chem. Thermodyn. **6:** 325.
22. Chang, S. S. Unpublished data.
23. Warfield, R. W. 1974. Makromol. Chem. **175:** 3285.
24. Johari, G. P. & M. Goldstein. 1970. J. Chem. Phys. **53:** 2372.
25. Johari, G. P. & M. Goldstein. 1971. J. Chem. Phys. **55:** 4245.
26. Day, D. E. & J. M. Stevels. 1974. J. Non-Cryst. Solids **14:** 165.
27. Chen, H. S., H. J. Leamy & M. Barmatz. 1970–1971. J. Non-Cryst. Solids **5:** 444.
28. Eisenberg, A. & S. Reich. 1972. *In* Amorphous Materials. R. Douglas and B. Ellis, Eds.: 79–87. John Wiley & Sons, New York, N.Y.
29. Turnbull, D. & D. E. Polk. 1972. J. Non-Cryst. Solids **8–10:** 19.

PHYSICAL AGING IN AMORPHOUS GLASSY POLYMERS*

L. C. E. Struik

Centraal Laboratorium TNO
Delft, The Netherlands

Introduction and Summary

This paper deals with the changes in physical properties (aging) caused by amorphous glassy polymers not being in thermodynamic equilibrium.[1] The approach towards equilibrium is gradual and slow and persists over periods of many years.

We have studied this physical aging for some 35 plastics and other organic glasses, and for a variety of mechanical properties. Aging appears to be very important; it often dominates the mechanical behavior in the practical temperature range. Further, nearly all aspects of aging can be explained from the free-volume concept. Finally, the aging behavior and the small-strain mechanical properties turned out to be very similar for all polymers. Even many nonpolymeric materials behave similarly.

Basic Aspects of Aging

In outline, we shall now derive the basic aspects of aging from the free-volume concept, and show that the deductions agree with experiment; for details see Kovacs[1] and Struik.[2,3]

The free-volume concept (Figure 1A) states that in every system of particles, molecules, and so forth, the transport mobility M primarily depends on the degree of packing, or in other terms, on free volume v_f. For polymers, M should be identified with the segmental mobility—the rate factor for changes in chain configuration.

Figure 1B illustrates what happens when a polymer is cooled from above to below its glass temperature T_g. Above T_g, both M and v_f are large. On cooling, v_f decreases, simply because the molecules attract one another, and M will decrease simultaneously. However, the rate of change of v_f is determined by M, so M cannot decrease without limit. At a certain temperature (T_g), M becomes so small that v_f (and M) can no longer follow the changes in temperature. During further cooling, v_f will, to a first approximation, remain constant; M may still decrease slightly because segmental motion also is thermally activated.

Suppose, now, that after cooling, the polymer is kept at $T_1 < T_g$ (Figure 1B). Here, mobility M will not be zero. For a decrease in M, v_f must be decreased, but this decrease requires some mobility. Therefore, M cannot become zero in a finite time; the state of zero mobility can only be approached asymptotically. The finite value of M implies that v_f will slowly decrease towards its equilibrium value.

*Most of the work reported here was sponsored by the following companies: Akzo, ANIC, BP Chemicals, DSM, Hüls, Montedison, Philips, Rhône-Progil, Shell, and Solvay.

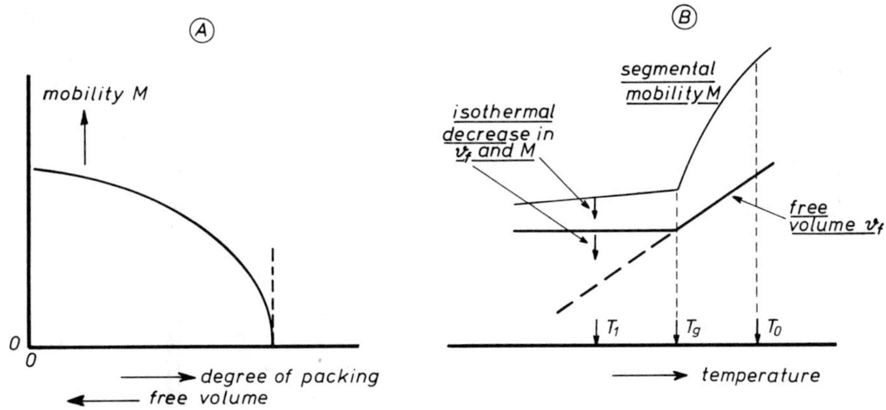

FIGURE 1. Illustration of the free-volume concept.

Mobility M and all other properties somehow depending on it will change simultaneously.

The basic aspects of this process, which we define as aging, are listed and explained below.

(1) Aging primarily affects relaxation times. This is obvious from FIGURE 1. Thus, creep or stress-relaxation curves will be shifted along the logarithmic (loading) time scale, the more so the longer the aging time. This was confirmed for all materials. Examples are given in FIGURES 2 and 3.

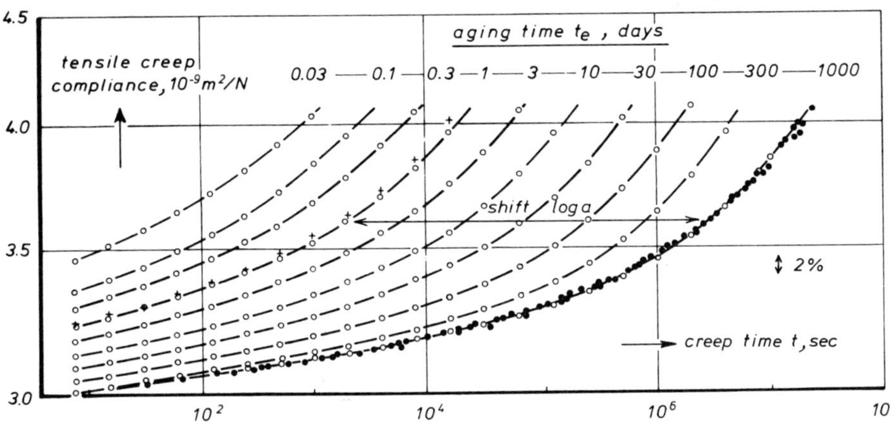

FIGURE 2. Small-strain tensile creep curves of rigid PVC quenched from 90°C (i.e., above T_g) to 20°C and further kept at 20°C. The different curves (○) were measured for various values of the time t_e elapsed after the quench. The master curve (●) gives the result of a superposition by almost horizontal shifts; it shows that aging primarily affects the retardation times, all in the same way. The crosses were found, when after 1000 days of aging, the sample was reheated to 90°C, requenched to 20°C, and remeasured for a t_e of 1 day; they show that this aging is thermoreversible.

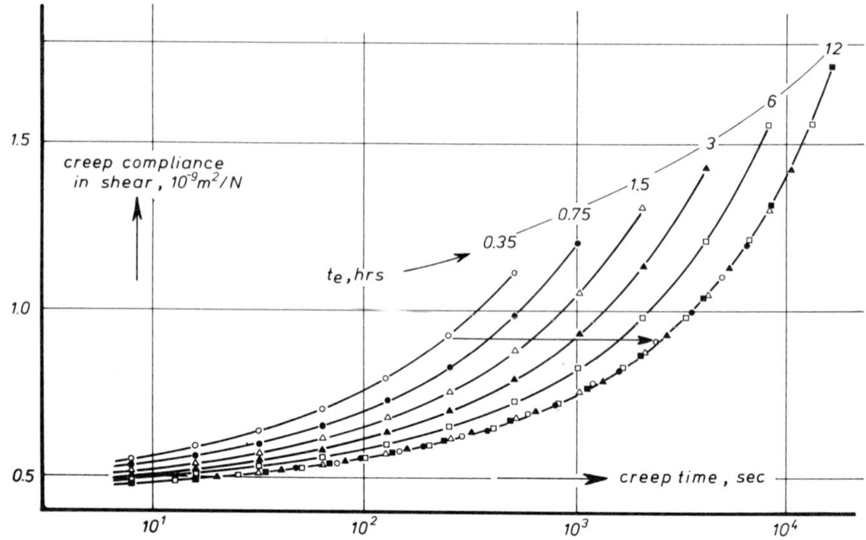

FIGURE 3. Same as FIGURE 2, but now for the torsional creep of amorphous sugar quenched from 43° to 22°C ($T_g \sim 40$°C).

(2) Aging is thermoreversible. On heating the material to above T_g, it readily reaches thermodynamic equilibrium. The history of the sample has, by definition, been "forgotten," any previous aging being erased. Aging therefore is a thermoreversible process that is reproducible an arbitrary number of times with the same sample (compare FIGURE 2).

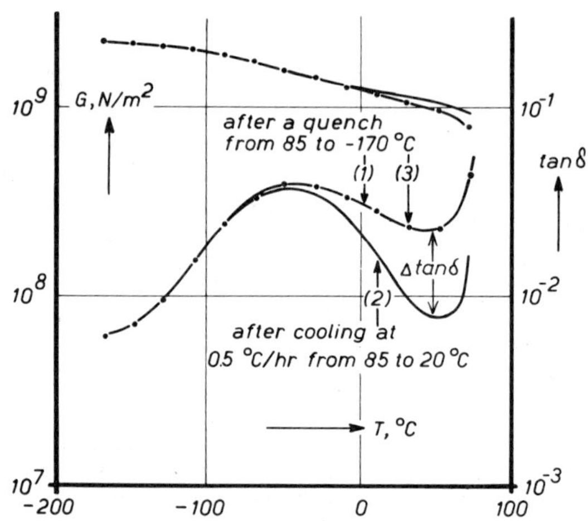

FIGURE 4. Shear modulus and damping at 1 Hz for rigid PVC, measured during heating from −170° to +65°C at a rate of two-thirds °C/min. Tests (1), (2), and (3) refer to different thermal histories (see diagram), and were done in succession on one sample. The results of Test (3) again show that the effects are thermoreversible.

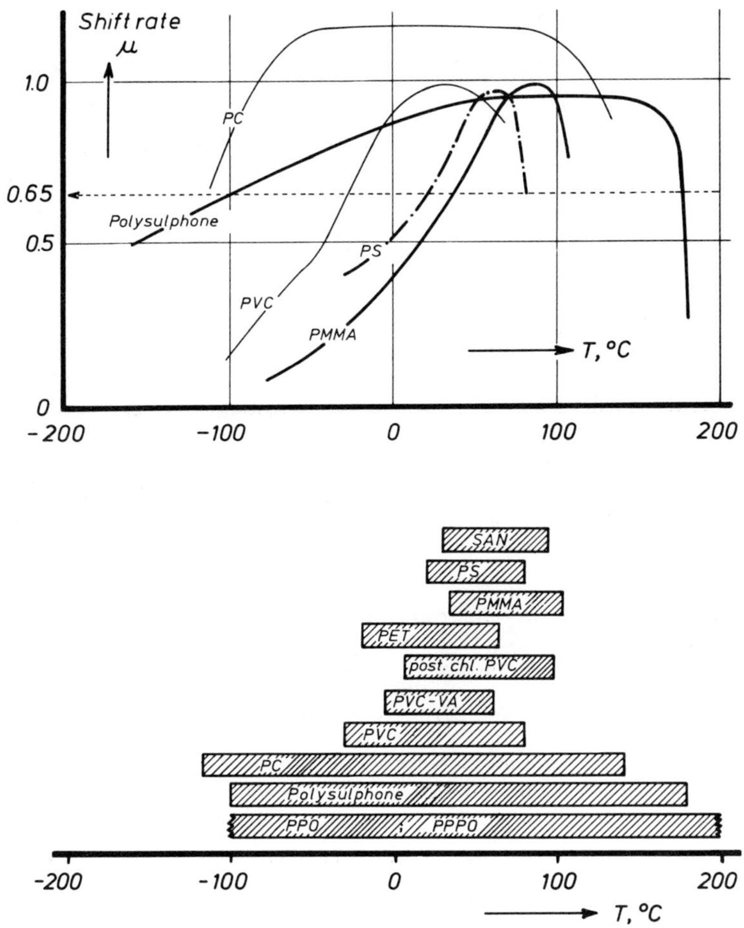

FIGURE 5. Shift rate $\mu = d \log a / d \log t_e$ (FIGURE 2 and Equation 2) vs temperature for various polymers (top); regions of strong aging ($\mu > 0.65$) (bottom).

(3) Aging does not affect secondary relaxations. Below T_g, v_f shrinks to a value at which segmental motion just becomes strongly hindered. In general, secondary motions require much less space, and v_f therefore always is sufficiently large to allow these. This was verified for 22 polymers. An example of the results is given in FIGURE 4, in which the changes in v_f were achieved by quenching and slow cooling rather than by isothermal aging.

(4) Aging is confined to a temperature range, called aging range, that is generally bounded by T_g and the highest secondary transition, T_β, below T_g. At T_β the flexibility of the chain segments decreases, since secondary motion becomes frozen. Between T_β and T_g, v_f has decreased so much that the motion of the still flexible segment just becomes hindered. Therefore, segmental motion and aging will disappear below T_β. This temperature thus is the lower limit of the aging range, T_g obviously being the upper limit. Experimental results confirming this conclusion are found in FIGURES 4 and 5 (for T_g and T_β values see Reference 4).

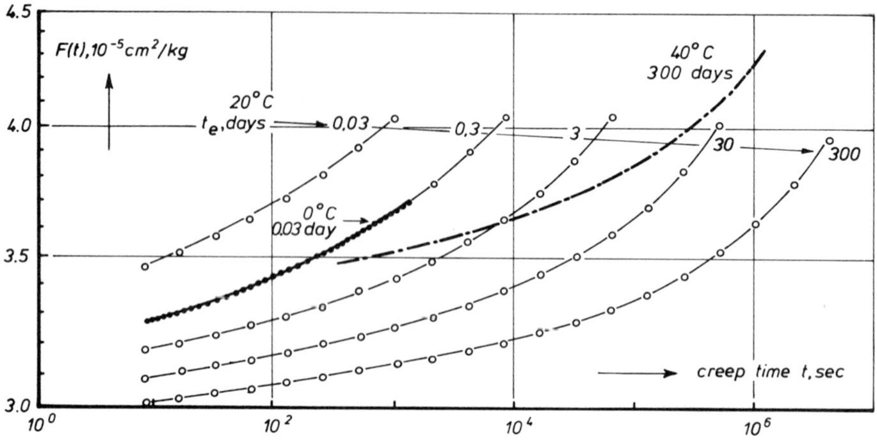

FIGURE 6. Comparison of the effects of aging and temperature on the small-strain tensile creep of rigid PVC. The curves were measured as described in the caption to FIGURE 2, i.e., after quenches from 90° to 0°, 20°, and 40°C. Note that after prolonged aging the creep rate at 40°C can become smaller than that at 0° or 20°C.

(5) In the aging range the shift rate μ is approximately unity for all polymers. Aging is a self-delaying process (FIGURE 1). For such a process, it can be derived[2] that, as long as the self-delaying effects are strong,

$$Mt_e \sim \text{constant.} \tag{1}$$

The relaxation times therefore increase proportionally to aging time t_e. The creep curves will shift at a constant double-logarithmic rate and this rate μ will be unity (compare FIGURE 2).

$$\mu = \frac{d \log a}{d \log t_e} = -\frac{d \log M}{d \log t_e} \sim 1. \tag{2}$$

FIGURES 2 and 5 reveal that this is indeed the case; in the aging range all polymers age in the same way.

(6) Aging is a general phenomenon. According to FIGURE 1, aging is a basic feature of the glassy state. It will be found in all glassy materials, and Equations 1 and 2 are expected to hold generally. The present work has confirmed this. Very similar aging effects were found in all polymers, as well as in materials such as sugar, cheese, bitumen, and shellac. That inorganic glasses age similarly is known from the literature.[1]

(7) The aging process persists over very long periods of time. The time t_∞ required for the attainment of equilibrium at $T < T_g$ can be estimated from the free-volume theory.[1,2] It follows that t_∞ increases exponentially with $T_g - T$, roughly by a factor of 10 per 3°C; at no more than 20°C below T_g, t_∞ reaches a value of 100 years.

It is difficult to check this conclusion [tests on ancient (in)organic glassy materials?]. However, FIGURE 2 at least shows that for PVC at 20°C the aging rate is constant over the first three years, and that there is no indication for a change in rate in the near future.

(8) In the aging range, aging time is the most relevant material parameter. During aging, the retardation times change by orders of magnitude. To produce similar effects by changes in, e.g., the temperature, we need changes of many tens of °C; compare FIGURE 6.

(9) In the aging range the small-strain behavior of all polymers is almost identical. To explain the meaning of this, we consider creep tests that are short compared to the aging period preceding the test. Such tests yield the "short-time" or "momentary" creep properties (compare FIGURES 2 and 3); in longer tests the creep behavior will be different, since it becomes accompanied with simultaneous aging. Suppose we measure such short-time creep curves for a number of temperatures, aging times, and polymers. If we plot the results in a double-logarithmic diagram, we observe that all creep curves have almost the same shape. They can be superimposed to a single master curve (FIGURE 7). The individual creep curves can be derived from the master curve by horizontal and vertical shifts.

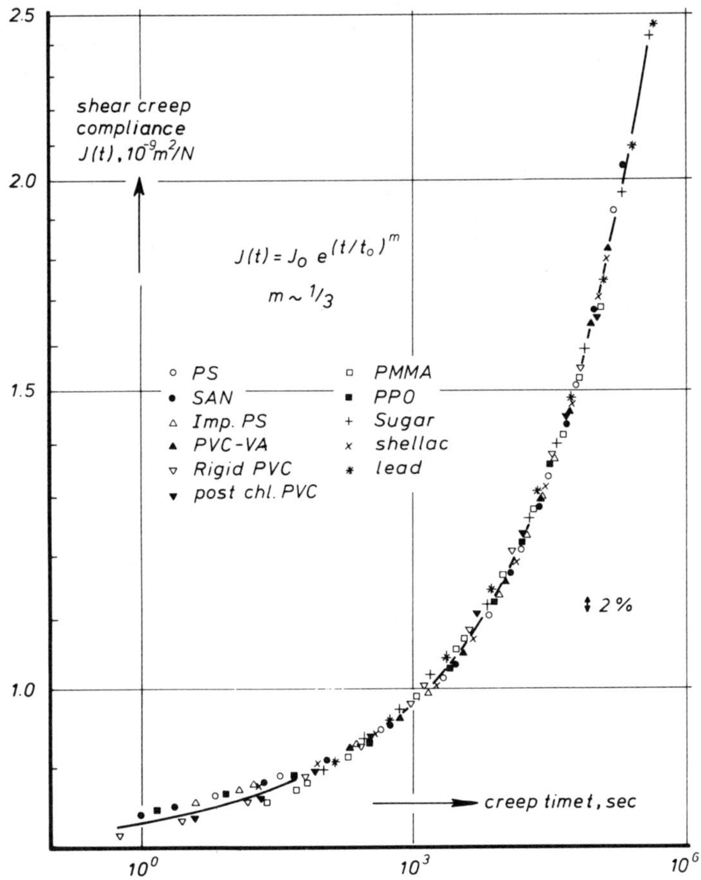

FIGURE 7. Master curve obtained by superposition (using horizontal and vertical shifts) of creep curves measured on various materials at various temperatures and aging times.

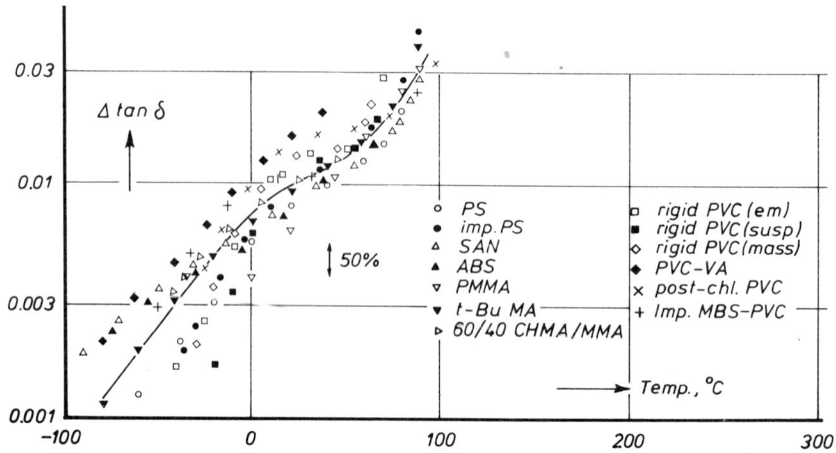

FIGURE 8. Effect of thermal history on the 1-Hz damping of various polymers. Quantity Δ tan δ is defined in FIGURE 4.

A simple formula for the creep curve is inserted in FIGURE 7; parameters J_0 and t_0 are related to the vertical and horizontal shift factors.

Linear viscoelastic theory teaches that this result can be generalized. Since the creep curves of all polymers have almost the same shape, the same must hold for stress-relaxation curves, curves of dynamic moduli vs frequency, and so forth.

An explanation of the existance of a general creep equation has not yet been found. Its wide applicability (polymers, bitumen, sugar, shellac, lead) suggests that the creep mechanism must be of a very general nature, and is not primarily determined by the polymeric or glassy structure of the material. Possibly, the equation describes how, below the softening point, a solid starts to collapse and gradually becomes a fluid.

The same generality of behavior has been discussed by Kubát.[5] At least for the case of stress-relaxation at small strains, his formula (Equation 1 of Reference 5) can be derived from ours.

DISCUSSION

In the preceding section, we considered only some of the basic aspects of aging. More results can be obtained already by combining some of the aspects. From among various possibilities, we will here give one example dealing with thermal history effects. FIGURE 4 shows that after slow cooling the damping is lower than after quenching. This is caused by the aging during the slow cooling. The aging only occurs in the aging range (Aspect 4). But within this range, aging as well as mechanical behavior are similar for all polymers (Aspects 5, 6, and 9). We therefore have to expect that the thermal history effects will be very similar too. FIGURE 8 shows that this is indeed the case for a number of polymers with roughly the same T_g.

Further, the present paper has been confined to aging effects on the small-strain properties after a simple thermal history, viz., a quench. How aging occurs after more complicated thermal histories, or at large stresses (nonlinear creep, yielding, impact) has also been investigated; the results will be reported in the near future.

Aging has important practical implications. Aspect 8 implies that aging time has to be included as a parameter in the testing methods; Aspect 9 implies that these methods can be simplified (all polymers behave similarly). Moreover, we have to revise the methods for predicting long-term behavior from short-time tests. For the case of small-strain creep, such revised methods have been developed.[2]

The most intriguing point remains the wide applicability of the creep equation of FIGURE 7. It suggests that a true understanding of the creep mechanism lies ready to hand.

ACKNOWLEDGMENTS

The author wishes to express his thanks to Dr. J. Heijboer, Dr. F. R. Schwarzl, Miss C. Zoeteweij, Miss H. C. J. Tetteroo, Mr. J. Seffelaar, and many others who substantially contributed to the present work.

REFERENCES

1. KOVACS, A. J. 1964. Fortschr. Hochpolym. Forsch. **3:** 394–507.
2. STRUIK, L. C. E. 1976. Transactions of the VIIth International Congress on Rheology, Gothenburg. To be published.
3. STRUIK, L. C. E. 1966. Rheologica Acta **5:** 303–311.
4. MCCRUM, N. G., B. E. READ, G. WILLIAMS. 1967. Anelastic and Dielectric Effects in Polymeric Solids. Wiley. London.
5. KUBÁT, J. 1965. Nature **204:** 378–379.

A CLASSIFICATION OF THE KINDS OF ORDER PARAMETERS

Edmund A. DiMarzio

National Bureau Standards
Washington D.C. 20234

It is worthwhile to reexamine the idea of order parameters in an attempt to classify them. Within the framework of the order parameter description of a system, one requires that in the high temperature equilibrium phase the order parameters Z_i adjust themselves to minimize the Gibbs free energy; this condition can usually be satisfied if

$$\frac{\partial G}{\partial Z_i} = 0 \qquad i = 1,2,\ldots.$$

This set of equations defines the order parameters in terms of temperature and pressure (for glasses the high-temperature phase is the liquid phase and we denote these Z_i as Z_{li}):

$$Z_{li} = Z_{li}(T, P).$$

The low-temperature phase is separated from the high-temperature phase by a transition line $T_2(P)$. There are both kinetic and thermodynamic interpretations on how the transition occurs. These interpretations lead to two distinct classifications of order parameters: Class I, kinetic (history-dependent), and Class II, thermodynamic (history-independent).

The history of the low-temperature phase (the glass phase) can be described in terms of the formation pressure P_2 and the time scale of the experiment τ_e. The dependence of the glass order parameters Z_{gi} on P_2 and τ_e results in a further division of Class I:

$$\text{Class Ia, } Z_{gi}(T, P; P_2\, \tau_e) = c_i(\tau_e), i = 1.$$

$$\text{Class Ib, } Z_{gi}(T, P; P_2, \tau_e) = h_i(P_2, \tau_e), i = 1,2,\ldots.$$

The usual notion of order parameters is that they are constants that only depend on the rate of formation of the glass (Class Ia), but in general one should allow for the order parameters to depend on the formation pressure (Class Ib). Below we will show that Class Ia can only include the case $i = 1$; i.e., two or more order parameters are not possible in Class Ia.

Thermodynamic order parameters (Class II) can be invoked whenever the transition occurs and the time scale of the experiment τ_e is much greater than the characteristic relaxation time for the system to come to equilibrium (an infinite τ_e would guarantee this condition). Under these conditions the order parameters would be history independent and are state functions:

$$\text{Class II, } Z_{gi}(T, P; P_2, \tau_e = \infty) = f_i(T, P), i = 1,2,\ldots.$$

A single-component, single-phase system only has two degrees of freedom (phase rule); therefore, specification of T and P completely determines the thermodynamic state of the system. Now if we impose an equation of constraint on the system, a degree of freedom will be lost (either T or P). *One equation of constraint will define a line $T(P)$ in the T-P plane while two equations of constraint would define a point in the T-P plane.* Three or more equations of constraint constitute an over-determined system of equations and do not have physical meaning. Examples of constraint equations are for one of the Z_i to be set equal to a constant or for the sum of the Z_i to be equal to a constant. Either of these conditions would define a $T(P)$ line. The salient point to be made is that it is physically meaningless to assert that two or more independent order parameters have some fixed or constant values along the transition line. Thus, Class Ia can only include systems that are described by *one order parameter*. If two or more kinetic order parameters are required to describe the transition, then they must belong to Class Ib.

The order parameters (f, n_0) of the Gibbs-DiMarzio theory belong to Class II. Above the $T_2(P)$ line (the liquid region) f and n_0 adjust themselves so as to minimize the free energy. The equation of constraint in this case is

$$S_l(f, n_0) = 0,$$

where S_l is the configurational entropy. This equation of constraint is very complicated, but it nevertheless establishes a well-defined $T_2(P)$ line.* Moreover, n_0 and f vary below the $T_2(P)$ line (the glassy region) in a manner that minimizes the free energy but subject to the condition that the entropy remain constant (zero).

The above classification of order parameters depends on the idea that above the transition line the relaxation time to reach equilibrium is much smaller than the experimental time scale τ_e while below the transition line the relaxation times are much longer than τ_e. Experiments characterized by a finite τ_e will, in general, lead to Class Ib order parameters even if the transition has a thermodynamic basis characterized by Class II order parameters.

The basic physical reality behind the concept of order parameters is that they are variables over which we sum when we evaluate the partition function of a system. By use of the relation

$$G = -kT\ln Q,$$

we see that the maximum term method of evaluating Q is equivalent to minimizing G,

$$\frac{\partial G}{\partial Z_i} = 0.$$

The classification of order parameters that we have made is easily interpreted in terms of the above view of the nature of order parameters. Class I arises when the equations of motion describing the time evolution of the Z_i are the determinants of Z_i rather than equilibrium.* Class II arises when pure equilibrium is obtained: Changes in the functional form of G arising from phase transition phenomena result in changes in the functional form of the Z_i.

Another possibility that we have not considered for the Z_i is that the maximum term method loses its validity over a range of some temperatures and pressures. Then presumably we can make the same arguments for expectation values of Z_i.

*DiMarzio, E. A., J. H. Gibbs, P. D. Fleming, III & I. C. Sanchez. 1976. The effects of pressure on the equilibrium properties of glass forming systems. Macromolecules. In press. This paper has a more extensive discussion of the classifications of order parameters.

APPLICATION OF HOLE THEORY TO ESTIMATE THE PRESSURE-INDUCED DENSIFICATION OF POLYMERS

John E. McKinney

Institute for Materials Research
National Bureau of Standards
Washington, D.C. 20234

Forming a glass by isobaric cooling at an elevated pressure produces a larger density than that obtained by cooling at the same rate at atmospheric pressure. Simple phenomenological theory is used to obtain a relation to estimate the densification from glass transition properties obtained by experiment. It is shown how the hole theory of Simha and Somcynsky may be used to facilitate the estimation of densification through the application of a universal reduced function that replaces the quantity most difficult to obtain experimentally in this relation.

Introduction

This short paper may be regarded as an extension of the one given by Professor Robert Simha earlier in this conference. He presented the results on the application of the generalized equation of state derived from the hole theory of Simha and Somcynsky[1] to liquid (equilibrium) and glassy states. In this paper a model is presented which utilizes the equilibrium equation of state to facilitate the estimation of "permanent" densification resulting from glass formation at elevated pressures.

The pressure induced densification rate is defined as

$$\kappa' = -(1/V)(\partial V/\partial P')_{T,P} \tag{1}$$

where V is the volume at temperature T and pressure P, and P' is the pressure during glass formation at isobaric cooling at constant rate k. The argument k is not included implicitly in Equation 1 because the discussions in this paper apply to only one rate of cooling. Note that the above definition for κ' is analogous to the one for isothermal conpressibility,

$$\kappa = -(1/V)(\partial V/\partial P)_{T,P'},$$

except that P and P' are interchanged.

The meaning of Equation 1 may be realized from the schematic volume-temperature diagram shown on FIGURE 1. Volume V_A in the glass is reached by isobaric cooling at a constant rate k at atmospheric pressure commencing in the melt at volume V_0. V_B is reached by pressurization in the melt followed by isobaric cooling at the same rate at an elevated pressure $P' = \Delta P$, and finally depressurizing at the same temperature corresponding to V_A. Since the same cooling rate is used in both cases, the intersection of the corresponding liquid and glass PVT surfaces gives the $T_g(P)$ line along which the mean relaxation time is assumed to be constant. In order to apply the analysis given in this paper it is important to choose the temperature at V_0 sufficiently above T_g for initial equilibrium to be assured at V_0 and maintained after pressurization ΔP. Also to obtain "permanent" densification the terminal temperature must be chosen sufficiently below T_g, where the

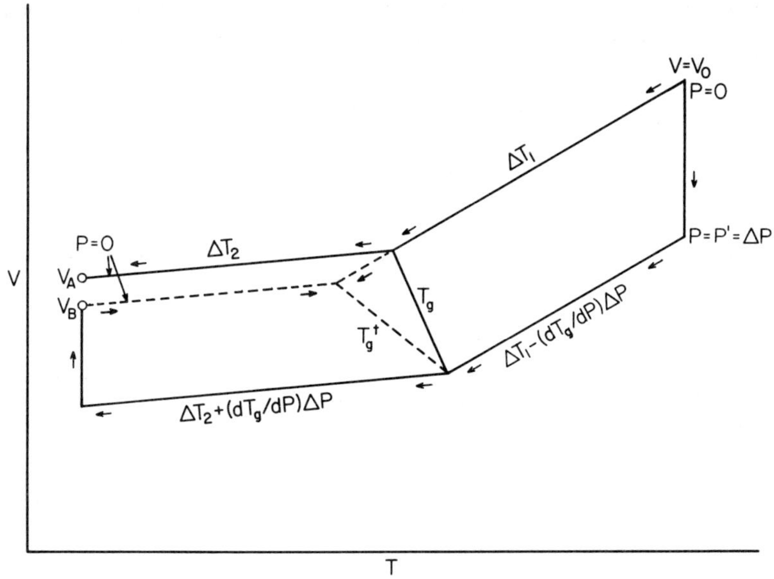

FIGURE 1. Schematic volume-temperature diagram illustrating the densification procedure and the distinction between T_g and $T_g^\dagger$.

mean viscoelastic relaxation time is very large in comparison to the expected observation time.

Professor Simha has alluded to a second kind of transition line designated $T_g^\dagger$, which is also an intersection of the liquid and glass PVT surfaces except the glass surface corresponds to only one formation pressure. This intersection is indicated by the dashed lines on FIGURE 1. Here the glass is formed by isobaric cooling at P' (which may be atmospheric) with subsequent pressure changes being made in the glass at temperatures sufficiently below T_g that no significant viscoelastic relaxation is possible during the course of the measurement. As evident from FIGURE 1, the T_g and $T_g^\dagger$ lines will coincide when $V_A = V_B$, i.e., no densification. With densification ($V_A > V_B$) the two transition lines will intersect at a temperature for which $P = P'$. From purely geometrical considerations it has been shown[2] that the Ehrenfest-like equation

$$\mathrm{d}T_g^\dagger/\mathrm{d}P = \Delta\kappa/\Delta\alpha \tag{2}$$

is valid, where κ and α are isothermal compressibility and thermal expansion coefficient, and the Δs indicate the differences in the respective quantities between liquid and glass. For further discussions on the meaning of T_g and $T_g^\dagger$, see References 2 and 3.

Phenomenological Relationships

We desire to obtain a relationship between κ' and other quantities that are more commonly obtained by experiment or those that may be evaluated with sufficient reliability by molecular theory. Assuming linear dependence of volume on temperature and pressure, which on FIGURE 1 is approximated for sufficiently small values of ΔT (above and below T_g) and ΔP, the initial and terminal volumes are related by

$$V_A = V_0(1 - \alpha_l \Delta T_1 - \alpha_g \Delta T_2),$$

$$V_B = V_0\{1 - \kappa_l \Delta P - \alpha_l[\Delta T_1 - (\mathrm{d}T_g/\mathrm{d}P)\Delta P] - \alpha_g[\Delta T_2 + (\mathrm{d}T_g/\mathrm{d}P)\Delta P] + \kappa_g \Delta P\},$$

where the subscripts l and g pertain to liquid and glass. In terms of FIGURE 1 the definition of the densification rate (Equation 1) may be rewritten as

$$\kappa' = -(V_B - V_A)/(V_0 \Delta P),$$

which is a good approximation for small ΔT and ΔP. After substituting the explicit expressions above for V_A and V_B into this equation, the desired relation is obtained:

$$\kappa' = -\Delta\alpha[\mathrm{d}T_g/\mathrm{d}P - \Delta\kappa/\Delta\alpha]. \quad \mathbf{(3)}$$

From Equation 3 it is apparent that if the first Ehrenfest equation (applied to T_g),

$$\mathrm{d}T_g/\mathrm{d}P = \Delta\kappa/\Delta\alpha, \quad \mathbf{(4)}$$

is obeyed, there is no densification. Positive densification is tantamount to the inequality

$$\mathrm{d}T_g/\mathrm{d}P < \Delta\kappa/\Delta\alpha, \quad \mathbf{(5)}$$

a relation that, as indicated from vast experimental evidence, appears to hold in general. Since the second Ehrenfest equation,

$$\mathrm{d}T_g/\mathrm{d}P = TV\Delta\alpha/\Delta C_P, \quad \mathbf{(6)}$$

where C_P is the heat capacity at constant pressure, appears to be a good approximation,[4] the analogous argument (using the temperature and pressure history shown in FIGURE 1) applied to the entropy predicts a single entropy surface with respect to formation pressure in contradistinction to the manifold of surfaces observed for the volume. This argument, of course, depends upon the validity of the assumption that $\mathrm{d}T_g/\mathrm{d}P$ for volume and entropy are the same.

Direct determination of κ' for glass forming substances from the displacement of the PVT surfaces of glasses pertaining to different formation pressures was apparently first undertaken by Shishkin.[5] In order to determine κ' through Equation 3, $\Delta\alpha$ is obtained simply by volume-temperature measurements through T_g. Although $\mathrm{d}T_g/\mathrm{d}P$ is more difficult to determine, there are alternatives that appear to be in good agreement. These include PVT measurements employing isobaric cooling at one constant rate through T_g at different pressures, and time-temperature-pressure superposition of frequency-dependent dielectric and mechanical data, including ultrasonic data at elevated pressures. Another possible way to determine $\mathrm{d}T_g/\mathrm{d}P$ is suggested through the apparent validity of Equation 6. Although there is some question with respect to the general application of this equation to the glass transition, there is the distinct advantage that the data used to determine $\mathrm{d}T_g/\mathrm{d}P$ may be obtained at atmospheric pressure only.

The most difficult quantity in Equation 3 to determine experimentally is $\Delta\kappa$. The usual and most direct method is to obtain the proper *PVT* surfaces for liquid and glass, for which the latter pertains to only one formation pressure. A glass formed by this history is called a constant formation glass ($P' = \text{const}$) applicable to a single physical substance in contrast to the variable formation glass ($P' = P$) formed at different pressures by the procedure mentioned in the previous paragraph.

Application of the Hole Theory to Estimate Densification

In this section it will be shown how the hole theory of Simha and Somcynsky[1] may be used to estimate the quantity $\Delta\kappa/\Delta\alpha$ appearing in Equation 3, which, in turn, may be used to facilitate the estimation of κ'.

Gee[6] has shown for a single ordering parameter Z which freezes in the glass at T_g, that

$$\Delta\kappa/\Delta\alpha = (\partial T/\partial P)_Z.$$

From Equation 2 the above equation is seen to be t[illegible]mount to

$$dT_g^\dagger/dP = (\partial T/\partial P)_Z. \tag{7}$$

Since with the hole theory, as applied by Simha and cowor[illegible], [illegible] ordering parameter h, which is the hole fraction, is not necessarily frozen, Equation (7) may not be valid. In order to obtain the extension of Equation 7 for the more general case, consider the single valued function $V = V(T, P, h)$, from which by the usual definitions,

$$-\kappa = (\partial \ln V/\partial P)_T = (\partial \ln V/\partial P)_{T,h} + (\partial \ln V/\partial h)_{T,P}(\partial h/\partial P)_T,$$

$$\alpha = (\partial \ln V/\partial T)_P = (\partial \ln V/\partial T)_{P,h} + (\partial \ln V/\partial h)_{T,P}(\partial h/\partial T)_P.$$

Since the derivatives with two fixed arguments (subscripts) are the same for liquid and glass, the differences become

$$-\Delta\kappa = (\partial \ln V/\partial h)_{T,P}[(\partial h/\partial P)_{T,l} - (\partial h/\partial P)_{T,g}]$$

$$\Delta\alpha = (\partial \ln V/\partial h)_{T,P}[(\partial h/\partial T)_{P,l} - (\partial h/\partial T)_{P,g}].$$

Applying Equation 2 to the above equations and using the rule for the ratio of partial derivatives, the ratio $\Delta\kappa/\Delta\alpha$ is

$$dT_g^\dagger/dP = (\partial T/\partial P)_h(F_P/F_T),$$

where the freezing fractions F_{X_i} are defined as

$$F_{X_i} = 1 - (\partial h/\partial X_i)_{X_{j,g}}/(\partial h/\partial X_i)_{X_{j,l}}, \quad i \neq j$$

as defined in Reference 7. As pointed out by Simha during this conference, F_P and F_T are nearly equal for the only two substances for which both of these quantities have been evaluated. With $F_P = F_T$, Equation 8 coincides with Equation 7 obtained by Gee also for a single ordering parameter, but which freezes in the glass.

Assuming that Equation 7 is a valid approximation, we may then estimate

$\Delta\kappa/\Delta\alpha$, appearing in Equation 3, from the hole theory for which

$$\Delta\kappa/\Delta\alpha \approx (\partial T/\partial P)_h = (T^*/P^*)(\partial\tilde{T}/\partial\tilde{P})_h, \tag{8}$$

where T^* and P^* are the scaling factors applicable to each substance, and $(\partial\tilde{T}/\partial\tilde{P})_h$ is a universal reduced function of temperature and pressure derived from the simultaneous solution of Equations 1 and 4 in the paper by Simha at this conference. Since Equation 8 applies to the $T_g^\dagger$ boundary, equilibrium theory may be used. Although the scaling factors, T^*, V^*, and P^*, are defined in the theory, they are normally obtained by superposition of equilibrium PVT data with respect to the theoretical universal surface.

Replacement of $\Delta\kappa/\Delta\alpha$ in Equation 3 by the right hand term in Equation 8 gives the final relation

$$\kappa' = \Delta\alpha[(T^*/P^*)(\partial\tilde{T}/\partial\tilde{P})_h - \mathrm{d}T_g/\mathrm{d}P] \tag{9}$$

for which the estimation of κ' involves a combination of quantities derived from theory and experiment. If $\mathrm{d}T_g/\mathrm{d}P$ for a given substance is determined from thermal expansion and heat capacity data employing Equation 6, there will not be sufficient information to determine P^*. For this purpose the empirical equation[8]

$$P^* = (T^*/V^*)\exp(1.139 - 1.493 \times 10^{-4}\,T^*), \tag{10}$$

where T^* and V^* may be determined from equilibrium volume-temperature measurements, seems to be a good approximation for many substances; however, some exceptions have been noted.

Owing to the lack of experimental data, mostly on $\Delta\kappa$, there are only a few substances for which Equation 9 may be tested. With the amorphous polymers tested[9] the standard deviation of the residuals of κ' determined directly from the definition of κ' (Equation 1) and from Equation 9 is 17%, which is about the same as that for the residuals of the experimental values and the average on data from different sources on one polymer.

Equation 9 was used to evaluate κ' on about 20 different polymers. Of these poly(dimethyl siloxane), abbreviated PDMSi, reveals a paradoxical result for which a negative value of κ' is predicted. In this case, however, there is insufficient experimental data available to obtain a reliable estimate. Since PVT data on this polymer is available only above $T_g \approx 150$ K, thermal expansion and heat capacity data above and below T_g were used to determine $\mathrm{d}T_g/\mathrm{d}P$ using Equation 6, which may not hold in general. Another potential source of error is the fact that the hole theory does not seem to apply to PDMSi. According to Prof. Simha, the agreement between the experimental and theoretical equations of state are not nearly as good for PDMSi as for the other polymers tested.

From Equation 3 it is clear that negative densification is tantamount to the reverse in Inequality 5. Assuming the validity of Equation 6, this behavior implies that the Prigogine-Defay ratio

$$R = \Delta\kappa\Delta C_p/[TV(\Delta\alpha)^2]$$

is less than unity (when κ' is negative). To my knowledge no values of $R < 1$ have been reported in the literature, and furthermore, according to Goldstein,[2] the condition $R > 1$ is assured from thermodynamic stability.* Accordingly, since the

*The condition $R > 1$ is consistent with that obtained by eliminating $\mathrm{d}T_g/\mathrm{d}P$ in Inequality 5 and Equation 6.

condition $R > 1$ is expected to hold, it appears from this argument alone that one cannot apply either the hole theory or Equation 6 to PDMSi. On the other hand, since the validity of Equation 6 is not assured, the condition $R > 1$ is insufficient to ensure the validity of Inequality 5, which is tantamount to positive densification. Consequently, the argument based on thermodynamic stability does not preclude the possibility of κ' being negative, a possibility that still seems to be an open question.

Aside from the paradox noted above for PDMSi, the densification model works reasonably well for the amorphous polymers with sufficient data to apply the test and seems to give reasonable values for the others considered. A manuscript giving the detailed results of this evaluation is presently under preparation.[9]

[NOTE ADDED IN PROOF: Since submission of this manuscript an alternative treatment of PDMSi data revealed positive densification for this polymer. For details, see Reference 9.]

References

1. SIMHA, R. & T. SOMCYNSKY. 1969. Macromolecules **2**:342.
2. GOLDSTEIN, M. 1973. J. Phys. Chem. **77**:667.
3. MCKINNEY, J. E. & M. GOLDSTEIN. 1974. J. Res. Nat. Bur. Stand. **78A**:331.
4. O'REILLY, J. M. 1962. J. Polym. Sci. **57**:429.
5. SHISHKIN, N. I. 1960. Sov. Phys. Solid State Phys. **2**:322.
6. GEE, G. 1966. Polymer **7**:177.
7. MCKINNEY, J. & R. SIMHA. 1974. Macromolecules **7**: 894.
8. OLABISI, O. & R. SIMHA. 1975. Macromolecules **8**: 211.
9. MCKINNEY, J. & R. SIMHA. 1976. J. Res. Nat. Bur. Stand., Sect. A. To be published.

MECHANICALLY ENHANCED AGING OF GLASSY POLYMERS*

F. A. Myers, F. C. Cama,† and S. S. Sternstein‡

Materials Engineering Department
Rensselaer Polytechnic Institute
Troy, New York 12181

Glassy polymers are known to exhibit spontaneous changes in their physical properties for long times following vitrification. Specific volume[1] and enthalpy[2] relaxation measurements have demonstrated conclusively that these materials may exist in metastable equilibrium for periods of many years. Although reports[3,4] have appeared that indicate that viscoelastic properties are likewise affected by the spontaneous relaxation, only recently has there been an attempt to investigate the interaction between the spontaneous processes and those resulting from the imposition of mechanical stress or strain.[5-8]

Our studies indicate that the spontaneous relaxation of a glassy polymer's thermodynamic reference state is significantly accelerated by a mechanical stress or strain. This is illustrated in FIGURE 1, where the spontaneous decay of specific volume or free energy is illustrated schematically at two temperatures T_1 and $T_2 > T_1$, both of which are below the glass transition temperature. If the imposition of a mechanical stress or strain at some time t_1 on a sample at temperature T_1 results in an acceleration of the aging process, then the reference state of the sample will change at a rate commensurate with some higher temperature T_2. Thus, during an interval under stress or strain of time Δt, the sample's reference state specific volume or free energy will change by an amount Δ over and above the change which would have occurred without the acceleration due to the mechanical stress or strain. This process is referred to as mechanically enhanced aging, and can be studied by comparison of stress relaxation or creep rates on samples subjected to cyclic load or strain histories at various times after vitrification relative to stress relaxation or creep rates of samples previously undeformed and at equivalent times after vitrification.

The stress relaxation behavior of a quenched polymethyl methacrylate (PMMA) sample subjected to four cycles each of 500 minutes of 0.5% strain followed by 1000 minutes of stress free recovery is shown in FIGURE 2. It is clear that the relaxation behavior of the quenched sample is approaching that of a slow cooled sample on each progressive cycle. However, it is not clear from this figure whether the aging process is due solely to spontaneous (time) aging or is due in part to the mechanical history.

The first cycle, $Q(I)$, shown in FIGURE 2 commenced at 900 minutes after quenching the sample and the four cycles requires $4 \times (500 + 1000)$ or 6000 minutes to complete. A second quenched sample was similarly tested but with the first cycle commencing at 9000 minutes after quenching. The first cycle stress relaxation curve was found to be only slightly slower than $Q(I)$ of FIGURE 2 and the remaining three cycles were effectively indistinguishable from those shown in

*This work was supported principally by the National Science Foundation (Grant No. GH 37249) and also by the B. F. Goodrich Chemical Co. and the Shell Foundation.

†Present affiliation: Mobay Chemical Co., Pittsburgh, Pa.

‡To whom correspondence should be sent.

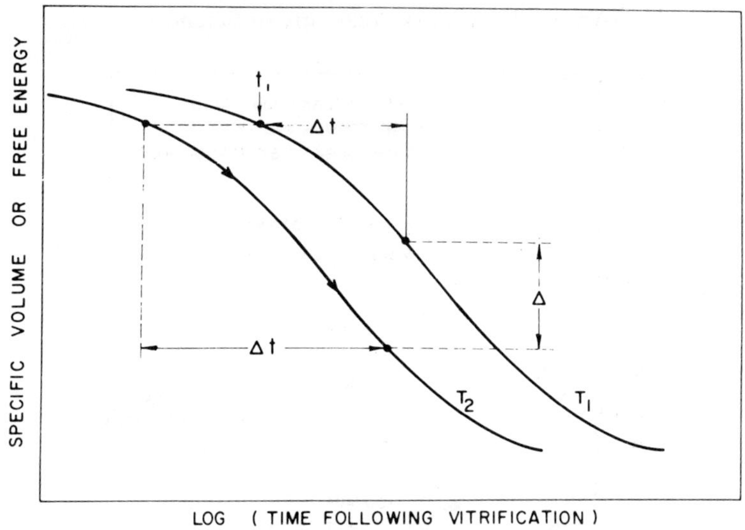

FIGURE 1. Schematic of the spontaneous relaxation of free energy or specific volume in a glassy polymer at two temperatures T_1 and $T_2 > T_1$. The quantity Δ represents an additional degree of aging due to mechanical enhancement by a stress or strain applied at time t_1 for a duration Δt.

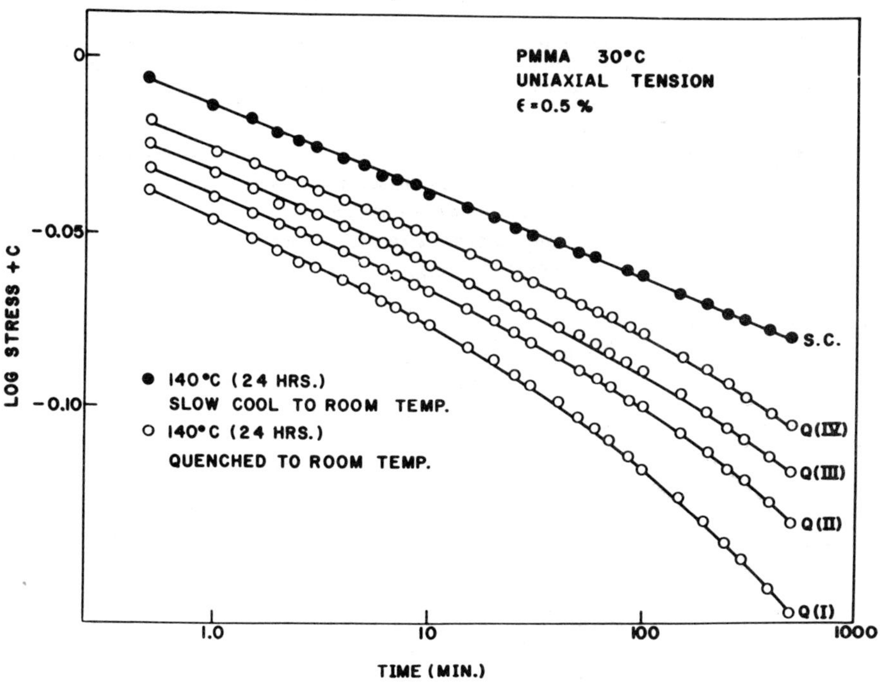

FIGURE 2. Repetitive cycle stress relaxation in glassy PMMA for quenched and slow cooled samples.

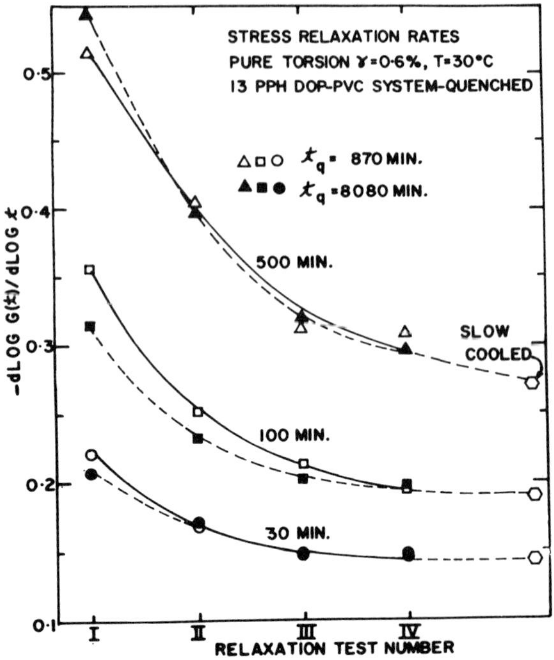

FIGURE 3. Logarithmic stress relaxation rates versus strain cycle for two quenched samples of PVC each held a different time t_q before commencement of the first cycle. The times on the curves are measured with respect to the beginning of the respective cycle.

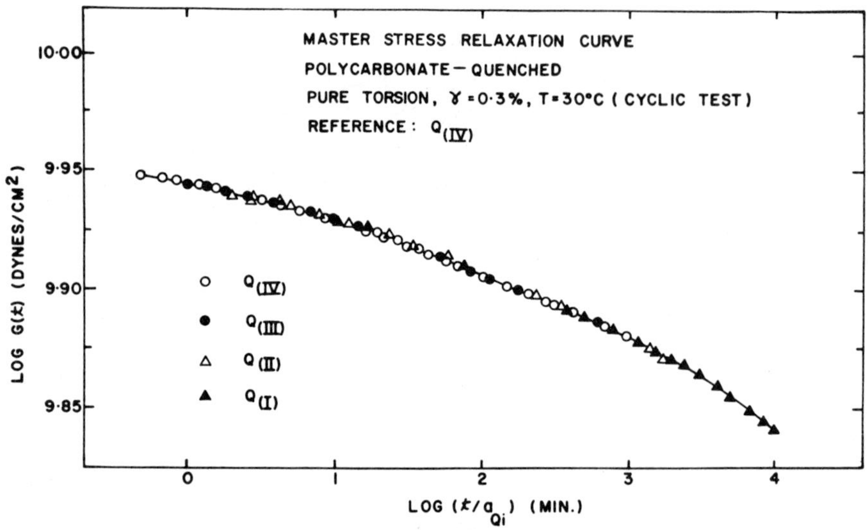

FIGURE 4. Master stress relaxation curve obtained for polycarbonate by time shifting a series of repetitive stress relaxation tests on a single quenched sample.

FIGURE 2 for the 900 minute sample, even though the sample is 8100 minutes older at each point in the strain history. Thus, it appears that the aging rate of PMMA at 30°C is significantly enhanced by a mechanical strain relative to the aging rate due to spontaneous (stress or strain free) time effects.

Mechanically enhanced aging has been observed in unplasticized polyvinyl chloride (PVC), both dioctyl phthalate (DOP) and tricresyl phosphate (TCP) plasticized PVC, and polycarbonate. For example, results on a 13 PPH/DOP-PVC sample are shown in FIGURE 3 where the ordinate is the logarithmic stress relaxation rate (basically the slope of curves such as given in FIGURE 2). The relaxation rate is given for each cycle of strain at various isochronous times measured with respect to the beginning of each strain cycle. Data for two samples are shown, one whose first strain cycle commenced at 800 minutes after quenching and one 8000 minutes after quenching. It is clear that the decrease in stress relaxation rate due to

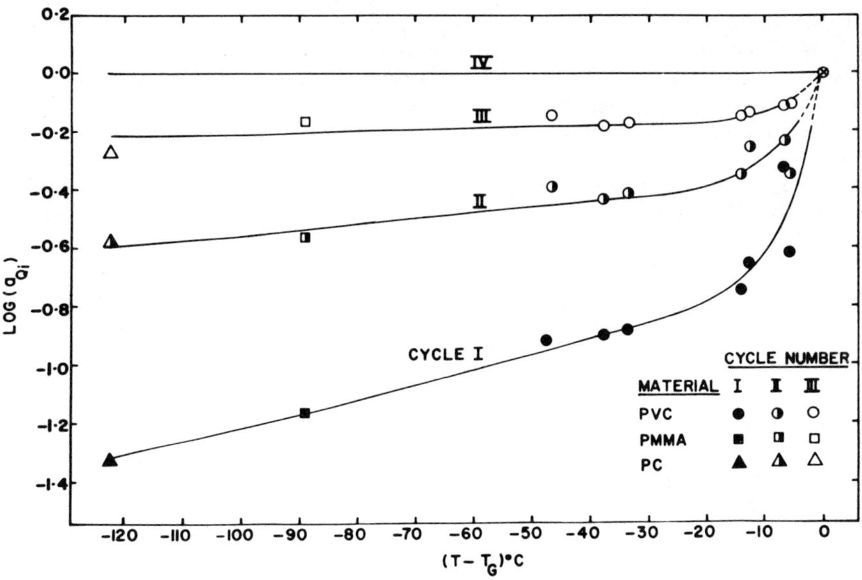

FIGURE 5. Time shift factors versus degree of supercooling for each cycle of stress relaxation and several polymers.

7200 minutes of time is small compared to that due to a strain cycle of 0.6% strain for 500 minutes.

The stress relaxation curves such as shown in FIGURE 2, when plotted as log stress relaxation modulus versus log time, are found to superpose when shifted on the log time axis. An example is given in FIGURE 4 where the master stress relaxation curve for bis-phenol A polycarbonate is shown. This curve is made up of data obtained from four stress relaxation tests performed on a single quenched sample at 30°C. The shift factors required to obtain superposition of the repetitive stress relaxation curves on all of the samples studied are shown in FIGURE 5. It appears that the mechanically enhanced aging process depends primarily on the degree of supercooling and is independent of polymer chemical structure. In FIGURE 5, it should be noted that the reference curve used to construct the master curve for each polymer (i.e., the curve for which the time shift factor is unity) is the fourth cycle stress relaxation curve for that polymer.

The results presented thus far are reported elsewhere[5-7] and were obtained on a static torsion balance relaxometer[7] and a biaxial stress relaxation apparatus.[5,6] More recently, a servo-controlled viscoelastic tester of original design has been used to obtain additional data. This instrument can control stress or strain to 1 part in 10,000 and can be digitally programmed to obtain any desired mechanical history. The step function rise time of the instrument is less than 20 milliseconds with no overshoot; consequently, stress relaxation or creep curves can be extended to times as short as 100 milliseconds. In addition, data may be obtained in tension or compression.

Results of experiments with this apparatus indicate that mechanically enhanced aging occurs at about the same rate in tension and compression and in stress relaxation and creep. It follows that the process is governed primarily by distortional (deviatoric) strain *energy* and is not due to, e.g., the dilatation present in uniaxial tension. Thus, the accelerated aging process is not due to free volume effects. Since the strain energy at zero time is proportional to the square of the stress or strain (elastic behavior at small times is assumed), the mechanical aging process should be quite sensitive to the stress level in a creep test or strain level in a relaxation test. We are currently investigating this prediction which appears to be correct.

It has also been observed that the short time data do not superpose as did the longer time data (e.g., FIGURE 4). An example is given in FIGURES 6 and 7 where it

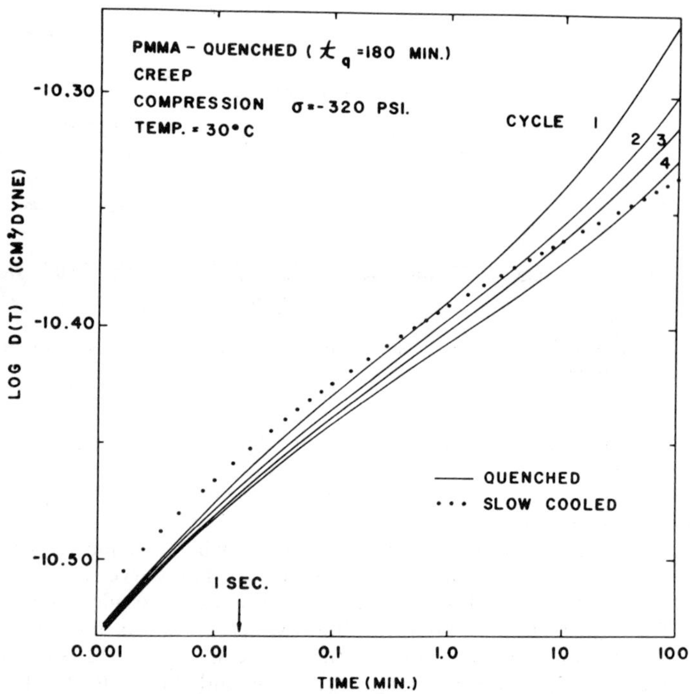

FIGURE 6. Compression creep compliance of a quenched sample of PMMA subjected to four cycles of creep and recovery.

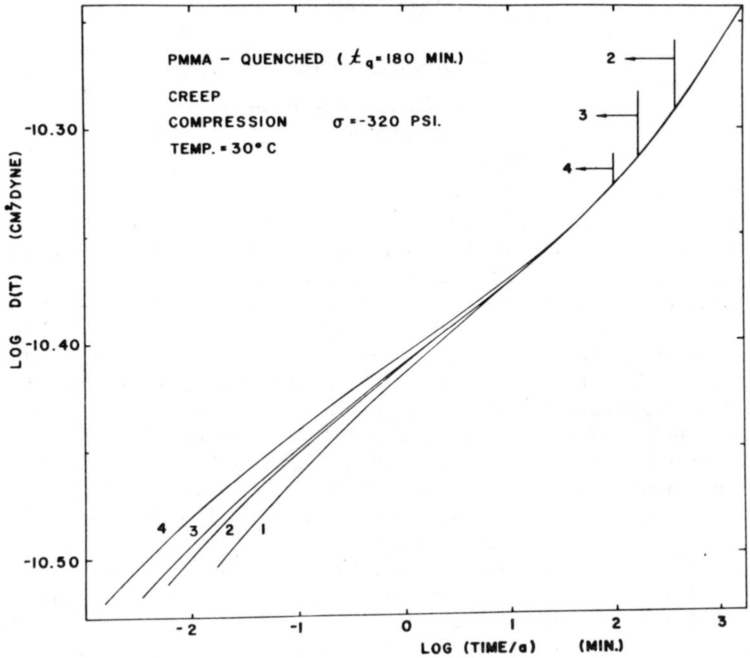

FIGURE 7. The curves of FIGURE 6 shifted to obtain a master curve at long times. Note the absence of superposition at short times.

is evident that superposition of cycles 1–4 at longer times can be accomplished but that the short time data do not lie on the master curve. It is found from tension and compression creep and relaxation that the short time data are essentially unaffected by the aging process but that the longer time behavior is as described in FIGURES 1–5.

These results have important applications to the engineering properties of glassy thermoplastics, especially in relation to impact strength (a short time process) and slow strain rate ductility or creep (long time processes). From a theoretical viewpoint our results suggest that mechanically enhanced aging is primarily involved with long-range cooperative chain motions generally associated with yielding phenomena and the glass transition.

References

1. KOVACS, A. J. 1958. J. Polym. Sci. **30:** 131.
2. PETRIE, S. E. B. 1972. J. Polym. Sci. A-2 **10:** 1255.
3. KOVACS, A. J., R. A. STRATTON & J. D. FERRY. 1963. J. Phys. Chem. **67:** 152.
4. STRUIK. L. C. E. 1966. Rheo. Acta **5(4):** 303.
5. HO, T. C. 1973. Biaxial stress relaxation of polymethylmethacrylate in the glassy state. Ph.D. thesis. Rensselaer Polytechnic Institute. Troy, New York.
6. STERNSTEIN, S. S. & T. C. HO. 1972. J. Appl. Phys. **43(11):** 4370.
7. CAMA, F. J. 1974. Stress relaxation of plasticized and unplasticized poly(vinyl chloride) in the glassy state. Ph.D. Thesis. Rensselaer Polytechnic Institute. Troy, New York.
8. MYERS, F. A. & S. S. STERNSTEIN. To be published.

DISCUSSION

E. A. DiMarzio, *Moderator*

National Bureau of Standards
Washington, D.C.

K. L. DeVries (*National Science Foundation, Washington, D.C.*): My remark is directed primarily to Dr. Struik and his very interesting presentation. It has always bothered me a little bit to see investigators extrapolate their predictions of mechanical response and aging out to a thousand years or more. I am a bit concerned that in length of time some chemical aging might take place. I was wondering whether you might comment on this aspect of polymer behavior. To illustrate my point may I, (somewhat tongue in cheek) use your own example of Dutch cheese. Some years ago I lived in Holland and became very fond of your cheese. Inadvertently, I performed some "experiments" somewhat akin to some of the studies you outlined. I enjoyed toasted cheese sandwiches made with old cheese. The "annealing operation" associated with toasting did not convert the old cheese to young cheese, at least according to my sense of taste. This would indicate to me that some chemical changes had taken place that were not reversed by annealing. Since I didn't measure mechanical properties of the cheese, I can't comment on whether or not these chemical changes effect modulus, strength, etc. I also note that Dr. Struik's measurements were conducted on "dried" cheese and perhaps these changes do not occur in the absence of moisture. It appears reasonable to me, however, that in some polymers chemical changes may occur and with time these may eventually affect mechanical response. I believe I know of polymer systems in which cross-linking increases with time and others where some chain scission occurs with age. If these occur at either a rapid enough rate or over a long enough period of time, one might expect them to be reflected in changing mechanical properties. I don't think this reflects on the validity of your very interesting results and observations on the essentially reversible nature of physical aging that occurs in the polymers you studied, but I wonder if they tell a complete story? In any of your studies have you seen evidence of chemical aging resulting in irreversible changes in response? Do you feel that if you waited long enough (i.e., hundreds of years) one might expect degradation and other chemical changes to effect the properties you have measured?

Struik: There are, or may, of course, be chemical changes in the polymer, especially when we consider periods of many years. What I intended to say was that, apart from the well-known chemical aging, there also exists a physical type of aging. This kind of aging is thermoreversible; i.e., it can be erased by a short heating to just above T_g (compare Figure 2). The reversibility observed in Figure 2 certainly does not prove the complete absence of chemical aging in PVC at 20°C. It might well be that the chemical changes have no effect on the tensile creep properties.

You asked whether in my studies I have seen any evidence of chemical aging resulting in irreversible changes in response. My aging experiments were generally performed in the dark and in a dry nitrogen atmosphere. Under these conditions, I have never observed any irreversible changes in the creep, yielding, and impact properties, at least when I started with dry specimens, free of internal stresses.

S. Matsuoka (*Bell Laboratories, Murray Hill, N.J.*): I wish to point out that there is a substantial difference in mechanical relaxation behavior of polymeric glasses near T_g (about 15°C below T_g) and at much lower (50°C or more below T_g) temperatures.

In the first or the high temperature range, or 15°C or so below T_g, the relaxation process at small deformation is essentially linearly viscoelastic, and the spectrum follows a Rouse or Zimm-like distribution. This is the temperature range most convenient to study the effect of thermal history. We have studied relaxation processes in this temperature range and obtained the similar history dependence of the relaxation spectra for polystyrene, PVC, and ABS. I might add that the time dependence of the shift of relaxation time can be interpreted in terms of Kovacs's exponential integral type function, which is the solution of the differential equation for the isothermal rate of decay of free volume in polymeric glasses for a wide range of temperatures.

In the second or the lower temperature range, the nonlinearity of the viscoelastic behavior becomes markedly more pronounced. The relaxation modulus shifts along the logarithmic time axis in a very drastic manner at 0.5 to 2% strain range. In this range the Poisson ratio decreases to ~0.35 from 0.45 in the higher temperature range mentioned above. Craze-yielding is a form of ultimate deformation accompanying the decrease of the apparent density. Because of these aspects, we proposed the structural interpretation of this nonlinear behavior to be associated with "reactivation" of free volume by the tensile strain-induced dilatation. The shift of relaxation times has been found to follow the exponential function of the inverse of the strain-induced fractional free volume increase, or the Doolittle type dependence in short. From the strain-dependent relaxation modulus, one can construct the stress-strain curves by the convolution integral. When this is done, one finds that there is a maximum stress at typically 2% or 3% strain, beyond which the solid is no longer able to sustain the stress because of the strain-shortened relaxation time. This was interpreted as the time-dependent yield stress. This yield stress agrees with the data on craze-yields, which depend on different rates of strain, thermal history, and hydrostatic pressure in the completely consistent manner.

The only shortcoming of the dilatational model for the nonlinear behavior is the dependence of the shear strain, and the shear yield under hydrostatic pressure. We are now attempting to study the volume change under shear, which should not be automatically assumed as zero or even negligible for nonlinear solids.

STRUIK: We studied the nonlinear behavior, viz., that of PVC and PC, over wide temperature ranges below T_g. However, we performed creep tests instead of stress-relaxation measurements, and this may strongly influence the results.

We found an acceleration of the creep by high stresses. The acceleration was of the Eyring sinh-type, but turned out to be almost independent of temperature. Thus, a stress of 200 kg/cm^2 accelerates the creep of PVC at 50°C by roughly the same amount as it does at −20°C. Nor does a change from tensile creep to shear (torsion) creep produce any large effect on the acceleration function. This, I think, points in the same direction as Dr. Matsuoka's final remark, viz., that in the nonlinear range a shear deformation will be accompanied by changes in free volume. Such volume effects in shear are known for set powders, and I believe that careful tests on sheared glasses will also reveal them.

G. P. JOHARI (*National Research Council of Canada, Ottawa, Can.*): The vanishing part of the excess entropy, S_{vp}, in a number of disorder-frozen-in crystalline solids shows a temperature dependence that is remarkably similar to that reported in ordinary glasses by Goldstein. The configurational fraction for several orientationally disordered crystals is less than 0.5, as given in TABLE 1 below. The con-

TABLE 1

SOME THERMODYNAMIC QUANTITIES* FOR SEVERAL ORIENTATIONALLY DISORDERED SOLIDS AND ONE LIQUID

Substance	T'_g °K	T_2 °K	$\Delta C_p(T_g)$ J°K^{-1} mol^{-1}	$\Delta S(T_g)$ J°K^{-1} mol^{-1}	ΔS_0 J°K^{-1} mol^{-1}	R
Cyclohexanol	148	128	24	14.9	4.7	0.32
Cycloheptanol	140	100	32	3.9	0.7	0.18
2,3-Dimethylbutane	76	65	51	19	7.4	0.39
Molecular compound of 2,3- and 2,2-dimethylbutane	69	52	56	18	10	0.55
cis-1,2-Dimethyl cyclohexane	94	82	63	17	8.6	0.50
Isopropylbenzene (liquid-glass)	126	106	72	21	12	0.57

The glasslike transition temperature, T'_g; the Adam-Gibbs temperature, T_2; the decrease in the heat capacity, ΔC_p, at T'_g; the difference between the entropy of the stable crystalline phase and the disorder-frozen-in crystalline phase, $\Delta S(T_g)$ at T_g, and ΔS_0 at 0°K; and the configurational fraction, $R = \Delta S(0°\mathrm{K})/\Delta S(T_g)$.

tribution to heat capacity due to the anharmonicity of vibrations in these crystals is likely to be very small.

It is also worth mentioning that a similar temperature dependence of S_{vp} has been found also in vitreous methanol and vitreous ice obtained from vapor phase deposition of the solids, but their configurational fraction is much smaller than that of any other amorphous material.

Some indication of the contribution to heat capacity due to the anharmonicity of vibrations can be obtained from the temperature dependence of the limiting high frequency dielectric permittivity, ϵ_∞. $\epsilon_\infty = n_D^2 + \Delta\epsilon_{\mathrm{ir}}$, where n_D is the refractive index for the Na-D line and $\Delta\epsilon_{\mathrm{ir}}$ is the contribution to permittivity due to the infrared polarization.

$$\Delta\epsilon_{\mathrm{ir}} = \Delta n^2 + 2n_D\Delta n, \tag{1}$$

and

$$\Delta n = \frac{1}{2\pi^2}\int_{\mathrm{band}} \frac{K(\nu)}{\nu^2}\,\mathrm{d}\nu \tag{2}$$

where ν is the wavenumber of the radiation. The absorptivity, K, is defined by the relation,

$$K(\nu) = x^{-1}\log_e(I/I_0),$$

I and I_0 being the intensity of radiation after and before travelling the distance x in the sample.

If the $\Delta\epsilon_{\mathrm{ir}}$ remains constant with temperature, the ϵ_∞ generally has a negative temperature coefficient, as given by the Clausius-Mossotti equation. The anharmonicity of vibrations causes the frequency, integrated intensity, and half-width of a particular normal mode to depend upon temperature and these changes alter the temperature dependence of ϵ_∞. In particular, the anharmonicity of lattice vibrations causes the ν in Equation 2 to decrease with increasing temperature and this in turn may cause the ϵ_∞ of a material to increase with temperature. Any significant contribution from the anharmonicity of lattice vibrations would produce a positive temperature coefficient of ϵ_∞. In most polymers the ϵ_∞ is known to have a negative temperature coefficient and, therefore, it would seem that in some of the amorphous substances discussed by Simha and Goldstein the contribution to the excess thermodynamic properties (expansivity, heat capacity, etc.,) due to the anharmonicity is small. Their discussion of the excess expansivity and heat capacity of a glass in terms of configurational changes would seem to be valid.

BRAWER: I would like to talk about something that was mentioned by Dr. Angell and Dr. Goldstein this morning, and that is that as you plot the entropy of the glass minus the entropy of the solid as a function of T extrapolated below T_g, the glass transition temperature, it is generally concluded that this line cannot cross zero, and I would like to know why not. The only thing that can't cross zero is the free energy, but the entropy certainly can cross zero, and in fact it is quite conceivable that it would. It is possible for the vibrational entropy of the glass to be smaller than that of a corresponding crystal. For example, in some crystals (e.g., quartz) a large density of low-frequency modes occurs because, in a sense, there is only a weak resistance to atomic motions in certain directions. One can have, for example, all SiO_4 tetrahedra rotating at the same time, and this is possible because of the regular crystal structure. The Si—O distance remains approximately constant during such a vibration, as do the O—Si—O angles. However, when the glass is formed, no such collective motion is possible and rotating an SiO_4 tetrahedron will change the Si—O or the O—Si—O angles and such changes will be resisted by strong force constants. For this case the vibration entropy may be smaller in the glass than in the crystal. The same principle can be applied to other glasses, and it's conceivable that you can find some glasses that actually will have a lot of low-frequency modes frozen out, whereas the crystal doesn't.

The idea of freezing out the low-frequency vibrations can perhaps be directly tested in certain cases by measuring the infrared absorption of glasses of various transition temperatures T_g. If the low-frequency modes freeze out, the absorption should decrease with decreasing T_g.

GOLDSTEIN: The curves of glass entropy (or "glassy crystal" entropy) minus crystal entropy shown here by Dr. Johari and by me seem to show the opposite: The disordered phase has a higher vibrational entropy than the ordered phase. The substances we examined do not, unfortunately, include SiO_2.

I would also like to note that conclusions about order parameters disagreeing with DiMarzio's have appeared or are about to appear in the literature: References 17–19 in the paper by Angell and Sichina.

MOLECULAR ORIGIN OF RELAXATIONS IN POLYMERS

J. Heijboer

Centraal Laboratorium TNO
Delft, The Netherlands.

Types of Molecular Motion Giving Rise to Loss Peaks

Relaxations in polymers are connected with molecular mobility, and therefore we shall consider what types of molecular motion are possible in the glassy state, and how these motions manifest themselves in the mechanical behavior.

When a polymer is cooled and passes its glass transition T_g the *cooperative motions of large parts of the main polymer chain* are frozen in. This process is a gradual one that is determined by the change in free volume. Below T_g, therefore, smaller parts of the main chain retain a residual mobility that gives rise to mechanical losses. In other words, the damping peak accompanying the glass transition has a low-temperature tail that very strongly depends on the remaining free volume. In the previous paper, Struik[1] has shown how the damping and creep properties in this region depend on aging properties, that is, on the preceding decrease in free volume.

An example is given in FIGURE 1, which shows the modulus and damping at 1 Hz of poly(ethylene terephthalate), PET, as a function of temperature for different thermal histories of the sample. The thin line gives the properties of a sample quenched from 75° to −170°C; the thick line gives the same properties of a sample slowly cooled from 75° to 25°C. A marked change is seen in the damping on the low-temperature side of the glass transition.

To show that this behavior is thermoreversible, we also present the data for the same specimen, which, after having passed the slow cooling and measuring cycle, is again quenched from 75° to −175°C (filled points). It is seen that the data coincide with those of the measurement on the first quenched sample. The effect of annealing has obviously been erased.

The second type of motion we shall consider is the *local main-chain motion*. This is a motion of main-chain segments smaller than those associated with the glass transition. Such a local main-chain motion is the only possible molecular mechanism causing a secondary loss peak in a polymer possessing no side groups that can move independently of the main chain. (We here assume that the secondary loss peak does not depend on molecular weight. This means that the motions of the chain ends do not contribute significantly to the losses.) This type of loss peak is rather general; it is found in, e.g., polycarbonates, polysulphones, polyesters, but also in poly(vinyl chloride), PVC.[2] The exact molecular mechanism is difficult to establish[3]; from a comparison of mechanical and dielectric losses, an impression is gained of the participation of polar groups.

FIGURE 1 gives the large β peak of amorphous PET; it is seen that slow cooling has practically no influence on the height of this peak. This insensitivity of the peak height to cooling rate has been noted for a series of secondary loss peaks of amorphous polymers; this means that these peaks are not sensitive to changes of free volume. This is qualitatively understandable: at the glass transition the cooperative motions of large parts of the chain require a considerable free vol-

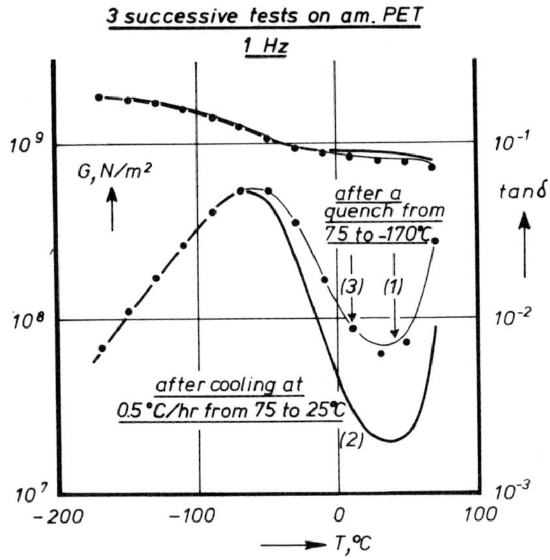

FIGURE 1. Shear modulus G′ and damping tan δ at 1 Hz as functions of temperature of amorphous poly(ethylene terephthalate) for different thermal histories.

ume; the motion of the much smaller groups that are responsible for the secondary transitions, require only a small free volume and after the freezing in of the cooperative motion of the larger segments, this small volume always remains. It is also understandable that the aging stops at temperatures below that of secondary loss peaks. The immobilization of the smaller groups renders the main chain stiffer, and a still larger volume would be required to accommodate large parts of the main chain in a new position.

Interestingly, the loss peak of the local main-chain motion and that of the glass transition are clearly separate. There is no gradual transition from a local mode motion to the glass transition by a gradual enlargement of the moving group with increasing temperature. It follows that there is a distinct difference between the two types of motion responsible for respectively the secondary loss peak and for the glass transition.

In my opinion this difference in molecular mechanisms also makes it doubtful whether we can expect a constant ratio of T_β/T_g.[4] This can be illustrated by the damping of three polyesters,[5] shown in FIGURE 2. These esters have about the same T_g, in spite of which their T_β values lie widely apart. The explanation is that the barrier opposing the rotation of phenylene groups with a carbonyl group in between governs the location of the β maximum. If this location were determined by intermolecular interactions, one would also expect large differences between the T_g values since it is intermolecular interactions which to a large extent determine the value of T_g.

Another interesting feature of the local mode relaxation is its sensitivity to antiplasticization; the β maxima of both polycarbonate[6,7] and PVC[8,9] can be depressed by addition of plasticizers.

A third type of motion to be discussed is a *side group motion with some cooperation of the main chain,* e.g., a partial rotation of the side group about the bond linking it to the main chain. The β maximum of poly(methyl methacrylate), PMMA, is

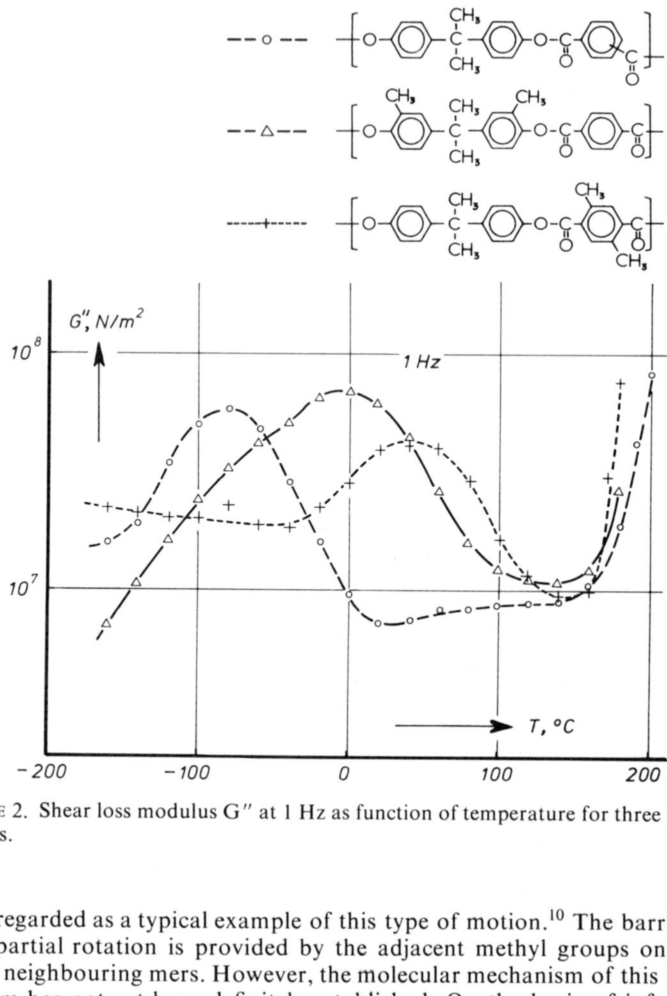

FIGURE 2. Shear loss modulus G″ at 1 Hz as function of temperature for three amorphous polyesters.

usually regarded as a typical example of this type of motion.[10] The barrier opposing the partial rotation is provided by the adjacent methyl groups on the main chain of neighbouring mers. However, the molecular mechanism of this secondary maximum has not yet been definitely established. On the basis of infrared data, Havriliak and Roman[11] suppose that the β maximum of PMMA is due to a main-chain motion, and the α maximum usually called the glass transition, to side chain motions. In a recent paper[12] I tried to reconcile Havriliak's infrared data with the usual ideas about the molecular mechanisms of the β and α maxima of PMMA. I also presented further arguments for this molecular interpretation. It must be admitted, however, that the extent to which the main chain takes part in the side group motion is not sufficiently quantified. The β maximum can best be separated from the glass transition by measurements of creep. These showed[12] that the temperature location of the maximum does not change in the series of poly-(*n*-alkyl methacrylates) from methyl to *n*-butyl. I regret that this result does not agree with that obtained by Haldon and Simha,[13] who determined the location of the transition by thermal expansion. However, I am afraid that the latter method is not sensitive enough for accurate determination of the temperature location of secondary transitions: what we see is a gradual change in linear coefficient of expansion, α, with only the derivative of α with respect to temperature showing maxima. However, the loss modulus itself shows a distinct maximum. To make our results more convincing, we present the experimental points in FIGURE 3.

Our results are in good agreement with those of Hideshima *et al.*[14] who observed by dielectrical and mechanical measurements that the β relaxations of PMMA, PEMA, and poly(*n*-propyl methacrylate), PnPrMA, lie at nearly the same temperature. Moreover, Wada *et al.*[15] observed by dielectrical measurements a constant temperature of the β maximum in a series of copolymers of MMA and *n*-butyl methacrylate (nBuMA).

As in the series of esters in FIGURE 2, structural changes affect the secondary transition in a completely different way from the glass transition. The ratio T_β/T_g for the β transition in poly(methacrylates) is not a constant either.

The effect of the addition of the external plasticizer dibutyl phthalate also affects T_g and T_β in different ways. T_g decreases whereas T_β remains constant.[12]

Substitution of hydrogen for the methyl groups on the main chain (by copolymerization of MMA with methylacrylate, MA) decreases the stiffness of the main chain as well as the barrier to rotation of the side group. In that case T_g as well as T_β decreases, as is shown in FIGURE 4.

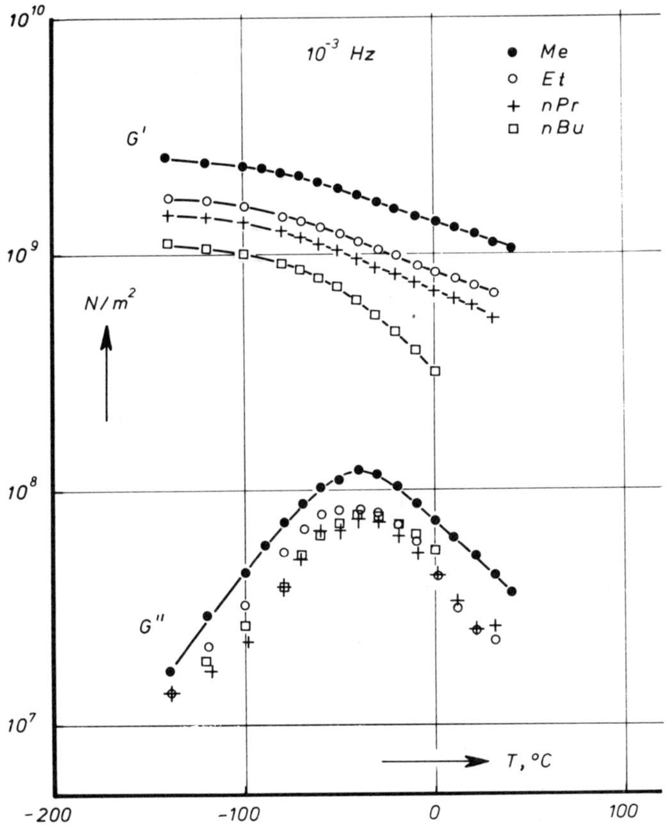

FIGURE 3. Shear storage modulus G′ and shear loss modulus G″ at 10^{-3} Hz as functions of temperature for poly(methyl methacrylate), poly(ethyl methacrylate), poly(*n*-propyl methacrylate) and poly(*n*-butyl methacrylate).

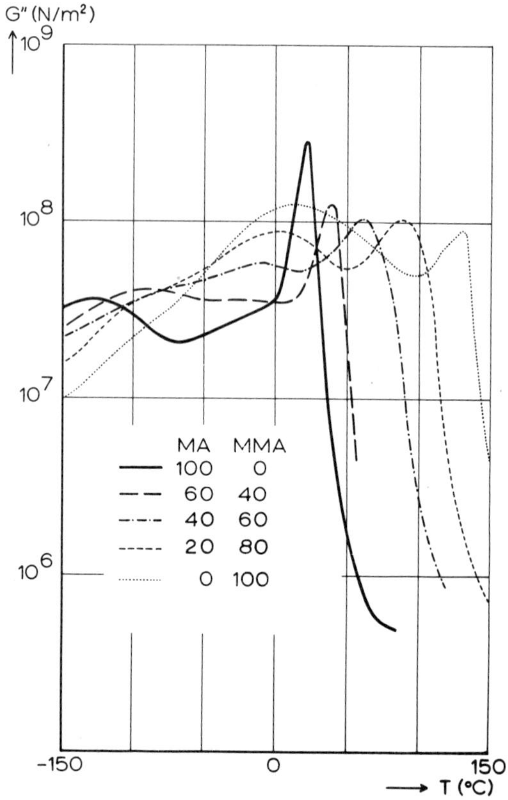

FIGURE 4. Loss modulus G″ as a function of temperature for a series of copolymers of methyl acrylate (MA) and methyl methacrylate (MMA). Composition in weight percent.

A fourth type of motion is an *internal motion within a side group* without interference by the main chain. Typical examples are the internal motions within R of the –COOR group of polymethacrylates.[16] A multitude of these compounds have been investigated; some R groups showing distinct mechanical loss peaks are: *n*-propyl, *n*-butyl, 2-hydroxyethyl,[17,18] 2-chloroethyl,[16,19] and cycloalkyl.[20,21] A few examples from outside the group of poly(methacrylates) are: the oxymethyl group in poly(4-oxymethylstyrene),[22] and the alkyl group in 2-methyl-6-alkyl substituted poly(phenylene ethers).[23] This list is by no means exhaustive.

It could be shown that the location of many of these loss peaks is determined by the barrier within the side group, the internal barrier. For some loss peaks[23,24] there is evidence that interactions between groups are also of importance. Obviously the ratio T_β / T_g for these loss peaks cannot be expected to be constant.

We disagree with Janacek,[25] who suggests that the absolute temperatures of loss peaks have values with ratios of integers. Already from the difference between the frequency dependence of a glass transition and that of a secondary transition, it follows that this assumption has no physical basis.

A fifth type of motion is the *motion of, or taking place within, a small molecule dissolved* in the polymer. This can be a motion within a plasticizer molecule, e.g., the *n*-butyl group in dibutyl phthalate. It is sometimes difficult to decide whether it is the entire molecule, or only a part of it, that moves.

FIGURE 5 shows a typical example of two relaxations due to motions of small molecules; for the phenyl-substituted molecule the maximum is due to the flipping motion of the six-ring. The maximum of the unsubstituted molecule lies at a considerably lower temperature, and is probably due to a rotation or oscillation of the molecule about its longitudinal axis. This molecule has no cyclohexyl maximum, probably because its frequency of rotation is higher than that of the flipping motion. When the molecule is anchored in the medium by the large phenyl ring, the cyclohexyl loss peak returns.

The loss peak of a cyclohexyl group contained in a polymer molecule lies at the same temperature as the loss peak of a cyclohexyl group of a small plasticizer molecule embedded in a polymer matrix.[26] Therefore internal barriers in small

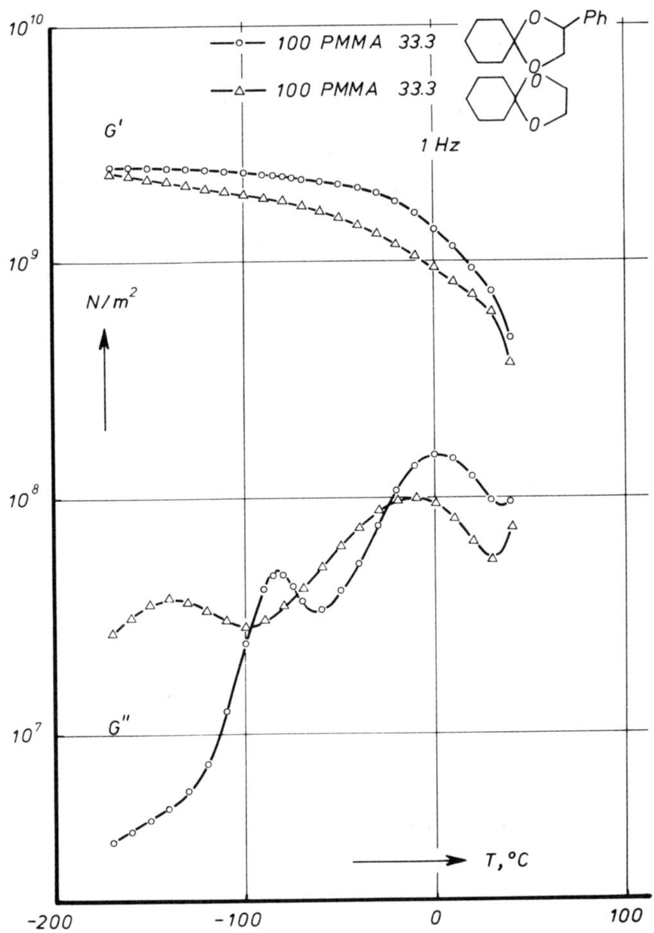

FIGURE 5. G′ and G″ at 1 Hz of solid PMMA solutions containing 25% (wt/wt) 1,4-dioxaspiro[4, 5] decane and 25% (wt/wt) the 2-phenyl derivative of the same.

molecules can be studied by mechanical or dielectrical measurements on solid solutions of such molecules in a polymer matrix.[27,28]

We found that the quantitative contribution of a cyclohexyl group to the mechanical damping is the same, no matter whether the group is in the plasticizer or in the polymer molecule.[26,29] I think that this observation is important for the understanding of the mechanism by which mechanical stress interacts with molecular motions.

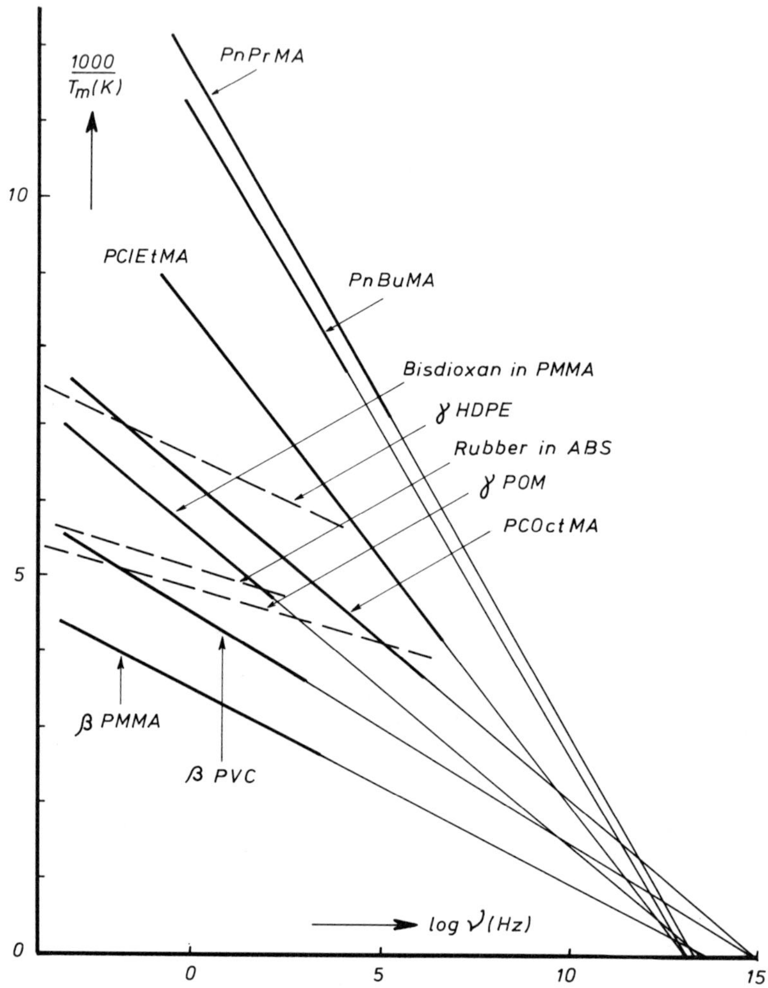

FIGURE 6. Arrhenius plots of secondary maxima. The thick parts of the lines indicate the region of the measurements; the thin parts are extrapolations. Explanation of abbreviations in the text.

Dependence of Secondary Maxima on Frequency

We shall now consider the frequency dependence of the temperature of the secondary maxima. FIGURE 6 shows Arrhenius graphs in which the reciprocal of the absolute temperature T_m of the maximum is plotted against the logarithm of the frequency ν. T_m is obtained from a plot of the losses at constant frequency as a function of temperature.

The following examples are shown:

(a) the β maximum of poly(vinyl chloride) (PVC), resulting from a local main-chain motion;

(b) the β maximum of poly(methyl methacrylate) (PMMA), caused by a side-group motion with some cooperation of the main chain;

(c) the peak of poly(cyclooctyl methacrylate) (PCOctMA)[21]; this is caused by an internal motion within the eight-membered ring;

(d) the γ maximum of poly(2-chloroethyl methacrylate)[19] (PClEtMA), also stemming from an internal motion within a side group;

(e) the γ maxima of poly(*n*-butyl methacrylate)[30] (PnBuMA) and poly(*n*-propyl methacrylate)[19] (PnPrMA), both arising from motions within the *n*-alkyl groups;

(f) a loss peak of a 40% (wt/wt) solution of bisdioxan in PMMA. This peak is caused by a flipping motion of the six-rings of bisdioxan, viz., an internal motion within a small molecule dissolved in a polymer matrix. The formula of bisdioxan (2, 4, 8, 10-tetraoxaspiro[5.5]undecane) is

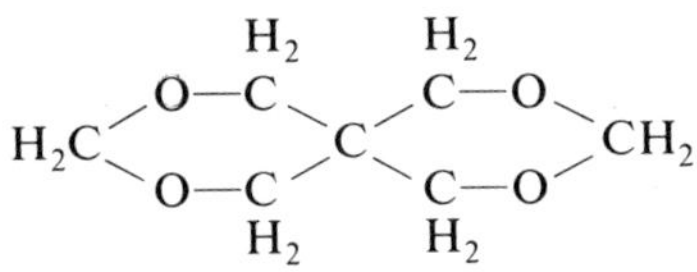

For comparison the following are also shown:

(g) the loss maximum of the rubber phase of an acrylonitrile butadiene styrene rubber (ABS); this maximum is a glass transition;

(h) the γ transition of polyoxymethylene (POM)[30] from a main-chain motion in a semicrystalline polymer;

(i) the γ transition of high density polyethylene (HDPE),[30] also caused by a main-chain motion in a semicrystalline polymer.

The measured values fit the Arrhenius equation

$$\ln \nu = \ln \nu_0 - E_a/RT_m \tag{1}$$

or

$$\log \nu = \log \nu_0 - 0.4343\, E_a/RT_m$$

where E_a is the activation energy and R the gas constant. When we first exclude the transitions in the crystalline polymers (h) and (i), and the glass transition (g), we see that the lines extrapolate to

$$\log \nu_0 = 13 - 15 \quad \text{for } 1/T_m \rightarrow 0.$$

The great majority of secondary loss peaks of amorphous polymers investigated at CL-TNO extrapolate to $\log \nu_0 = 13.5 \pm 1$.

10^{13} Hz is a reasonable frequency for a molecular vibration. The molecular picture behind an activated process described by an Arrhenius equation, is as follows: Suppose the mechanism is one involving two potential wells separated by a barrier much higher than kT. Each of the groups is vibrating at its molecular frequency in a well, and sometimes it jumps across the barrier to the other position. If entropy differences between the two positions are neglected, the relative numbers of the groups in each of the two positions in the state of equilibrium are determined by Boltzmann's equation. Application of a stress causes the differences in depth of the two wells to change; the equilibrium is disturbed and a redistribution of the groups over the two positions starts. The rate of redistribution is determined by the temperature and by the height of the barrier, which is therefore the activation energy E_a. When during the time of redistribution the stress field changes its direction, energy is dissipated. This molecular picture implies that the location of *the secondary loss peak is determined by the local barrier within the molecule.*

It is clear that Equation 1 neglects entropy contributions. It is therefore not unexpected that the PVC maximum and the cyclooctyl-ring maximum extrapolate to slightly higher values. For the local main-chain motion of PVC a larger entropy contribution might be expected than for the flipping motion of the six-membered ring. The internal motion of the eight-membered ring is not a simple flipping, as in the six-membered ring; the number of transition states probably is greater. From an Eyring-type of equation the activation entropy is found to be $\Delta S^* = 9.4 \pm 1.6$ cal/mole K, whereas for poly(cyclohexyl methacrylate) $\Delta S^* = 2.8 \pm 0.4$ cal/mole K).[26]

It is immediately clear that the glass transition of the rubber phase in ABS shows a behavior completely different from that of the secondary transitions in the amorphous polymers: the curve is much less steep. The slopes of the curves for the γ maxima of POM and HDPE are also much smaller; in their frequency dependence they behave like glass transitions.

When we assume, in a first approximation, that in Equation 1 $\log \nu_0 = 13$, we can estimate the activation energy E_a (in kcal/mole) from the maximum T_m at 1 Hz by the simple equation

$$E_a = 0.060\, T_m \qquad (1\ \text{Hz}). \tag{2}$$

For other frequencies we get

$$E_a = (0.060 - 0.0046 \log \nu)\, T_m(\nu),$$

where $T_m(\nu)$ is the absolute temperature of the maximum for a frequency ν.

The validity of this estimation has been investigated for a series of maxima measured at our laboratory. The result is illustrated in FIGURE 7. A distinction has been made between main-chain motions, side-chain motions and motions within dissolved molecules. Some literature data have been included, but only in so far as they refer to determinations of E_a from data over a frequency range of at least three decades.

Obviously the glass transition of the rubber phase in ABS and the γ maxima of PE and POM exhibit a behaviour completely different from that of the side chain maxima as well as from the local main-chain maxima. Nearly all side-chain motions and motions within dissolved molecules obey Equation 2 to within 10% whereas local main-chain motions of amorphous polymers obey the equation to within 20%.

Data obtained by Eisenberg *et al.*[22] on poly(phenylene ethers) deviate by more than 20% only for the motion of the longest alkyl side group. Roe and Simha[34] take log ν_0 = 14 and then obtain a somewhat better correlation of the experimental and calculated activation energies than with our log ν_o = 13. Indeed, when there is a considerable activation entropy, the Roe and Simha's formula is a better

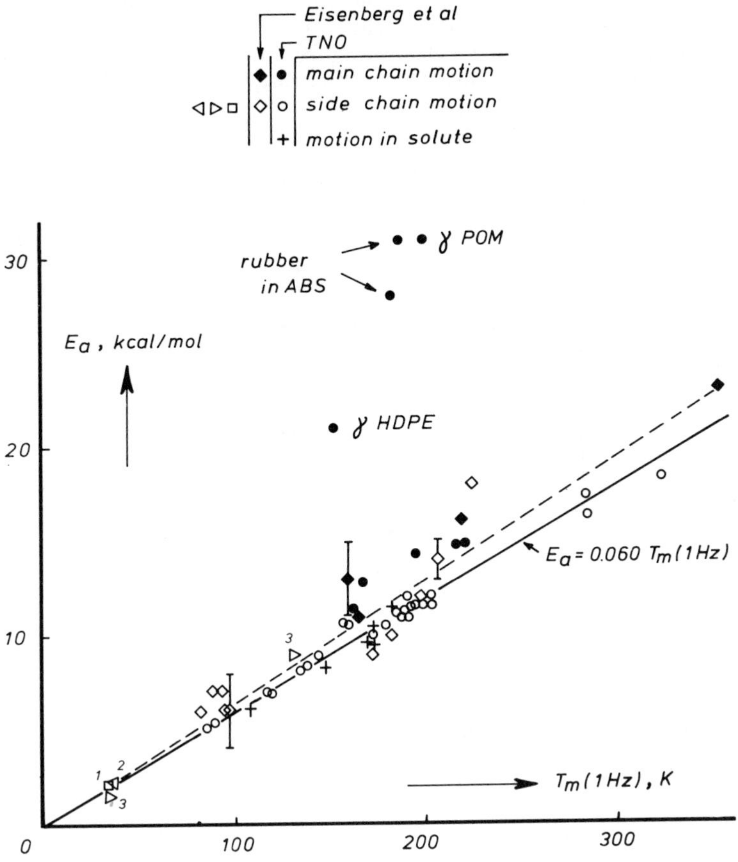

FIGURE 7. Activation energy E_a as a function of the temperature T_m of the mechanical loss maximum at 1 Hz. Filled symbols: main-chain motions; open symbols: side-group motions; crosses: motions within molecules dissolved in the polymer matrix; squares: Eisenberg *et al.*,[23] (1) PEtMA–Wada *et al.*,[31] (2) PS–Sauer and Saba,[32] and (3) PS–Yano and Wada[33]; dotted line: Roe and Simha.[34]

approximation than Equation 2. However, since Equation 2 applies very well to most side-group motions, we prefer to use this equation, keeping in mind that an appreciable entropy contribution will give rise to a deviation. This equation probably gives a more accurate value of E_a than does a determination from measurements over a narrow frequency range (say 1 decade).

Intermolecular vs Intramolecular Interaction

Johari and Goldstein[35–40] emphasized that the presence of secondary relaxations in the glassy state does not require specific *intra*molecular mechanisms for their existence. They state that *inter*molecular interactions are clearly sufficient to provide the barrier for β relaxations as well.

We do not deny that intermolecular interaction alone can produce the barrier for a secondary loss peak; the mechanical relaxation caused by the motion of a dissolved molecule as a whole is a clear example of the operation of intermolecular interactions only. Brot[41] explains why in this case a temperature dependent activation energy should be expected: the potential barrier is of repulsive origin, and so it should decrease with increasing temperature as a consequence of the thermal expansion.

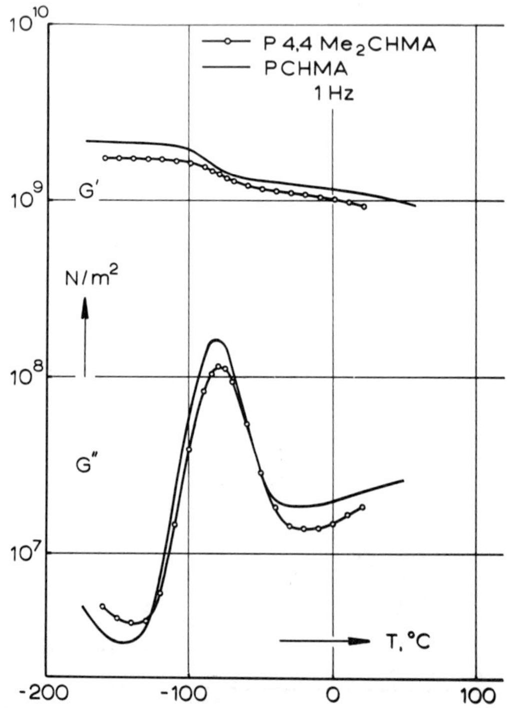

FIGURE 8. Shear storage modulus G′ and shear loss modulus G″ at 1 Hz for poly(cyclohexyl methacrylate) and for poly(4,4-dimethylcyclohexyl methacrylate).

When intermolecular interaction is important, a strong effect on the loss peaks of the remaining free volume, that is of quenching and annealing, is to be expected. On this basis Boyer[4,42] arrives at an intermolecular contribution to the mechanism of the polystyrene loss peaks. On the other hand, Struik[1] did not observe any effect of annealing on a series of secondary loss peaks of other polymers. To these loss peaks intermolecular mechanisms do not significantly contribute.

Strong arguments for such intermolecular contributions are available for the γ maxima of 2-methyl-6-alkyl-substituted poly(phenylene ethers)[23] and for poly(2-hydroxyethyl methacrylate).[24] For the former the temperature of the loss peak increases by elongation of the alkyl side chain, for the latter this temperature decreases by copolymerization with MMA.

Enlargement of the moving group provides an insight into the importance of intermolecular contributions to the energy barrier. A larger group is generally thought to need a higher activation energy.[42] This holds for the alkyl group in the above-mentioned poly(phenylene ethers). However, for the β maximum of PMMA,[12] as well as for the cyclohexyl maximum[26,29] this idea proved to be incorrect. The β maximum of poly(*tert*-butyl methacrylate) lies at the same temperature as that of PMMA, only it is lower. Introduction of one or two methyl groups in the 4-position of the ring does not shift the cyclohexyl maximum to a higher temperature either. This is illustrated for the dimethyl derivative in FIGURE 8. The small decrease of the height of the maximum can be nearly completely explained by the decrease in cyclohexyl concentration.

Enlargement of the side groups therefore has a different effect on these secondary transitions than on the glass transition.

Another way of studying the intra vs inter-molecular barrier is to add plasticizers. With dibutyl phthalate the secondary maximum of PMMA remains at the same temperature,[12] as does the cyclohexyl maximum.[26,29] Though plasticizers decrease the glass transition temperature, the temperature of the secondary loss peak remains constant.

Conclusions

The behavior of secondary maxima in glassy amorphous polymers is different from that of glass transitions:

(a) They obey an Arrhenius relationship over a broad frequency range.

(b) For other than local main-chain motions the activation energy E_a of the molecular processes underlying the loss maximum, can be calculated from $E_a = 0.060\ T_m$ (1 Hz) with an accuracy of 10%. For local main-chain motions, E_a usually is slightly higher, say 20%.

(c) For many secondary maxima the origin of E_a is mainly *intra*molecular.

(d) By plasticization the temperature of a secondary maximum is shifted much less than that of a glass transition.

References

1. STRUIK, L. C. E. 1976. Physical aging in the glassy state. Ann. N.Y. Acad. Sci. This volume.
2. MCCRUM, N. G., B. E. READ & G. WILLIAMS. 1967. Anelastic and Dielectric Effects in Polymeric Solids. John Wiley & Sons. London.
3. For PET: SACHER, E. 1971. J. Macromol. Sci. Phys. **B5:** 739.
4. BOYER, R. F. 1975. J. Polymer Sci. Polym. Symp. **50:** 109.
5. BUSSINK, J. & J. HEIJBOER. 1965. *In* Proc. Int. Conf. Physics Non-Crystalline Solids, W. Prins, Ed.: 388. North Holland Publishing Co. Amsterdam.
6. PETRI, S. E. B., R. S. MOORE & J. R. FLICK. 1972. J. Appl. Phys. **43:** 4318.
7. WYZGOSKI, M. G. & G. S-Y. YEH. 1973. Polymer J. **4:** 29.
8. IKEDA, S., N. KINJO, T. KOMATSU & T. NAKAGAWA. 1974. Rep. Progr. Polymer Phys. Japan **17:** 335.

9. Pezzin, G., G. Ajroldi & C. Garbuglio. 1967. J. Appl. Polymer Sci. **11:** 2553.
10. Heijboer, J. 1965. *In* Proc. Int. Conf. Physics Non-Crystalline Solids. W. Prins, Ed.:231. North Holland Publishing Co. Amsterdam.
11. Havriliak, S. & N. Roman. 1966. Polymer **7:** 387.
12. Heijboer, J. 1975. Secondary loss peaks in glassy amorphous polymers. Midland Macromolecular Meeting. To appear in Intern. J. Polymeric Mater.
13. Haldon, R. A. & R. Simha. 1968. J. Appl. Phys. **39:** 1890.
14. Kakizaki, M., K. Aoyama & T. Hideshima. 1974. Rep. Progr. Polymer Phys. Japan **17:** 379.
15. Kawamura, Y., S. Nagai, J. Hirose & Y. Wada. 1969. J. Polymer Sci. **A-2 7:** 1559.
16. Hoff, E. A. W., D. W. Robinson & A. H. Willbourn. 1955. J. Polymer Sci. **18:** 161.
17. Janacek, J. 1973. J. Macromol. Sci-Rev. C **9:** 1.
18. Kolarik, J. 1972. Intern. J. Polymeric Mater. **1:** 125.
19. Waterman, H. A., L. C. E. Struik, J. Heijboer & M. P. van Duijkeren. 1970. *In* Amorphous Materials, Int. Conf. Phys. Non-Crystalline Solids, R. W. Douglas and B. Ellis, Eds.:29. Wiley. New York, N.Y.
20. Frosini, V., P. Magagnini, E. Butta & M. Baccaredda. 1966. Kolloid-Z. **213:** 115.
21. Heijboer, J. 1968. J. Polymer Sci. **C 16:** 3413.
22. Baccaredda, M., E. Butta, V. Frosini & S. de Petris. 1968–69. Mater. Sci. Eng. **3:** 157.
23. Cayrol, B., A. Eisenberg, J. F. Harrod & P. Rocanieri. 1972. Macromolecules **5:** 676.
24. Kolarik, J. 1971. J. Macromol. Sci-Phys. B **5:** 355.
25. Janacek, J. 1974. Poly. Lett. **12:** 569.
26. Heijboer, J. 1972. Doctoral Thesis, Leiden, C. L.-Communication:435.
27. Davies, M. & J. Swain. 1968. Chem. Phys. Lett. **2:** 42.
28. Heijboer, J. 1960. Kolloid-Z. **171:**7.
29. Heijboer, J. 1975. Molecular origin of the cyclohexyl loss peak. Midland Macromolecular Meeting. To appear in Intern. J. Polymeric Mater.
30. Struik, L. C. E. & H. A. Waterman, Personal communication.
31. Shimizu, K., O. Yano, Y. Wada & Y. Kawamura. 1973. J. Polymer Sci.-Phys. **11:** 1641.
32. Sauer, J. A. & R. G. Saba. 1969. J. Macromol. Sci.-Chem. A **3:** 1217.
33. Yano, O. & Y. Wada. 1971. J. Polymer Sci. **A2 9:** 669.
34. Roe, J. M. & R. Simha. 1974. Intern. J. Polym. Mater. **3:** 193.
35. Goldstein, M. 1969. J. Chem. Phys. **51:** 3728.
36. Johari, G. P. & M. Goldstein. 1970. J. Phys. Chem. **74:** 2034.
37. Johari, G. P. & M. Goldstein. 1970. J. Chem. Phys. **53:** 2372.
38. Johari, G. P. & M. Goldstein. 1971. J. Chem. Phys. **55:** 4245.
39. Goldstein, M. 1972. *In* Amorphous Materials R. W. Douglas & B. Ellis, Ed.:23. Wiley. New York, N.Y.
40. Johari, G. P. 1973. J. Chem. Phys. **58:** 1766.
41. Brot, C. 1969. Disc. Faraday Soc. **48:** 213.
42. Boyer, R. F. 1974. J. Macromol. Sci.-Phys. B **9:** 187.

GLASS TRANSITION AND SECONDARY RELAXATIONS IN MOLECULAR LIQUIDS AND CRYSTALS

G. P. Johari

Glaciology Division
Department of the Environment
Ottawa, K1A OE7 Canada

Introduction

It has been known for many years that substances in the glassy state retain some degree of molecular mobility that is detectable by a dielectric or a mechanical relaxation, or by an NMR experiment. These relaxations have been termed secondary or β relaxations and they occur on a time scale many times shorter than that of the main relaxation responsible for the glass transition itself.[1] The presence of such relaxations has generally been associated with the motion of a side group attached to a polymer chain, or with a certain type of movement of the chain itself, and has been explained in terms of hindered internal molecular modes of motion that remain active even when the molecule as a whole is frozen in place in a glassy matrix.[1]

Several years ago we studied a number of glasses made from molecular liquids[2] lacking either a side chain or any other internal degree of freedom capable of giving rise to a relaxation traditionally invoked for polymers and network glasses. The study revealed a remarkable similarity in the dielectric relaxations of these glasses to those of polymers, and a surprisingly uniform pattern of behavior. The main conclusion drawn from the study was that the molecular mobility seen as β relaxations is intrinsic to the nature of the glassy state. It became apparent then that a theory for the structure of grossly disordered solids must necessarily consider such relaxations as arising from a motion over the potential energy barriers similar in origin to those involved in the glass transition itself.

There is, however, another approach to the study of grossly disordered solids, such as glasses. One may start from a perfect crystal, relatively well understood both theoretically and experimentally because the translational symmetry allows enormous simplification of the algebra, and approach the glassy state gradually. An orientationally disordered or plastic crystal is intermediate between a perfect crystal and a glass in that, although there is a long-range order of molecular positions, there is no long-range order in the molecular orientations.

This paper presents a brief review of the progress made in the study of relaxations of molecular liquids near and below the glass transition temperature in the context of present theories of glass structure, as well as some new results on the relaxation of rigid molecular liquids and plastic crystalline solids, and the implication these results have for the concepts of the glass transition phenomenon.

Relaxations in Molecular Glasses

General Features

The molecular liquids showed two maxima[2] when the dielectric loss factor tan δ or the dielectric loss ϵ'' was plotted against temperature at a constant fre-

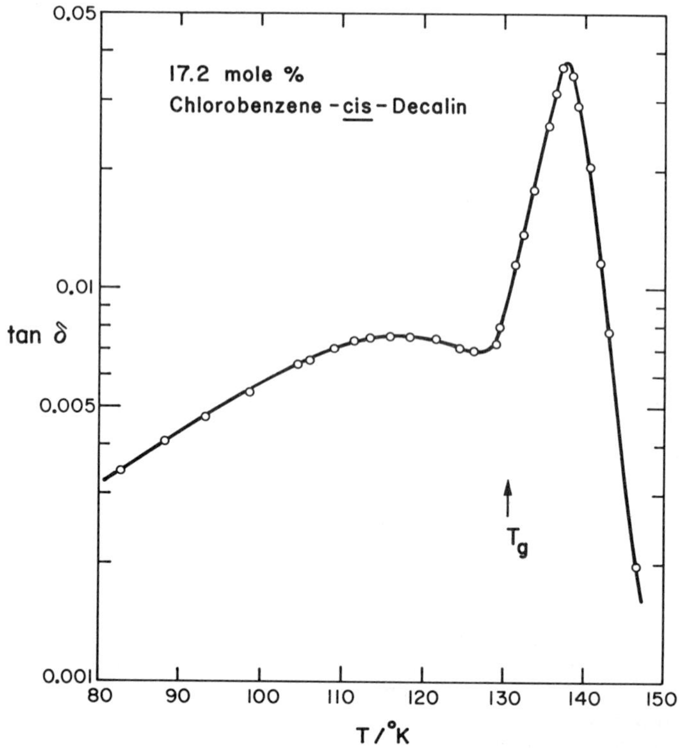

FIGURE 1. The dielectric loss factor, tan δ, of 17.2 mole% chlorobenzene/*cis*-decalin mixture at 1 kHz plotted against temperature, showing the temperature of the α and β relaxation peaks.

quency. One maximum occurred at a temperature above the glass transition and the other, which was 1–2 orders of magnitude lower, occurred at several tens of degrees below the glass transition temperature T_g. A typical plot showing the two maxima is given in FIGURE 1, where tan δ of 17.2 mole% solution of chlorobenzene in *cis*-decalin is plotted logarithmically against temperature at 1 kHz. Dilute solutions of halogen-substituted benzenes and naphthalenes in nonpolar solvent, *cis*-decalin,[2] approximately 40 mole% mixtures of toluene, substituted benzenes and naphthalenes in pyridine[2] and in tetrahydrofuran, pure liquids, e.g., *iso*-propylbenzene,[2] *o*-terphenyl,[2] methyl-substituted heptanols,[3] dialkyl phthalates,[3] insulating oils,[4] calcium nitrate tetrahydrate, and glucose–water mixtures of several compositions,[5] all showed similar peaks in tan δ–temperature plots.

The peak at temperatures below T_g could not be detected in a few substances, namely in a mixture of chloronaphthalene in tetrahydrofuran,[2] propylene carbonate,[2] *iso*-butanol,[3] 1,2-propanediol,[3] 45 mole% $Ca(NO_3)_2KNO_3$,[2] and in glycerol,[6] but the secondary relaxation could be clearly seen in a plot of tan δ against the logarithm of frequency at temperatures below T_g in the chloronaphthalene–tetrahydrofuran mixture.[2] The secondary relaxation could be clearly observed also in glycerol on the application of a few kilobars.[6] In other substances it can probably be either detected at high pressures or resolved (although less convincingly) by a suitable analytical method as in ice.[7]

Without implying a similarity in their molecular mechanisms to the loss peaks seen in amorphous polymers, the relaxation observed above T_g is referred to here as α relaxation and that observed immediately below T_g as β relaxation.

The spectral features of the two relaxations were quite apparent. In the majority of substances, the plots of ϵ'' against the logarithm of frequency for α relaxation were asymmetric and had a half-width of 2–3 decades of frequency, which is many times higher than 1.40 decades for a single relaxation time. The frequency of

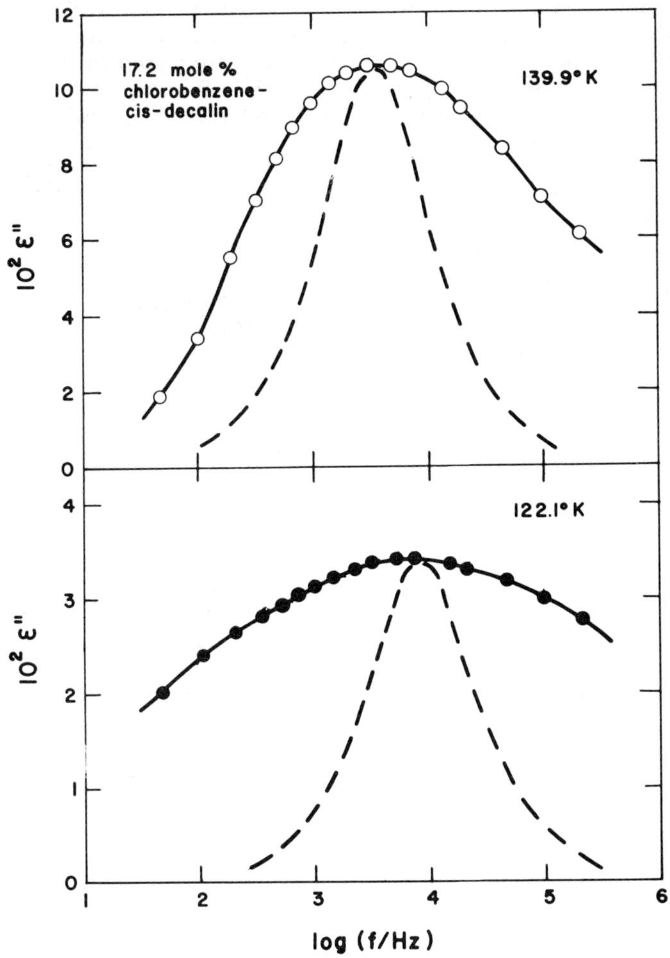

FIGURE 2. The dielectric loss ϵ'' of 17.2 mole % chlorobenzene/*cis*-decalin mixture plotted logarithmically against frequency at 139.9°K (○) and 122.1°K (●). The top curve is the α relaxation and the bottom curve the β relaxation region. The dashed curves are for a Debye-type single relaxation time.

maximum loss, f_m, was strongly dependent upon temperature and pressure and, when plotted logarithmically against the reciprocal temperature, showed, in most cases, a non-Arrhenius behavior with a formal "activation energy" increasing from 20 kcal mole^{-1} to 100 kcal mole^{-1} as the T_g was approached from higher temperatures. Plots of the logarithm of f_m, obtained from results in Reference 6 against pressure, also showed strong curvature indicating a several-fold increase in the volume of activation as the pressure of glass transition, P_g, was reached.

The plots of ϵ'' against $\log f$ for the β relaxation were also asymmetric and had a half-width of 4–6 decades of frequency. This is interpreted as indicating a broad distribution of relaxation times. The frequency of maximum loss, when plotted logarithmically against reciprocal temperature, showed an Arrhenius behavior with an "activation energy" between 5–10 kcal mole^{-1} for various substances. The f_m, when plotted logarithmically against pressure,[6] also showed a linear dependence with an activation volume of 4 ml mole^{-1} for glycerol at 202.9°K.

Typical plots for molecular glasses are shown in FIGURE 2, where ϵ'' is plotted against the logarithm of frequency at 139.9° and 122.1°K, showing the α and β

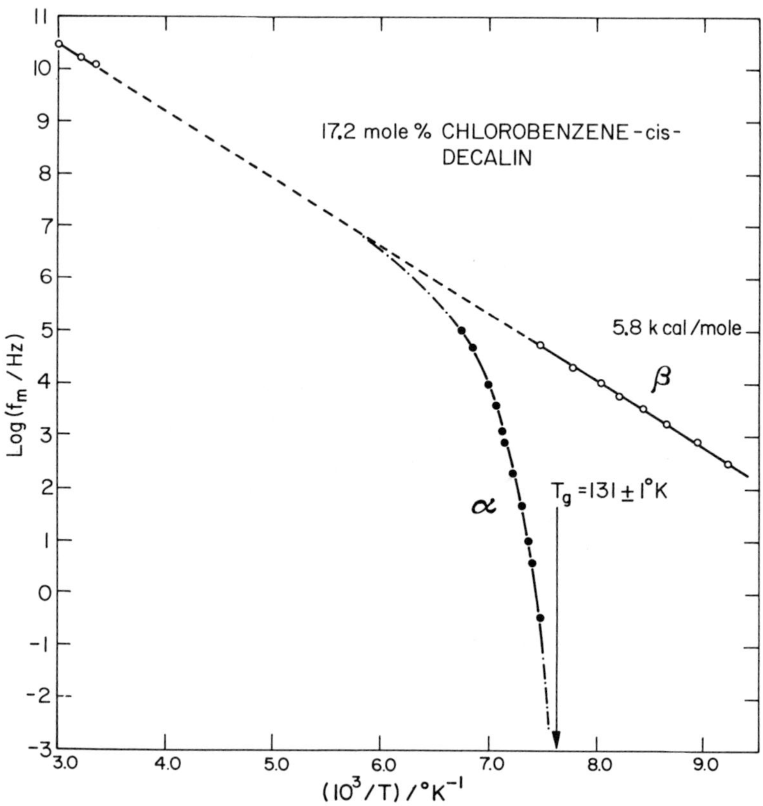

FIGURE 3. The frequency of maximum loss, f_m, plotted logarithmically against reciprocal temperature for 17.2 mole% chlorobenzene/*cis*-decalin in the liquid and the glassy states. The data points at frequencies above 10 GHz are from measurements at microwave frequencies.

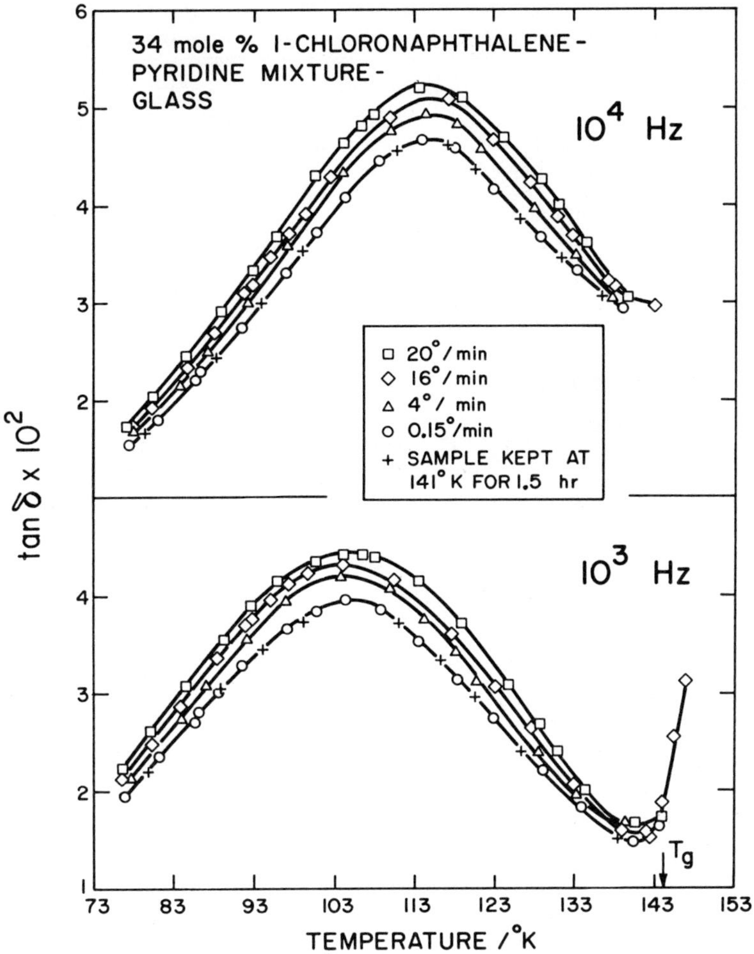

FIGURE 4. The dielectric loss factor tan δ of 34 mole% 1-chloronaphthalene-pyridine glass at 1.0 and 10.0 kHz plotted against temperature. The plots show the effect of the rate of cooling during vitrification of a substance on the strength of the β relaxation.

relaxation in 17.2 mole% chlorobenzene–*cis*-decalin solution. The plots of the logarithm of f_m against reciprocal temperature for the α and β relaxation are shown in FIGURE 3. The f_m for the α relaxation could be fitted to the Vogel–Tamman–Fulcher equation:

$$f_m = A \exp -\left(\frac{B}{T - T_0}\right) \tag{1}$$

where A, B, and T_0 are empirical constants. For 17.2 mole% chlorobenzene–*cis*-decalin solution, $A = 19.46\ \text{sec}^{-1}$, $B = 186.3°\text{K}$, and $T_0 = 125°\text{K}$. The f_m

TABLE 1

EQUILIBRIUM DIELECTRIC PERMITTIVITIES OF RIGID MOLECULES IN DECALIN SOLUTIONS*

Temperature °K	ϵ_0	ϵ''_m	$\epsilon_{\infty,1}$	ϵ_S	$\Delta\epsilon_\alpha$ $(\epsilon_0 - \epsilon_{\infty,1})$	$\Delta\epsilon_\beta$ $(\epsilon_{\infty,1} - \epsilon_S)$	$\mu(\Delta\epsilon_\alpha)$ D	$\mu(\Delta\epsilon + \Delta\epsilon_\beta)$ D	f_m kHz
12.1 mole% Chlorobenzene, T_g = 133°K, μ_{lit} = 1.51 D									
135.9	2.970	0.071	2.54	2.347	0.430	0.193	1.20	1.48	0.08
138.9	2.965	0.072	2.56	2.345	0.405	0.215	1.17	1.49	0.70
139.9	2.958	0.074	2.57	2.344	0.385	0.226	1.15	1.48	2.0
143.0	2.950	0.074	2.59	2.342_5	0.360	0.250	1.12	1.50	15.0
143.3	2.938	0.078	2.61	2.342	0.328	0.270	1.07	1.49	20.0
11.1 mole% Bromobenzene, T_g = 134°K, μ_{lit} = 1.50 D									
144.4	2.840	0.076	2.53_5	2.341	0.305	0.194	1.14	1.49	70.0
18.0 mole% Toluene, T_g = 128°K, μ_{lit} = 0.43 D									
135.1	2.414	0.005	2.385	2.347_5	0.029	0.037	0.27	0.41	30.0
7.9 mole% Tetrahydrofuran, T_g = 130°K, μ_{lit} = 1.69 D									
135.6	2.806	0.017	2.690	2.347	0.116	0.343	0.78	1.62	0.70
2.6 mole% Fluoronaphthalene, T_g = 139°K, μ_{lit} = 1.42 D									
146.0	2.439	0.006	2.395	2.340	0.0440	0.055	0.93	1.40	0.30
10.8 mole% 1-Chloronaphthalene, T_g = 140°K, μ_{lit} = 1.58 D									
145.1	2.872	0.067	2.450	2.341	0.422	0.109	1.39	1.58	0.05
7.4 mole% 1-Bromonaphthalene, T_g = 142°K, μ_{lit} = 1.59 D									
153.5	2.688	0.058	2.460	2.336	0.228	0.124	1.26	1.58	50.0
12.3 mole% 1-Methylnaphthalene, T_g = 148°K, μ_{lit} = 0.23 D									
159.6	2.445	0.014	2.374	2.338	0.071	0.036	0.19	0.23	20.0

*Equilibrium dielectric permittivity of the solution ϵ_0, and the solvent ϵ_S; the maximum loss ϵ''_{max}; the resolved contribution to permittivity, $\Delta\epsilon_\alpha$ and $\Delta\epsilon_\beta$ due to orientation polarization relaxing as the α and β processes, respectively; the frequency f_m corresponding to ϵ''_m; the extrapolated high frequency permittivity $\epsilon_{\infty,1}$; and the dipole moment, $\mu(\Delta\epsilon_\alpha)$, calculated for the α process and μ, that for the total polarization for rigid molecules in decalin solutions at several temperatures.

for the β relaxation could be fitted to the equation, $f_m = f_0 \exp(-E/RT)$, with $A = 1.398 \times 10^{14}\ \text{sec}^{-1}$ and $E = 5.8\ \text{kcal mole}^{-1}$.

The height of the β relaxation peak decreased, on annealing, with the molar volume of the glass under isothermal conditions.[2] This is evident in FIGURE 4 where the family of curves show the tan δ as a function of temperature at 1 and 10 kHz, measured after cooling a 34 mole% 1-chloronaphthalene-pyridine glass through the calorimetric T_g of 144 ± 1°K at rates 20°, 16°, 4°, and 0.15° min^{-1} The location of the β peak is independent of the cooling rates.

An additional important fact that emerged from this study is that the *secondary relaxations are a property of the equilibrium liquid state* above T_g. They have been observed in a number of liquid alcohols.[8-10] Several rigid molecular glasses[2] and a number of amorphous polymers[1] show at least the beginning of a secondary relaxation above their calorimetric T_g. From a calculation of the dipole moment μ using the equilibrium and the limiting high-frequency permittivity obtained from the complex plane plots of ϵ' and ϵ'', it was concluded that nearly 30%–40% of the total polarization in dilute solutions of rigid molecules in decalin[11] and nearly

10%–50% in dilute solutions in *o*-terphenyl[12] is due to the β process. Some of the data for dilute solutions in *cis*-decalin are given in TABLE 1, where the contribution to permittivity due to the α and β relaxations has been resolved and the dipole moment, calculated from the α relaxation, is given. The clear evidence for the occurrence of the α and β relaxation peaks above T_g is seen in FIGURE 5 where the dielectric loss of chlorobenzene–decalin and toluene–pyridine mixture[13] is plotted against frequency from 0.1–2 $\times$ 10^5 Hz. The α and β peaks are separated by about 4.5 orders of magnitude of frequency at a temperature several degrees above the calorimetric T_g.

An analysis of ϵ'' of decalin solutions[11] at temperatures above T_g shows that the distribution of relaxation times, when compared at constant f_m, slightly increased with the concentration of the rigid molecular solute. The effect is similar to that found in the dilute solutions of several polymers in nonpolar solvents[14] at frequencies above 10^7 Hz.

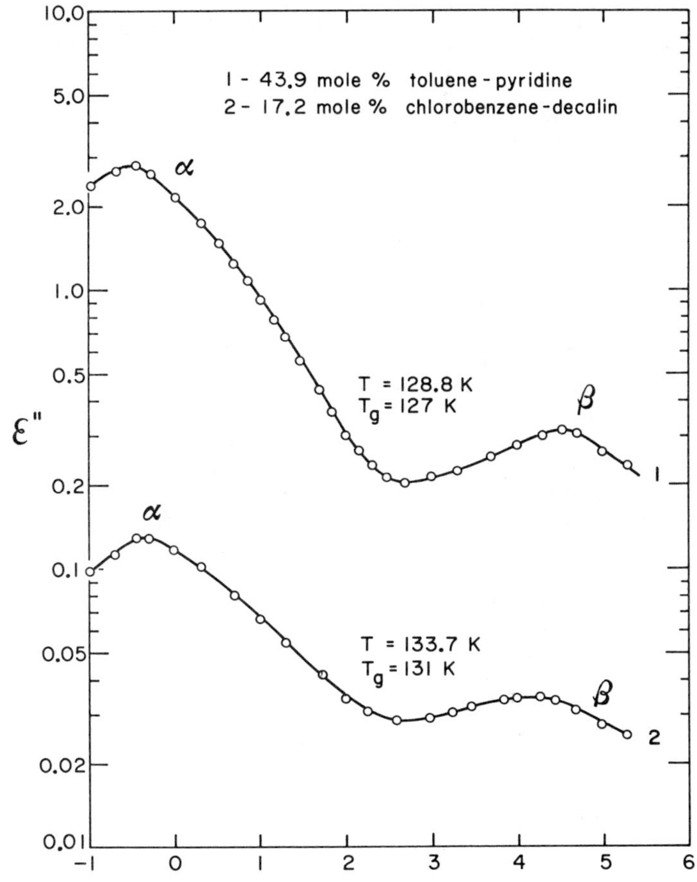

FIGURE 5. The dielectric loss, ϵ'', of two glass-forming liquids plotted against frequency on a logarithmic scale at a temperature several degrees above T_g.

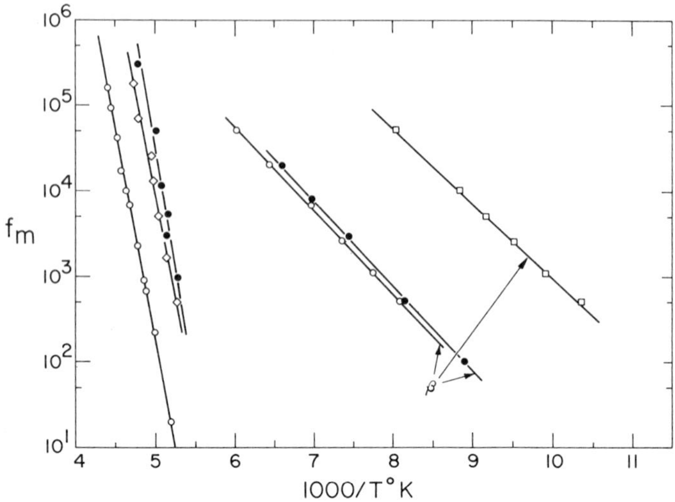

FIGURE 6. The frequency of maximum loss, f_m, of several alcohols plotted logarithmically against reciprocal temperature in the liquid and the glassy states. ○, 5-Methyl-3-heptanol; ◇, 4-methyl-3-heptanol; ●, 3-methyl-3-heptanol.

Unusual Features of the α Relaxations

The α relaxation in a number of alcohols showed several unusual features. The dielectric loss-frequency plots were symmetrical with a half-width of 1.40 decades of frequency, indicating a single relaxation time in the entire temperature range, an Arrhenius temperature dependence of the frequency of maximum loss and a low activation energy—in the range 8–16 kcal $mole^{-1}$ for different substances.[3,8-10,15] This is shown in FIGURE 6 where f_m of several alcohols is plotted logarithmically against reciprocal temperature. Contrary to the commonly held view, no definite correlation was found to exist between the characteristics of the α relaxation and the temperature dependence of the relaxation rate. These features are summarized in TABLE 2 where the calorimetric T_g and the dielectric $T_g(D)$, obtained from a linear extrapolation of Arrhenius plots to an f_m of 10^{-3} Hz, is also given. The last three entries are for the disordered crystalline phases, to be discussed in the next section. In a few cases $T_g(D)$ is about 10°–15° lower than T_g but for most cases they are nearly equal. The discrepancy between $T_g(D)$ and T_g can be qualitatively accounted for by the breakdown of the Arrhenius relation in the usual sense as T approaches T_g.

A tendency for supercooled liquids to return to an Arrhenius behavior at a temperature somewhere near T_g has, in fact, been reported in non-hydrogen bonded substances,[16-20] although the reasons may be more complex than have been predicted by the theories. If such a behavior is general, then the temperature at which the return of the Arrhenius behavior occurs is much higher for several alcohols than for other liquids.

It appears that the only relaxation process that has universal features is the secondary or β process, which, without an exception, has a broad distribution of relaxation times that increases with decreasing temperature, and has an Arrhenius temperature dependence of f_m with an "activation energy" ranging from 5–10 kcal $mole^{-1}$ for a variety of different types of glasses.

Relaxations in Orientationally Disordered Crystals

Thermodynamic Aspects

Although the glass transition is believed to occur in the supercooled liquid state, evidence has accumulated in recent years to indicate that some crystalline solids, in which the molecules possess a certain degree of rotational freedom, also show a behavior that is phenomenologically similar to the glass transition. These crystals show a decrease in the heat capacity in the supercooled metastable state at a certain temperature below the temperature of their transformation to a non-rotor phase, and have a definite residual entropy. According to Timmerman's classification, these solids are generally known as plastic crystals.

Plastic crystals are disordered with respect to the orientation of molecules but have a translational symmetry—and therefore are ordered—with respect to the center of gravity of the molecule. Such crystals have interesting characteristics; they are generally isotropic, have a cubic or hexagonal structure with lattice dimensions of 6–10 Å, have low entropy (1–5 cal $°K^{-1}$ $mole^{-1}$) and volume of fusion and a large diffusion coefficient near the melting point. A review of their physical properties is given elsewhere.[21] These crystalline solids undergo a transformation to different phases with ordered molecular orientations, analogous with the freezing of a liquid into an ordered crystal.

The glass-like transition in orientationally disordered solids can be conveniently illustrated by the thermodynamic behavior of cyclohexanol, the heat capac-

Table 2

Calorimetric and Dielectric Glass Transition Temperatures and the α Relaxation of Several Aliphatic Alcohols

Substance	Calorimetric T_g(°K)	Dielectric $T_g(D)$(°K)	Relaxation Characteristics	Reference
2-methyl-1-heptanol	144	135	Single-Arrhenius	15
4-methyl-1-heptanol	138	126	Single-Arrhenius	15
6-methyl-1-heptanol	140	125	Single-Arrhenius	15
2-methyl-3-heptanol	158	156	Spectrum-Arrhenius	8,9
3-methyl-3-heptanol	151	151	Spectrum-Arrhenius	8
4-methyl-3-heptanol	160	156	Spectrum-Arrhenius	8
5-methyl-3-heptanol	159	160	Single-Arrhenius	8,9
6-methyl-3-heptanol	159	162	Single-Arrhenius	8,9
1-phenyl-1-propanol	193.6	—	Single-non-Arrhenius	*
n-butanol	114	—	Single-non-Arrhenius	10
iso-butanol	116	—	Single-non-Arrhenius	10
1,2-propanediol	169	—	Spectrum-non-Arrhenius	3
neopentanol crystal	133	134	Single-Arrhenius	This work
neohexanol crystal	163	163	Single-Arrhenius	This work
cyclohexanol crystal	148	—	Single-non-Arrhenius	39

*Unpublished data of Johari and Dannhauser.

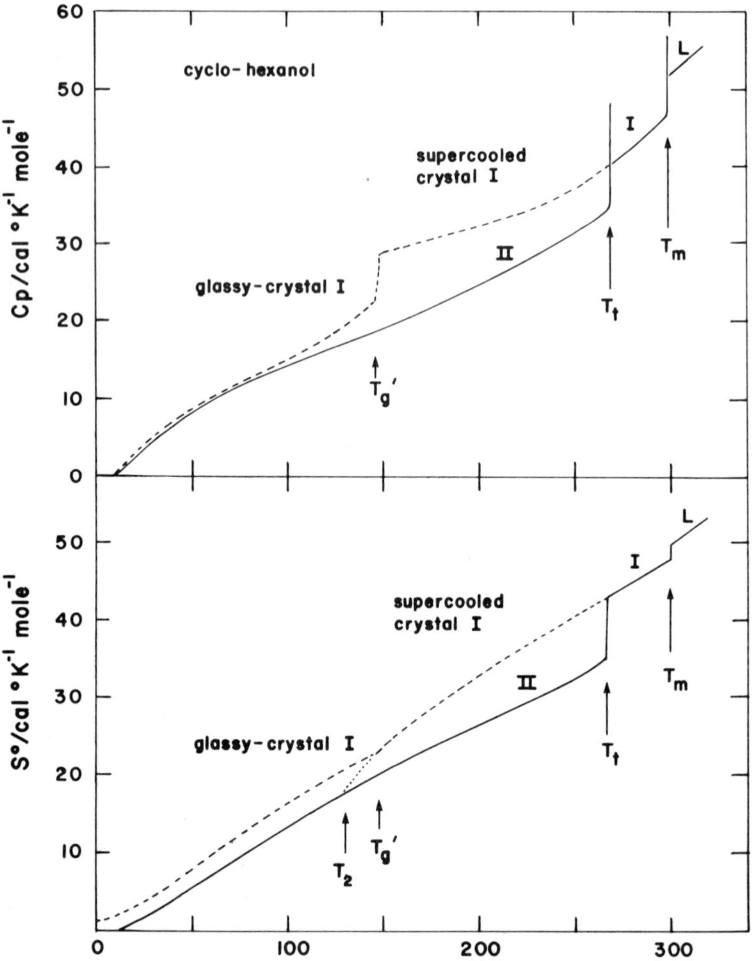

FIGURE 7. The heat capacity C_p and the entropy $S°$ of cyclohexanol in its liquid, supercooled solid and stable solid phases plotted against temperature. The entropy curves show the temperature T_2 at which the configurational entropy is anticipated to become zero.

ity of which has been studied in some detail by Kelly,[22] Otsubo and Sugawara,[23] and Adachi, *et al.*[24] The heat capacity C_p and the entropy $S°$ in the liquid, in both the stable and metastable supercooled states of the orientationally disordered phase and in the nonrotor phase, are plotted against temperature in FIGURE 7 from 10°K to 320°K. The C_p data are from the literature and $S°$ was calculated from the C_p data, or was taken from the data of Adachi *et al.*[24] Cyclohexanol freezes to an orientationally disordered, face-centered cubic solid,[25] crystal I, at 299.1°K. The crystal I has an equilibrium dielectric permittivity of 15, and a relaxation time of 10 nsec[26] at 295°K and, when cooled, undergoes a phase transformation at 265.5°K to an orientationally ordered or nonrotor solid, crystal II, whose equilibrium dielectric permittivity is about 3 or lower. The crystal I can be supercooled to a fairly low temperature and shows a decrease in C_p by about 6 cal °K^{-1} mole^{-1} at 148°K. At lower temperatures the C_p decreases monotonically and tends to approach the value for crystal II at 0°K. Measurements of enthalpy at several annealing temperatures have revealed that the temperature at which the decrease in C_p occurs depends upon the rate of both cooling and heating, and on the annealing time. The degree of freedom that ceases to contribute to C_p at 148°K is recognized to be the orientational mobility of the cyclohexanol molecule and this temperature, by analogy with that in liquids, has been termed the glass transition temperature.[27] It is perhaps more appropriate to use the term glass-like transition temperature T_g' in order to avoid a possible confusion with the commonly known liquid–glass transition. The temperature T_t at which the plastic crystalline cyclohexanol undergoes the phase transformation to a fully ordered nonrotor phase is analogous with the freezing point T_m of a liquid. At temperatures below T_g' the orientational disorder in crystal I is frozen-in and cyclohexanol retains a configurational entropy of 1.18 cal °K^{-1} mole^{-1} at 0°K.

The entropy of supercooled crystal I, plotted against temperature in FIGURE 7, shows the temperature T_2 where, according to the Adam and Gibbs theory,[28] the configurational entropy would become zero if crystal I were allowed to come to an internal thermodynamic equilibrium.

The heat capacity of a number of plastic crystals has been accurately measured at temperatures from about 15°K to about 300°K by Seki *et al.*, and a recent review by Suga and Seki[27] on the subject of glass transition in crystalline solids gives a list of substances they have studied during the last decade. Using the heat capacity data, they have been able to demonstrate that the temperature dependence of the entropy of an orientationally disordered crystal in the supercooled state

TABLE 3

HEAT PROPERTIES OF SEVERAL ORIENTATIONALLY DISORDERED CRYSTALS*

Substance	T_g' (°K)	T_t (°K)	T_g'/T_t	T_2 (°K)	T_g'/T_2	ΔC_p (cal mol^{-1} °K^{-1})	S_0 (cal mol^{-1} °K^{-1})	Reference
2,3-dimethylbutane	76	136	0.56	65	1.17	12.1	1.76	30
cis-1,2-dimethylcyclohexane	94	173	0.54	82	1.15	12.9	2.05	31
cyclohexene	81	140	0.58	—	—	—	—	27,32
cycloheptene	100	153	0.65	—	—	—	—	32
cycloheptane	84	135	0.62	—	—	—	—	32
cycloheptatriene	106	153	0.69	—	—	—	—	32
cyclopentanol	138	201	0.69	—	—	—	—	32
cyclohexanol	148	265	0.56	128	1.18	5.7	1.12	24
cycloheptanol	140	280.3	0.50	—	—	7.1	1.2	33
neopentanol	133	234.2	0.57	—	—	—	—	This work
neohexanol	163	183	0.89	—	—	—	—	This work
H_2O ice Ih	100	—	—	—	—	0.12	0.81	34
D_2O ice Ih	128	—	—	—	—	0.12	0.81	35
$SnCl_2 \cdot 2H_2O$	150	—	—	—	—	—	0.15	36
$SnCl_2 \cdot 2D_2O$	155	—	—	—	—	—	0.15	36

*The glass-like transition temperature, T_g'; the transformation temperature T_t from disordered to an ordered phase; the temperature T_2 at which the configurational entropy would become zero; the change in the heat capacity at T_g'; and the residual entropy.

presents a situation identical to the one known as Kauzmann's paradox[29] in the glassy state. They have also derived the Adam–Gibbs temperature T_2 at which the configurational entropy of an orientationally disordered crystal would become zero if the state of crystal were not to fall out of thermodynamic equilibrium.

The glass-like transition temperature T_g' of several substances is listed in TABLE 3. All values of T_g' were obtained either from measurement of the heat capacity or from the discontinuity observed in a differential thermal analysis during the warming of the disorder-frozen-in solid. Measurements of volume, isobaric expansivity, and isothermal compressibility near T_g' have not been made for these crystals. It would be interesting to see if a dilatomatric characterization of T_g' is possible in these solids. The derived Adam–Gibbs temperature T_2 the heat capacity change at T_g', ΔC_p, and the residual entropy S_0 of crystals for which the C_p data are available are also given in TABLE 3 where the source of data is indicated.

In Table 3 the ratio of T_g' to T_t ranges between 0.5–0.9. The values are comparable to the ratio of T_g to T_m, which is 0.7–0.8 for most liquid–glass transitions. The ratio (T_g'/T_2) for orientationally disordered crystals is 1.17 ± 0.02, a value which is comparable with the corresponding average value of 1.30 for many substances, including amorphous polymers and molecular liquids, given by Adam and Gibbs.[28] These observations further suggest the similarity between the molecular mechanisms responsible for a glass-like transition in orientationally disordered solids and the glass transition in liquids.

It is noteworthy that the glass-like transition in some orientationally disordered crystals occurs at nearly the same temperature as the glass transition in the liquid phase of the same substance. For example, water is thought to have a T_g of about 135°K, comparable to T_g of ice of about 100°K; the glass transition in liquid cyclohexene and the glass-like transition in its orientationally disordered crystal I both occur at 81°K[27]; and both the glass transition in liquid ethanol and the glass-like transition in its crystal II occur at about 97°K.[27]

Kinetic Aspects

The dielectric relaxation study of the orientationally disordered (or plastic) crystals in the supercooled metastable state near T_g' revealed features similar to those in molecular liquids and some aliphatic alcohols, despite the large difference in the molecular shape, size, charge distribution, and the degree of flexibility within the molecule. It is appropriate, therefore, to discuss the general features of relaxations in a typical substance, neohexanol, as an example. It should be mentioned that none of the disordered crystals studied here are molecularly rigid, but the movement of the dipolar —OH group in them, which largely contributes to the dielectric polarization, is greatly hindered by the steric effects of the alkyl groups attached to the neighboring carbon atom.

The dielectric loss factor of neohexanol at 1 kHz is plotted logarithmically against temperature in FIGURE 8. The plot shows two maxima, one at 143°K with a tan δ of 3.6×10^{-2} and the other at 198°K with a tan δ of 1.15. The tan δ for the main relaxation, seen above the T_g' of 163°K, is 32 times higher than that of the secondary relaxation seen below T_g'. There is clear evidence that the molecular mobility also exists in the orientational-disorder-frozen-in (or glassy) state of a crystal below T_g', but its magnitude, measured in terms of the dielectric loss, is much lower than that of the main relaxation, the cessation of which on the time scale of one's experiment, causes the glass-like transition.

Typical plots of ϵ'' against the logarithm of frequency for the main and secondary relaxations are shown in FIGURE 9. As evident, the loss curve for the main relaxation at 213.1°K is symmetric and has a half-width of 1.40 decades of frequency a feature characteristic of a single Debye-type relaxation. This has been confirmed by plotting ϵ' and ϵ'' in a complex plane.[37] The plots remain symmetric to the lowest temperature of our measurements, although the ϵ''_{max} increased with decreasing temperature. The loss curve for the secondary relaxation process, as seen in FIGURE 9, is asymmetric with a half-width of 3.5 decades of frequency at 147.1°K. The half-width increased to 5.5 decades at the lowest temperature of our

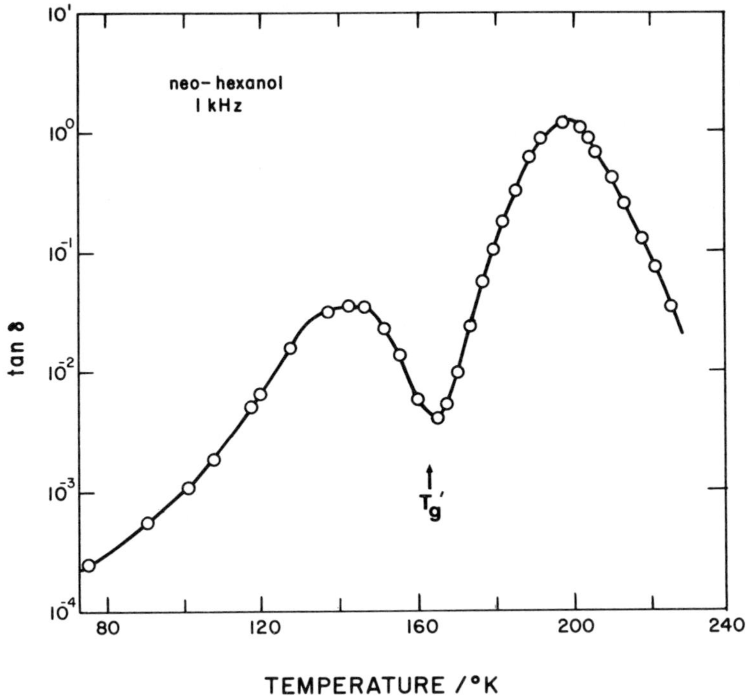

FIGURE 8. The dielectric loss factor, tan δ, of neohexanol at 1 kHz plotted logarithmically against temperature.

measurement. Clearly, the secondary relaxation has a distribution of relaxation times which increases with decreasing temperature. The ϵ''_{max} for the secondary relaxation decreased with temperature due partly to the spreading out of the relaxation and partly to a possible decrease in the magnitude of the fraction of the polarization that relaxes as the secondary process.

The relaxation rates are characterized in this paper by the frequency f_m of maximum loss rather than a cut-off frequency for asymmetric distribution of relaxation times.[38] The advantage of using f_m is that it does not presuppose any particular distribution of first order relaxation times. The values were obtained by interpolating from plots similar to those given in FIGURE 9. These values are

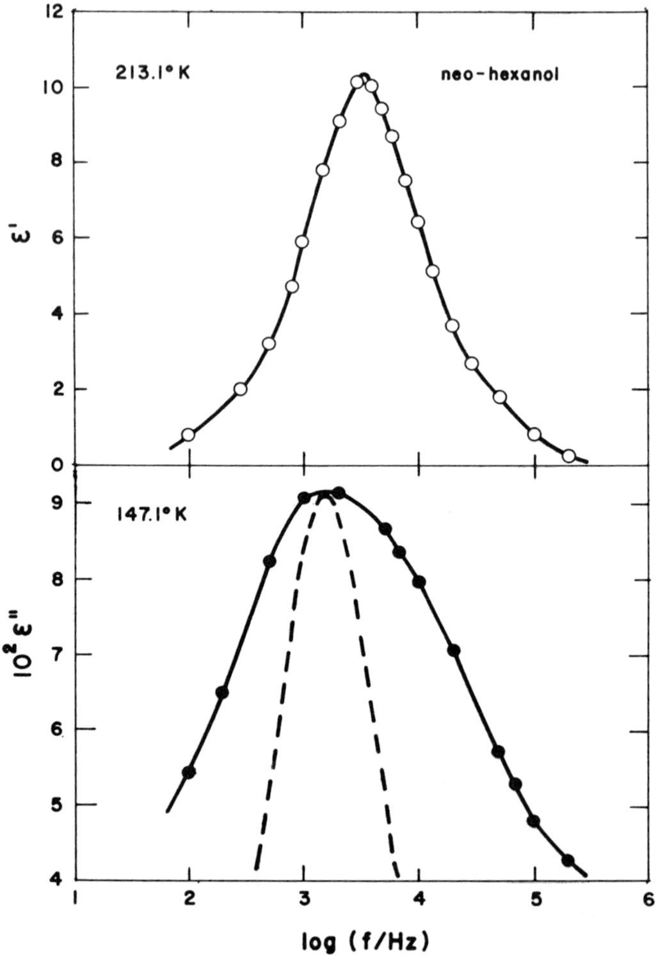

FIGURE 9. The dielectric loss ε'' of neohexanol plotted against the logarithm of frequency at 213.1° K (○) and 147.1°K (●). The glass-like transition temperature is 163°K. The dashed curve is for a Debye-type single relaxation time.

plotted logarithmically against the reciprocal temperature in FIGURE 10. As evident, the rate plots for both the main and secondary relaxation are linear and have an "activation energy" of 12.4 and 7.9 kcal $mole^{-1}$, respectively. The preexponential factor f_0 of the Arrhenius equation, $f_m = f_0 \exp(-E/RT)$, is 1.48×10^{16} sec^{-1} and 1.66×10^{15} sec^{-1} for the main and secondary relaxation, respectively.

Adachi *et al.*[39] have found a non-Arrhenius dependence of the rate of main relaxation in cyclohexanol near T_g' and have fitted their data to Equation 1. Their log f_m reciprocal temperature plot for cyclohexanol curves very steeply in the range 10^0–10^{-2} sec^{-1} but is linear in the range 10^2–10^6 sec^{-1}. The "activation energy" for the secondary relaxation is 5.7 kcal $mole^{-1}$ in cyclohexanol and 3.4 kcal $mole^{-1}$ in 2,3-dimethyl butane.[39] The main relaxation in 2,3-dimethyl butane above T_g' could not be studied because of phase transformation to a fully ordered state that occurred in the temperature range 85°–136°K.

The extrapolated relaxation rate at T_g', obtained from linear extrapolation of the Arrhenius plots of the main relaxation, is of the order of 10^{-4} sec^{-1}, as indicated in TABLE 2. This shows that the molecular degrees of freedom involved in dielectric relaxation are probably the ones whose freezing out causes a decrease in the heat capacity observed in a differential thermal analysis experiment.

GLASS TRANSITION IN A STABLE PHASE

The recognition of the molecular degrees of freedom, the freezing out of which causes the glass-like transition, is particularly important in the case of hexagonal ice, where a decrease in the heat capacity and a relaxation of enthalpy has been found to occur in the temperature range 110°–123°K for D_2O[40] and 90°–110°K for H_2O ice.[41] The dielectric relaxation time for the hexagonal ices in their respective temperature range is 10^3–10^4 sec, which is comparable to the time scale of a thermodynamic experiment. This indicates that the degrees of freedom involved in the relaxation of enthalpy are the same as in the dielectric relaxation. It seems, therefore, that the rotation of a water molecule in ice may involve some configurations that differ in energy from others, contrary to Pauling's statistical model[42] based

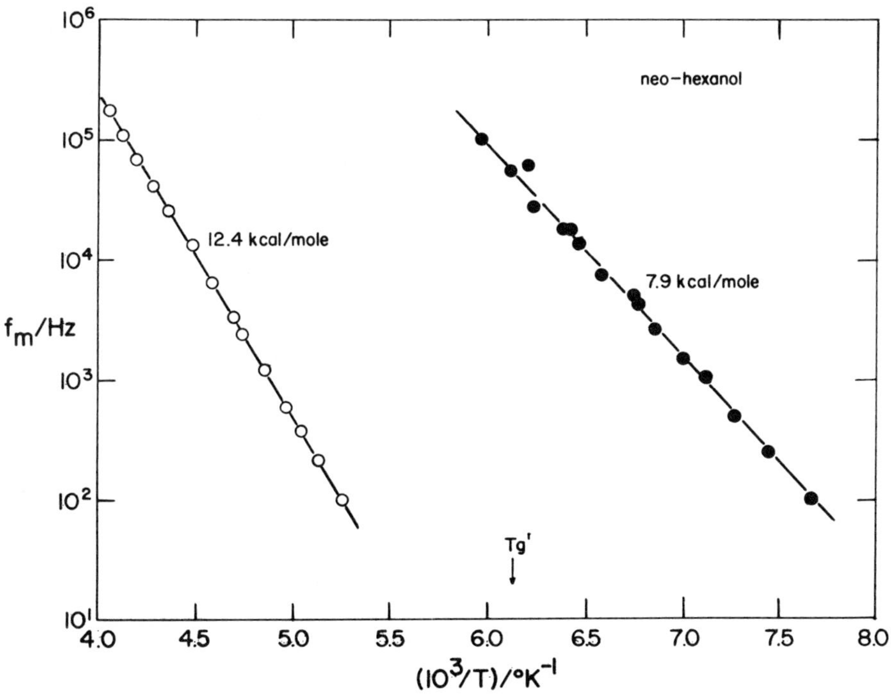

FIGURE 10. The frequency of maximum loss, f_m, plotted logarithmically against reciprocal temperature for neohexanol.

upon equal energy of all six orientations of a water molecule and consequently for all configurations in ice. Detailed calculations of the lattice energy of ice by Campbell *et al.*[43] have indeed shown that multipole interactions produce small, but significant, differences between the energy of the various configurations. These differences in the energy become comparable to kT near 100°K. Consequently, some configurations in ice at low temperatures would become more stable than others. The stabilized configuration may not necessarily be the one having complete orientational order resulting from a thermodynamic phase transformation.

It is noteworthy in this connection that a search for a phase transformation in ice[44-46] has not shown any evidence for a disorder–order transformation. No change in the limiting high frequency permittivity has been found on annealing ice for many months near 100°K,[46] and the equilibrium dielectric permittivity of H_2O ice at 98.1°K is 276,[45] a value that is consistent with Boltzmann's distribution of orientation and does not indicate a phase transformation to either a ferroelectrically, or an antiferroelectrically, ordered phase.

It is also important to mention here that hexagonal ice shows a distribution of relaxation times and a non-Arrhenius behavior[47] in its dielectric relaxation rate of the main process at temperatures above 100°K and indeed the relaxation rate for D_2O ice below 170°K can be fitted to Equation 1 with $A = 3 \times 10^{-16}$ sec^{-1}, $B = 828$°K, and $T_0 = 60$°K.[47]

Because of a small decrease in C_p of 0.12 cal °K^{-1} mole^{-1} at T_g' given in TABLE 3, a detailed analysis of the relaxation of enthalpy[40,41] in ice would not be unambiguous, and a situation similar to Kauzmann's paradox,[29] of course, cannot exist in hexagonal ice. However, in view of the results described earlier in this section it does seem that the long-known anomaly in the heat capacity of ice[34] near 100°K is due to the freezing out of the configurational degrees of freedom in a manner similar to that at the glass transition, as was also noted by Giauque and Stout[34] in 1935. If this view is accepted, then one observes that a glass-like transition can also occur in a *stable* phase of matter, namely the hexagonal ice.

This brings us to a further point of interest, which is that, contrary to the generally held view, and based upon our practical experience on the glass transition phenomenon, we believe there is no thermodynamic reason requiring that a glass transition must necessarily occur in the supercooled metastable state of a liquid or of a crystal. In an analysis of the relation between the relaxation rate, temperature, and pressure, it has been shown[6] that the melting curve of glycerol would cross the glass transition curve in a temperature pressure plane at negative 25 kbar, and that below this pressure the glass transition in glycerol would occur above its melting point. Such a high negative pressure is certainly well above the tensile strength of glycerol and is not attainable. The argument, however, does suggest that for substances in which the entropy of fusion is small or the volume of fusion is large, it may be possible to achieve a pressure, temperature condition at which the glass transition would occur in a stable phase above the freezing point of the liquid.

SIMILARITY IN THE FEATURES OF RELAXATIONS

Let us now summarize our conclusions from the dielectric relaxation studies of the substances in the glassy state. We have discussed that glasses made from a variety of substances show almost identical features in their main relaxations and in their secondary relaxations. These substances are (1) rigid molecular liquids, (2) nonrigid molecular liquids, (3) hydrogen-bonded liquids, (4) inorganic nitrates,

(5) orientationally-disordered crystalline solids, (6) organic polymers, and (7) inorganic silicates.

Measurements of transport properties of liquid by other experimental methods have also indicated a similarity of features. Barlow *et al.*[48] have found that the viscoelastic relaxation behavior of a number of molecular liquids and of several polymers at high temperatures conform to a standard pattern describable by their phenomenological equations. The NMR measurements of McCall and coworkers[49,50] show that the profile of spin-lattice relaxation time versus temperature in the molecular liquids is similar to that observed in polymers.

Mechanical measurements[51,52] on metallic glasses have shown the presence of regions of high mobility, and a strong similarity in their viscoelastic responses to low-molecular-weight polystyrene. Chen *et al.*[53] did not find a secondary relaxation in a Pd-Au-Si alloy glass, but Eisenberg and Reich[54] found secondary relaxations in Pd-Si and Pd-Au-Si alloys, the presence of which depended upon the thermal history of the sample.

The qualitative uniformity of the relaxation features of glasses has been recognized subsequently by Williams and coworkers,[12,55–58] who also found a quantitative similarity between the normalized plots of ϵ'' against the logarithm of frequency in a variety of molecular liquids and amorphous polymers. The exact origin of the distribution interpreted from the broad loss curves in FIGURE 2 is, however, still uncertain although current explanations pursue the possibility that movement of a unit dipole may not be completely independent of the movement of the neighboring dipoles. A correlation in angular positions between neighboring dipoles can effect the observed dipole moment per molecule and the time dependence of this correlation may cause a departure from a Debye-like relaxation behavior.

Williams and coworkers[12,57] have shown that the broad loss curves, such as those in FIGURE 2, may reflect a dipole moment autocorrelation function which has a natural nonexponential dependence upon linear time due to the cooperative molecular motion in the supercooled liquid state. Our ϵ'' data for 17.2 mole% chlorobenzene/*cis*-decalin mixture at 128.2°K agree reasonably well with the Williams-Watts equation,[57]

$$\left(\frac{\epsilon^*(i\omega) - \epsilon_\infty}{\epsilon_0 - \epsilon_\infty}\right) = \int_0^\infty \left[-\frac{\partial \gamma}{\partial t}\right] \exp(-i\omega t)\,dt,$$

and $\gamma(t) = \exp(-t/t_0)^{\bar{\beta}}$, with a value of $\bar{\beta}$ of about 0.55.

Molecular Origin of Relaxation in Glasses

The main conclusion from this study is that the molecular rearrangements giving rise to a secondary relaxation process are similar to those that are responsible for the glass transition itself. In the glasses made from rigid molecular liquids and in the orientational-disorder-frozen-in crystals, both the main and secondary relaxation process should involve major rearrangements in the position and/or orientation of at least one and probably several molecules in a certain local region. At temperatures above T_g, the molecular configurations in an ordinary liquid and in a disordered crystalline solid are generally random and any change in the configurational state no doubt involves a distribution of energy barriers. A distribution in the heights of potential energy barriers resisting the molecular jumps may indeed be responsible for the presence of some molecular mobility[59] in a glass, for only at very low temperature will the modes of motion, involving certain low energy barriers, freeze out. Rather than producing two separate maxima, the distribution would lead to a spreading out of the dielectric relaxation spectrum. For the appearance of a secondary relaxation that is distinct from the main relaxation it would be necessary to assume a form of the density-of-states vs energy relation that differs from that inferred from thermodynamics.[60]

The anisotropy of polarization in a special type of crystalline field, in which the dipole reorients, can also give rise to a somewhat broad distribution and even two loss peaks in the ϵ''–log (frequency) plots for single-axis rotators.[61] Obviously, this explanation cannot be offered for liquids. It is also not likely to be valid for disorder-frozen-in crystals because the height of potential barriers resisting the motion of a given molecule in the crystal would depend on the orientation of the near neighbors, which are already disordered and are time-dependent. The crystalline field is neither fixed nor well defined. The basic assumption that many potential energy minima are accessible to a molecule is, however, most useful and in a sense is similar to the consideration involved in the potential energy barrier picture[59] of glass transition that led to the prediction of molecular mobility in glasses.

Williams and Watts[57] and Williams[62] have suggested that a polymer or a rigid-molecular dipole may exist in a variety of different environments, and in a given environment may be partially relaxed by local motions in that environment. This local motion is reflected as the high-frequency, or secondary, relaxation. That portion of μ^2 that is not relaxed by local motions will be relaxed by the slower and grosser process of cooperative micro-Brownian motion of the environment and this is the α process. Thus the relaxation of the total dipole moment given by μ^2 is divided into two parts: local motions in a variety of environments partially relax μ^2, and the remainder of the μ^2 is completely relaxed by the micro-Brownian motion. As the temperature is increased the rate of micro-Brownian motion far exceeds that for local motions. Thus in the log f_m–temperature plots the α and β processes intersect at some high temperature. Their consideration in terms of equations for correlation functions leads to two relaxation processes, α and β, at low temperatures and a single $\alpha\beta$ or α at high temperatures.

A qualitative view of the origin of secondary relaxation has been offered elsewhere[13] and perhaps can be briefly given here. It is intuitively obvious that a number of statistically distributed regions of low density, in which molecules or atoms can sit with non-equivalent probabilities in many possible orientation sites, would exist in a glass. The secondary relaxation may then be envisaged as arising from noncooperative but hindered rotation of some molecules in these local regions which are encaged by large regions where the requirement for a concerted, or a cooperative, motion has made relatively immobile the arrangement of the majority of molecules. The motion of the molecules in these local regions is analogous with the motion of guest molecules in a clathrate compound[63,64] where the orientation of the host molecules forming the cage-like lattice are relatively fixed.

Let us now consider the possible consequences of our qualitative view of the origin of the β processes. Since the electrostatic field E determines the distribution of barrier heights through contribution of the form $\mu \cdot \mathrm{E}$, the presence of a broad distribution of electrostatic field and field directions imposed by the neighboring molecules surrounding a given local region would lead to a highly variable perturbation of the potential energy function that describes the short-range interactions. As there is no symmetry imposed by the rigid molecular matrix around a molecule in such a region, the orientations would become distinguishable from an isotropic reorientation. The dielectric relaxation of the β process would depart considerably from a Debye behavior. In addition, the potential energy contours in the different local regions would be far from identical, thus further causing a wide distribution of relaxation times in the β process. The asymmetry of the absorption in the β process appears to be mainly attributable to the effect of electrostatic field due to the surrounding molecules in lowering the barriers to rotation of molecules in the local region. For example, the electrostatic field would tend to lower the barrier between two orientations most favored by the field and to raise the barriers between those less favored. The effect is to increase the absorption at high frequencies more than that at low frequencies.

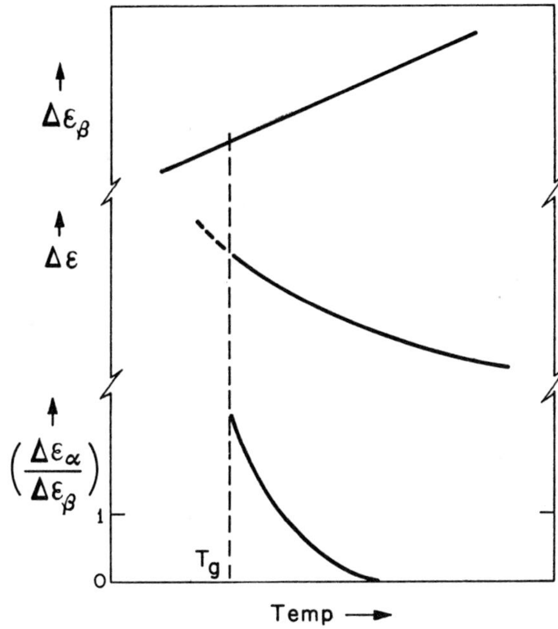

FIGURE 11. A schematic representation of the effect of temperature on the permittivity, $\Delta\epsilon$, due to the total orientation polarization; on the contribution to permittivity, $\Delta\epsilon_\beta$, due to the orientation polarization relaxing as the β process, and on the relative amplitudes of the permittivity due to the α and β processes.

The contribution to the secondary relaxation, $\Delta\epsilon_\beta$, would increase with temperature, for the orientations favored by the electrostatic field will become less populous as the kT increases. Furthermore, the number of such "islands of mobility" would increase with temperature because of a decrease in the size of the cooperatively rearranging regions. The increase in $\Delta\epsilon_\beta$ would occur at the expense of the contribution due to α relaxation, $\Delta\epsilon_\alpha$, and would be reflected in a decrease in the ratio of $(\Delta\epsilon_\alpha/\Delta\epsilon_\beta)$ with increasing temperature. This is schematically shown in FIGURE 11, where $\Delta\epsilon_\beta$, $(\Delta\epsilon_\alpha/\Delta\epsilon_\beta)$, and the permittivity due to total orientation polarization, $\Delta\epsilon$, is plotted against temperature. With increasing temperature, $\Delta\epsilon_\beta$ increases while both $\Delta\epsilon$ and $(\Delta\epsilon_\alpha/\Delta\epsilon_\beta)$ decrease.

Some idea of the temperature dependence of the magnitude of β relaxation can be obtained by examining TABLE 1, where $\Delta\epsilon_\alpha$ and $\Delta\epsilon_\beta$ for several rigid molecular substances are given. It is evident that $\Delta\epsilon_\alpha$ decreases and $\Delta\epsilon_\beta$ increases with increasing temperature. The ratio $\Delta\epsilon_\alpha/\Delta\epsilon_\beta$ decreases from 2.23 to 1.20 in the temperature range 135.9–143.3°K.

The number of loosely packed regions in a glass, where molecules can admit different orientations, would, under isothermal conditions, decrease with the molar volume and therefore with the fictive temperature of the glass. The strength of the β process would then be lower for an annealed glass than for one obtained by fast cooling. This is clearly seen in FIGURE 4 where the height of the β relaxation peak decreases on annealing the 34 mole% 1-chloronaphthalene-pyridine glass.

Insofar as the life of the "islands of mobility" is limited by the time scale of the cooperative rearrangement, and that this type of rearrangement occurs above T_g, the β process should exist in the liquid state above T_g, but at high frequencies. That a β process does exist above T_g is, of course, evident in TABLE 1 and FIGURE 5.

At some temperature above T_g, no cooperative rearrangement is required and the total dipolar reorientation would be hindered by the potential energy barriers that are different from those involved in the cooperative rearrangements. At very high temperatures, therefore, the secondary relaxation would be similar to that seen in liquids and in orientationally disordered crystals at the microwave frequencies. The frequency of maximum loss of 8.2 mole% chlorobenzene/*cis*-decalin mixture at 298°, 313°, and 333°K are included in FIGURE 3, where the dashed line indicates a possible extension of the rates of the α relaxation process. It is evident from FIGURE 3 that the relaxation rate of the β process in the glassy state extrapolates linearly to very close to the values of the relaxation rates at room temperature and above, with an Arrhenius energy of 5.8 kcal mole^{-1}. Although the extrapolation may not be entirely unambiguous, it is significant that the β process has about the same Arrhenius energy as the relaxation process seen in liquids at a viscosity as low as several centipoises and in disordered crystals near their melting points.

It appears then that in liquids, and in orientationally disordered crystals, both the cooperative and hindered type of molecular rearrangements occur at temperatures above T_g. A schematic representation of the dispersion and absorption at a temperature above T_g is shown in FIGURE 12. The relative contribution of the α and β process to the transport property varies with the temperature. As the liquid approaches T_g, there is an increasing proportion of cooperative molecular rearrangements. The consequent onset of the non-Arrhenius behavior separates the cooperative molecular process in the rate–temperature plane. This is the α process. The glass transition occurs at the cessation of this process on the time scale of one's measurement. The β process, which is due to the hindered rearrangement of the molecules, continues to exist through the complete temperature range of the liquid and the glass. The exact temperature at which the α process becomes predominant and separates from the β process in the rate temperature plane is not known. This temperature cannot be easily measured and an extrapolation has to be done to obtain it. The onset of the predominance of the cooperative rearrangements, which may give rise to a non-Arrhenius behavior, is also seen from studies of the effect on the rate of molecular processes. For example, the pressure coefficient of the volume of activation for the shear and the dielectric relaxation rates has been found to change from a negative or zero to a positive value as the glass transition pressure is approached.[6]

Let us now consider the situation shown in FIGURE 3 in terms of Goldstein's theory[59] of glass transition. In his view,[59] the configurational state of a glass is trapped in one deep minimum in the potential energy surface. This deep minimum, which represents an α configuration, has in it multiple "local" minima of varying depths separated by potential barriers smaller than those that separate the deep minima. The α configuration can be graphically represented as a deep well in the configurational space with a "rough and corrugated" bottom rather than a rounded one. The configurational changes involving the deep minima determine the rate of the α process and those involving the shallow local minima, the rate of the β process. An interpretation of the results in FIGURE 3 in Goldstein's view[59]

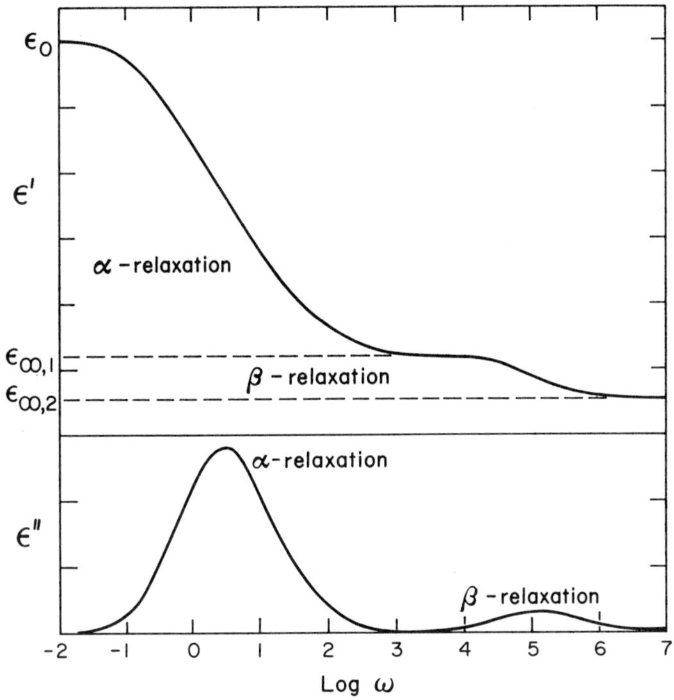

FIGURE 12. A schematic representation of the dielectric dispersion and absorption in a material near T_g showing α and β relaxations.

would mean that as a glass is heated the lower energy wells become accessible to its configurational state while local minima in a given configurational state remain largely unaltered. If this continued to occur on heating then at a certain temperature above T_g, there would no longer be a distinction between the respective minima involved in the molecular rearrangements that give rise to the α and β relaxation. This temperature would be the one at which the α and β processes apparently merge. Above this temperature the configurational states are likely to involve many minima separated by small potential energy barriers and changes between these states would be observed only as what appears to be the β process.

Molecular Mobility and the Structure of a Glass

The molecular mobility in glasses and in disorder-frozen-in crystals can be interpreted in two ways. The first is to suggest the presence of two types of environments, one in which the structure is relatively loose and where the molecules can undergo hindered rotation, and the other in which the structure is closely packed and a cooperative rearrangement occurs. In this interpretation only a fraction of the total number of molecules contribute to the secondary relaxation. The second interpretation is to suggest that all molecules arranged in a random network type of structure in a glass reorient by a small angle, which shows up as the secondary relaxation, and by a large angle which gives rise to the main relaxation, the small angle reorientation being a necessary prior step for the large angle jump. Unfortunately, it does not seem possible to resolve the relative merits of the two interpretations by an experimental method.

Structural studies on glasses have most often been interpreted in terms of an entirely random network model. Some recent evidence on the stability of small aggregates of particles[65,66] has raised an alternative possibility that glasses may be composed of aggregates of high density and low energy which lack the symmetry needed for long-range periodic packing. These aggregates are termed amorphous clusters. The structure of a glass consisting of such clusters would require relatively loose packing of atoms or molecules in the interstices between the amorphous clusters, a feature that can be graphically referred to as *glue* or *connective tissue*. In contrast to the random network model in which all the atoms or molecular units are in an essentially equivalent environment, the amorphous cluster model implies the presence of two different environments in the structure. Our results may lend support to the amorphous cluster model in which the α relaxation arises from the rearrangement of molecules in the small clusters and β relaxation from that of the molecules in the interstices between the clusters.

Possible Future Studies of Disordered Crystals

A number of experimental studies of the disordered crystalline state near the glass-like transition region should prove to be of great value in the progress towards a theoretical understanding of the nature of the glassy state. Among these, the dilatometric studies are the most important, for such studies would help in further clarifying the role that the free volume is thought to play in the glass transition phenomenon. The thermodynamic measurements of a substance, both in the supercooled metastable liquid and the disordered crystalline state, would be useful, because the difference between the heat capacity in the two different physical states would reflect largely the contribution to configurational entropy due to translational degrees of freedom that are present in the liquid but not in the crystal. Substances in which no change occurs in the characteristics of relaxation at T_m are particularly attractive for such a study.

Relaxation studies of rigid molecular, disordered crystals by various techniques would certainly be valuable in further elucidating the correlation between the thermodynamic and relaxational features of the molecular processes that occur in the disorder-frozen-in state. Spherical molecules such as *tertiary*-butyl halides and nitrates in the supercooled disordered crystalline state, for which the energetics of dipolar orientation is theoretically well understood, can also serve as model substances. Above all, the disordered crystals, by virtue of their relatively simple structure, may help in providing a general and hopefully more accurate statistical mechanical approach to the description of thermodynamic and relaxational features of the glass transition phenomenon in general.

Acknowledgments

I am indebted to Professor M. Goldstein of Yeshiva University, New York, for his stimulating discussions on the subject of the glass transition.

I would also like to express my thanks to Miss L. Lalonde for her expert typing and to my wife, Jean, for her help in editing this manuscript.

References

1. McCrum, N. G., B. Read & G. Williams. Anelastic and Dielectric Effects in Polymeric Solids. John Wiley and Sons, Inc. New York.
2. Johari, G. P. & M. Goldstein. 1970. J. Chem. Phys. **53:** 2372. J. Phys. Chem. **74:** 2034.
3. Johari, G. P. & M. Goldstein. 1971. J. Chem. Phys. **55:** 4245.
4. Hakim, R. M. 1973. J. Appl. Phys. **44:** 887.
5. Chan, R. K. & G. P. Johari. To be published.
6. Johari, G. P. & E. Whalley. 1972. Faraday Symp. Chem. Soc **6:** 23.
7. Johari, G. P. 1976. J. Chem. Phys. **64:** 3998.
8. Dannhauser, W. 1968. J. Chem. Phys. **48:** 1918.
9. Johari, G. P. & W. Dannhauser. 1969. J. Chem. Phys. **50:** 1862.
10. Dannhauser, W. & R. H. Cole. 1955. J. Chem. Phys. **23:** 1762.
11. Johari, G. P. & C. P. Smyth. 1972. J. Chem. Phys. **56:** 4411.
12. Williams, G. & P. J. Hains. 1972. Faraday Symp. Chem. Soc. **6:** 14.
13. Johari, G. P., J. Chem. Phys. **58:** 1766.
14. North, A. M. 1972. Chem. Soc. Rev. **1:** 49.
15. Dannhauser, W. & A. F. Flueckinger. 1970. Phys. Chem. Liquids **2:** 37.
16. Macedo, P. B. & A. Napolitano. 1968. J. Chem. Phys. **49:** 1887.
17. Weiler, R., S. Blaser & P. B. Macedo. 1969. J. Phys. Chem. **73:** 4147. (1969).
18. Bose, B., R. Weiler & P. B. Macedo. 1970. Phys. Chem. Glasses **11:** 117.
19. Uhlmann, D. R. 1972. In Amorphous Materials. R. W. Douglas & B. E. Ellis, Eds.: 205. John Wiley and Sons, Inc. New York.
20. Ambrus, J. H., C. T. Moynihan & P. B. Macedo. 1971. J. Electrochem. Soc. **119:** 192.
21. Chan, R. K. & G. P. Johari. 1975. Canad. J. Chem. Educ. **10:** 8, 10.
22. Kelly, K. K. 1929. J. Amer. Chem. Soc. **51:** 1400.
23. Otsubo, A. & T. Sugawara. 1955. Sci. Rep. Res. Inst. Tohoko Univ. **A7:** 583.
24. Adachi, K., H. Suga & S. Seki. 1968. Bull. Chem. Soc. Japan **41:** 1073.
25. Oda, T. 1945, 1948. X-rays **4:** 2. **5:** 26.
26. Corfield, G. & M. Davies. 1964. Trans. Faraday Soc. **60:** 10.
27. Suga, H. & S. Seki. 1974. J. Non-Cryst. Solids **16:** 171.
28. Adam, G. & J. H. Gibbs. 1965. J. Chem. Phys. **43:** 139.
29. Kauzmann, W. 1948. Chem. Rev. **43:** 219.
30. Adachi, K., H. Suga & S. Seki. 1971. Bull. Chem. Soc. Japan **44:** 78.
31. Huffman, H. M., S. S. Todd & G. D. Oliver. 1949. J. Amer. Chem. Soc. **71:** 584.
32. Adachi, K., H. Suga & S. Seki. 1970. Bull. Chem. Soc. Japan **43:** 1916.
33. Adachi, K., H. Suga & S. Seki. 1972. Bull. Chem. Soc. Japan **45:** 1960.
34. Giauque, W. F. & J. W. Stout. 1936. J. Amer. Chem. Soc. **58:** 1144.
35. Long, E. A. & J. D. Kemp. 1936. J. Amer. Chem. Soc. **58:** 1829.
36. Matsuo, T., H. Oguni, H. Suga & S. Seki. 1972, 1974. Proc. Japan. Acad. **48:** 237. Bull. Chem. Soc. Japan **47:** 57.

37. Dannhauser, W., L. W. Bahe, R. Y. Lin & A. F. Flueckinger. 1965. J. Chem. Phys. **43:** 257.
38. Davidson, D. W. & R. H. Cole. 1951. J. Chem. Phys. **19:** 1484.
39. Adachi, K., H. Suga, S. Seki, S. Kubota, S. Yamaguchi, O. Yano & Y. Wada. 1972. Mol. Cryst. Liq. Cryst. **18:** 345.
40. Haida, O., H. Suga & S. Seki. 1973. Proc. Japan. Acad. **49:** 191.
41. Haida, O., T. Matsuo, H. Suga & S. Seki. 1974. J. Chem. Thermodyn. **6:** 815.
42. Pauling, L. 1935. J. Amer. Chem. Soc. **57:** 2680.
43. Campbell, E. S., H. Gelerutner, H. Heinen & V. R. G. Moorti. 1967. J. Chem. Phys. **46:** 2690.
44. Johari, G. P. 1975. Phys. Lett. **53A:** 144.
45. Johari, G. P. & S. J. Jones. 1975. J. Chem. Phys. **62:** 4213.
46. Whalley, E. & A. Lavergne. 1974. As quoted in J. Chem. Phys. **61:** 4292.
47. Johari, G. P. & S. J. Jones. 1976. Proc. R. Soc. (Lond.). To be published.
48. Barlow, A. J., M. Day, G. Harrison, J. Lamb & S. Subramanian. 1969. Proc. Soc. (Lond.) **A309:** 497.
49. McCall, D. W., D. C. Douglass & D. R. Falcone. 1969. J. Chem. Phys. **50:** 3839.
50. McCall, D. W. 1971. Accounts Chem. Res. **4:** 223.
51. Chen, H. S. & T. T. Wang. J. Appl. Phys. **42:** 5338.
52. Chen, H. S. & M. Goldstein. 1972. J. Appl. Phys. **43:** 1642.
53. Chen, H. S., H. J. Leamy & M. Barmatz. 1970–71. J. Non-Cryst. Solids **5:** 444.
54. A. Eisenberg, & S. Reich. 1972. The Dynamic Viscoelastic Properties of Some Non-Crystalline Metals. *In* Amorphous Materials. R. Douglas & B. Ellis, Eds.:23. John Wiley and Sons, Inc. New York.
55. Cook, M., D. C. Watts & G. Williams. 1970. Trans. Faraday Soc. **66:** 2503.
56. Williams, G. & D. C. Watts. 1970. Trans. Faraday Soc. **66:** 80.
57. Williams, G. & D. C. Watts. 1971. Trans. Faraday Soc. **67:** 1971. NMR-Basic Principles and Progress **4:** 271.
58. Williams, G., D. C. Watts, S. B. Dev, & A. M. North. 1971. Trans. Faraday Soc. **67:** 1323.
59. Goldstein, M. 1969. J. Chem. Phys. **51:** 3728.
60. Goldstein, M. 1972. Faraday Symp. Chem. Soc. **6:** 7.
61. Hoffman, J. D. & B. M. Axilrod. 1957. J. Res. Nat. Bur. Stand. **58:** 61.
62. Williams, G. 1972. Faraday Symp. Chem. Soc. **6:** 45.
63. Dryden, J. S. 1953. Trans. Faraday Soc. **49:** 1333.
64. Davidson, D. W. 1971. Canad. J. Chem. **49:** 1224.
65. Turnbull, D. & D. E. Polk. 1972. J. Non-Cryst. Solids **8–10:**19.
66. Hoare, M. R. & P. Pal. 1972. J. Cryst. Growth **17:** 77.

DISCUSSION

A. Eisenberg, *Moderator*

McGill University
Montreal, Quebec
Canada

S. Moss (*University of Houston, Houston, Texas*): I was fascinated by Dr. Johari's description of these orientationally disordered crystals and the glass transition effect in them and I wondered if the ability to quench them implies a first order transition between state 1 and state 2, in other words, between the rotationally disordered state and the rotationally ordered state. Does that imply a first order transition?

The second question involves the canonical example of ammonium chloride in which the NH_4 goes between four possible corners of a cubic unit cell, and in ammonium chloride it's a rotational transition; and it's an Ising model because it's just these four or those four, yes or no, one or two, up or down. I thus wondered if the similarity between the orientationally disordered crystals that you're talking about and the above breaks down since you implied that the orientation can be any way and that it's random. Is that so or is it Ising-like?

Johari: The transition from rotational to a nonrotational state in cyclohexanol, as in the majority of disordered cyrstals, is a first order transition. There are, however, some materials, such as methane, whose heat capacity rises sharply near the transition region (15°–20°K). Interpretation of such a behavior have been in terms of a second order or a lambda transition.

With regard to your second comment, attempts to predict the entropy of transition in disordered crystals have been met with only a limited degree of success, and that also for tetrahedral molecules. One finds that the configurational entropy of the majority of orientationally disordered crystals cannot be entirely explained by the disappearance of an intuitively anticipated number of possible orientations.

Moss: What about diffraction? Because there will obviously be diffuse scattering arising from both the uncertainty of fluctuation and of orientation. One could follow this diffuse scattering, not only above the 1–2 transition but also in the vicinity of the glass transition in these crystals. It's fantastic, this is really interesting.

Johari: The x-ray diffraction patterns from the orientationally disordered crystals are not as well defined as ones from the corresponding ordered states. Furthermore, in the disordered state the reorientation of molecules occurs at such a high frequency that the x-ray measurements cannot distinguish between free rotation and random orientations. There is an added complication in the interpretation of such measurements because the diffraction studies are generally unable to distinguish between the time-averaged and space-averaged features of molecular structure.

In the vicinity of the glasslike transition temperature, one would anticipate a change in the x-ray or neutron diffraction and scattering, if such experiments were able to distinguish between the time- and space-averaged features of structure above T_g' and only the space-averaged features of the frozen-in structure below T_g'. Studies on hexagonal ice, the only case I know where both the diffraction and scattering measurements have been made near 100°K, remain inconclusive in this respect.

LEADBETTER: Dr. Moss, I think the answer to your second question is that there's a whole spectrum of these things from the case of the ammonium salts you mentioned, to these which are nearly completely orientationally disordered, but I know of no case (although there have been relatively few detailed diffraction studies), even the most disordered one, where the orientation is truly random. There are rather certain preferred positions, which may be 5 or a dozen or maybe more. And the other thing to emphasize about these materials of course in the high-temperature disordered crystalline phase, the orientational disorder is rapidly dynamic, the reorientation frequency is something like 10^{12} sec $^{-1}$.

MOSS: With x rays you couldn't tell; with neutrons presumably you can.

LEADBETTER: Well, with x rays the few studies that have been done have shown quite categorically that it's not totally random; there is some preferred set of positions, but the question of which are the preferred positions is a difficult one that has not often yet been answered.

D. W. MCCALL (*Bell Laboratories, Murray Hill, N.J.*): I substantially agree with what Johari told us this morning. It's a very interesting paper, but there are two points I think should be mentioned. One of them is that whereas the molecular mechanisms are basically consistent in most cases, as he pointed out, and they can be studied by a variety of different techniques that probe the molecules quite differently, there are some difficult cases outstanding. One of them is polyvinyl acetate for which he showed an Arrhenius plot. If you will notice, there are no NMR points on the beta curve for that polymer. We looked very carefully at polyvinyl acetate and I am vexed by that one because it is essentially an impossible result and you will discover a mysterious passage in our paper in this connection.

JOHARI: It's interesting to point out that the relaxations in clathrate compounds, particularly the relaxation of the guest molecules, encased in clathrate cavities, can be seen by NMR measurements and have indeed been. I think if a "self-enclathration" occurred in certain regions in the glassy state, the NMR studies might also be able to show the existence of a β process. Polyvinyl acetate seems to be rather exceptional in this regard.

MCCALL: In almost all cases it is true, but polyvinyl acetate is not the only example. You will recall that ortho-terphenyl is another example where we did not see a low-temperature transition in the NMR results.

Let me make a second comment here. The problem that you mentioned toward the end of your talk, of distinguishing between where a few molecules are reorienting or all of them are reorienting, I think can be studied from the depolarization of fluorescence. There were early papers on this subject, but the time is now right for a new look with modern techniques.

ANGELL: Dr. Johari, I had two points to make: One was to say I thought that last slide that you showed in which the temperature dependence of the β relaxation time and the temperature dependence of the oridinary dielectric relaxation up in the very high frequency range were the same, was of particular interest and I wanted to ask if that was found for more than one case? And, perhaps before you answer that, I wanted to make an addition to the comments of Professor Moss in connection with the interest content of these plastic crystals and their ability to undergo glasslike transitions.

There are a lot of these funny glasslike crystal phenomena buried in the chemical literature, some of them even more peculiar than the ones that we've seen here today. For example, I've seen a heat capacity versus temperature diagram for an organosulfur compound plastic crystal in which there's a glass transition immediately followed by a lambda-type transition imposed on top of it and separated only by a few degrees (MESSERLY, J. F., H. L. FINKE & S. S. TODD 1974. J. Chem. Thermodynamics **6:** 635–37). I think that there's probably a whole "spectrum" of intricate cooperative phenomena in which two types of transitions tend to blend in towards one another depending on the details of the nearest neighbor interactions. What would be nice would be to find one series of crystals in a binary system with solid solubility in which you could systematically convert a lambda transition into a glass transition. At Purdue we sought unsuccessfully to do this using the $NaNO_3$ + $AgNO_3$ system. I think that this sort of approach might help a lot in understanding our particular type of cooperative phenomenon, the glass transition. In particular, a system showing a continuous conversion from lambda to glasslike transition would help to bring out the important point, often discounted in discussion of the glass transition, that the interesting part of the glass transition from the standpoint of statistical thermodynamics, (viz., the rapid decrease of heat capacity at equilibrium necessary to resolve the Kauzmann paradox), is hidden by a kinetically imposed curtain below the experimental glass transition temperature. In the lambda-type transition the sharp configurational heat capacity maximum almost invariably appears at temperatures where equilibrium is rapidly achieved. In our hypothetical binary system, possibly to be found amongst materials of the type studied by Dr. Johari, change of composition would shift the maximum (and presumably change its shape) systematically from the short relaxation time region into the long time (and inaccessible) region.

JOHARI: The temperature dependence of the relaxation rates of the α and β processes similar to that seen in FIGURE 3 has also been observed in solutions of pyridine and chloronaphthalene in *cis*-decalin and in a number of aliphatic alcohols. Porter and Boyd (1971. Macromolecules **4:** 589.) have also observed a closely similar temperature dependence of dielectric relaxations in poly(ethylene oxide) at microwave frequencies. It seems that the merging of the α and β processes at high temperatures might be a general feature of glass-forming materials.

HEIJBOER: May I remark that the temperature dependence of β relaxation you showed fits the formula given in my paper.

JOHARI: It is remarkable particularly because your formula is valid for relaxations in organic polymers. It seems to serve as additional evidence in support of the similarity between the dielectric relaxation features of amorphous polymers and molecular glasses.

C. MOYNIHAN (*Catholic University, Washington, D.C.*): I want to make a very brief comment in support of Dr. Johari's conclusion that the glasslike transitions in these plastic crystals are phenomenologically quite similar to the ordinary glass transition of liquids. This fall at Catholic University we carried out some heat capacity measurements on one of these substances, cyclohexanol, as a function of heating and cooling rate of the sort that Prof. Macedo described yesterday, and combining this with some other thermodynamic data available from Suga and Seki we were able to conclude that phenomenologically and qualitatively there's no distinction between the kinetics of the transition you see in these plastic crystals and the kinetics of the glass transition in ordinary liquids in two respects:

First the kinetics are highly nonlinear. This means that the relaxation time at a given temperature depends strongly on how far you are from equilibrium. To put it in the language that some other people here seem to prefer, this means that the relaxation time is going to depend strongly on the free volume.

Second the relaxation kinetics seem to require a nonexponential correlation function, or to put it in other words, a very broad distribution of relaxation times.

So it would appear that to observe this sort of glass transition phenomenon it is not required that you have the positional disorder that you find in liquids.

JOHARI: I should, however, like to express that it is not quite clear as to how the concept of free volume could be applied to plastic crystals. One would certainly need to characterize the glasslike transitions in the crystals by dilatometric studies prior to explaining their relaxation behavior in terms of a free-volume theory.

STRUIK: I'd like to say that the merging of β and α transitions is probably a general phenomenon. It's not only known for low-molecular-weight materials; Mikhailov using dielectric relaxation found it in polymers, and if I remember well, Koppelmann found the same with mechanical measurements. I think that yesterday I have suggested an explanation for this phenomenon. The β relaxation is generally a prerequisite for the α relaxation. If you try to move through a crowded room, the losing of your internal flexibility will strongly increase your "relaxation time"; your mobility will decrease. If the experimental vibration time becomes smaller than the relaxation time of the β transition, the α motion becomes much more difficult and the α motion has to wait until the segment reorients internally. I think that is a very simple explanation for polymers.

JOHARI: The second comment regarding the beta relaxation is that even in such circumstances where there are pendent groups or side groups, the rotation of the side groups occurs in an environment that is intermolecular in nature. The intermolecular environment determines the potential energy function for the rotation of even a pendent group. So in a certain sense our conclusions that the β relaxations are dominated by the intermolecular potential energy barrier would be similar to the mechanism assumed for polymers if the people who have studied polymers are willing to think in terms of the importance of intermolecular forces.

RAVECHE: Relative to the plastic crystal data, has anyone ever observed the volume change at the ordering temperature in the plastic crystals? I suspect that this is quite small, a magnitude of a percent or so.

JOHARI: The volume change at the rotational ordering temperature in most plastic crystals ranges between 4%–10% of the molar volume. In cyclohexanol the change in volume is about 8 ml mole^{-1}, which is about 8% of the molar volume of the disordered phase at the transition temperature of 265.5°K.

H. BRAWER (*National Bureau of Standards, Washington, D.C.*): I think the analogy of the disorder in the plastic crystals to the Ising model is quite appropriate, and I seem to be aware from several people at Penn State who work in ferroelectrics that there's a tremendous amount of theoretical work done on time dependent Ising models. In other words you sort of say that the spins conflict, you give them a probability of flipping and the energy barrier depends on the interaction with neighboring spins. And I know that a lot of computer work has been done on one- and two-dimensional cases of such models. Similar models can be applied to glasses and they really ought to be because if these crystals have a glass transition then here's a model where you can calculate everything and compare the results to experiment.

JOHARI: Yes, I agree with you; the study of orientationally disordered solids would be of great value in understanding the glass transition.

GOLDSTEIN: Kikuchi and Sato have worked out treatments of the kinetics of ordering and disordering in Ising-type systems, and I believe are currently attempting to apply it to the same sort of relaxation behavior at the glass transition that Macedo described in his lecture.

MOSS: Just one comment about the existence of the glass transition as I'm still into the phase transitional aspects. I just want to point out something that happens in alloys which has to do with freezing out some things selectively. You have an alloy system of, say, aluminum and copper. A solid solution exists in the high-temperature region while at low temperatures there may be an ordered phase. While it's an ordered phase at a low temperature, slow diffusion prevents you from ever ordering (which happens in many alloys). Perhaps you have aluminum 10% copper and as you cool this alloy down there is short-range order where aluminum prefers copper as its first neighbors, and so forth. That short-range order follows the temperature down as you cool but, because diffusion has exponential behavior with temperature according to an activation energy, after a certain temperature you can no longer, with any quenching rate, achieve equilibrium. The alloy becomes frozen in a configurational state that is characteristic of some higher temperature. The atomic arrangements can no longer follow any quenching rate and so in the alloy you freeze in the short-range order characteristic of that temperature and then you continue to cool. What you've done is to freeze out configurational entropy or the configurations associated with the higher temperature.

Then in a specific heat experiment, if you've held it just above this fictive temperature for a long time you get a little specific heat bump and these things are frequently reported in the metallurgical literature. And people say, ah ha, it's a phase transition. It's not a phase transition. Just because you've frozen out the configurations characteristic of a higher temperature does not mean that when you go back and pick up diffusive motions that you have a phase transition. The orientational disorder that exists in the plastic crystals is like the configurational disorder in alloys when you heat up above a certain point. Call it a glass transition if you wish. It's not a particularly useful name but it is the configurational AB alloy analog of the plastic crystal orientational disorder, and there are many things wrong with it because the associated relaxation phenomena are very different from the relaxation phenomena in glasses. They have one thing in common, however, which is that there's a specific heat bump and it looks like a glass transition.

All that I want to say is that just because you have frozen out some configurational freedom does not mean you have a phase transition.

ANGELL: Well, nobody's going to disagree with that at all, but it misses the point of interest about the long time experiments in the case of the glass-forming liquids. The thermodynamic interest lies more in the *form* of the heat-capacity–temperature relation that would be observed under equilibrium conditions, than in the fact that a heat capacity change occurs when equilibrium is lost. Let's consider another example of a binary alloy C_p versus temperature relation that will help clarify the position, viz., the Fe—Co alloy studies long ago by Sato and Kaya (KAYA, S. & H. SATO. 1943. Proc. Phys. Math. Soc. Japan). These workers found, on cooling, a lambdalike C_p maximum followed only a little lower in temperature by the same sort of diffusion-limited structural freeze and consequent C_p drop that you have described. Now your Cu—Al system, but not the Sato Fe—Co system, has in common with the normal glass transition the circumstance that the interesting aspect of the order-disorder process, viz., the heat capacity (ΔC_p) maximum, has not yet occurred when equilibrium is lost. You imply, no doubt correctly for Cu—Al alloy, that in very long time measurements the system would yield the normal lambda form. But a supposed lambda-shaped C_p anomaly does not offer an acceptable resolution of the Kauzmann paradox for most glass-forming liquids. Regrettably, we have no equivalent of the Sato Fe—Co system to tell us exactly what sort of C_p maximum an appropriate statistical theory should yield. Very long relaxation times near the C_p maximum seem intrinsic to our phenomenon and we are always prevented from seeing the interesting part of the transition.

MOSS: That's exactly what I'm talking about.

ANGELL: O.K., but the interesting part is there even if buried, and the challenge *we* talk about in connection with the glass *transition* lies in accounting for the equilibrium form which definitely cannot, at least in most cases, be of the ordinary lambda type. In the Cu—Al case you have described you have every right to believe that the long time heat-capacity–temperature relation would be of the normal lambda form because (a) there exists a variety of analog systems that fall out of equilibrium at temperatures not only above the lambda point (as in your Cu—Al system) but also a little below it (the Fe–Co system of Sato and Kaya) and far below it (the most common case), and (b) there is no severe restriction placed on the form of the equilibrium C_p versus T function by the amount of excess entropy remaining when equilibrium is lost. Neither (a) nor (b) apply to systems undergoing what we call the glass transition. Thus we must rely on the formulation of a good partition function for the liquid based on a different sort of order-disorder process if we want to know what sort of equilibrium transition we are dealing with.

MOSS: That's exactly what I'm talking about and it is precisely not being able to follow the alloy down to its "lambda transition" because the diffusion stops.

ANGELL: Maybe the point to emphasise then is that in the case of the liquid → glass phenomenon we cannot be dealing with a suppressed lambda transition (in the ordinary sense) because the excess entropy remaining at T_g does not permit [because $S_{ex} = \int_0^{T_g} dT(\Delta C_p/T)$] the luxury of the characteristic long exponential C_p tail at the low-temperature end. In fact if you look at the experimental values of ΔC_p permitted below T_g by the S_{ex} at T_g, the "transition" looks more like the mirror image of an ordinary lambda transition. The limited supply of excess entropy, and the large value of ΔC_p at T_g simply forces you either to recognize this "new" C_p versus T form (some relevant data are given in my paper) or to deny the existence in principle of an equilibrium form (e.g., by establishing that the crystal nucleation energy barrier always vanishes for T not much less than T_g).

MOSS: In fact the systems would show a "lambda transition"—you can't stop it because it's only in the case of first order transitions that metastable equilibrium states can be observed.

B. HALPERIN (*Bell Laboratories, Murray Hill, N.J.*): The question arose as to studies of Ising systems with glasslike transitions. This has been studied fairly extensively. There have been a number of people interested in what kind of transition might occur in an Ising spin system with interactions of random signs, so that it is neither ferromagnetic nor antiferromagnetic. This model has been motivated in part by the existence of so-called spin glasses—dilute systems of magnetic impurities in a nonmagnetic host metal—in which the oscillatory Ruderman-Kittle interaction between the spins may be considered to have random sign. There are many very interesting phenomena that have been studied experimentally in these systems and there appears to be a phase transition that may or may not be related to the usual glass transition, with which this conference is concerned. The theory is in a very controversial stage and I won't attempt to present the different points of view here, but it is a very active field. There are also Monte Carlo type computer studies of these random Ising systems, but, as far as I know, the systems are too small to be of direct interest to the problems in the glass transition at least as yet.

G. D. PATTERSON (*Bell Laboratories, Murray Hill, N.J.*): The question of inter- or intra-molecular effects on the secondary relaxation was addressed during Dr. Johari's lecture when he put the pressure dependence of the secondary relaxation temperature up on the screen for us. If it were purely intramolecular there would probably be a much smaller pressure dependence to that transition temperature than is actually observed. It is much less than the glass transition but it's not zero, and it's a good deal larger than you would expect for simple molecules. So on that basis it can't be purely intramolecular even though it may be largely intramolecular. There must be an intermolecular contribution because it shows up in a fairly strong pressure dependence of the transition temperature.

JOHARI: The pressure dependence of the relaxation rates of both the main and secondary relaxation has been measured by Dr. G. Williams for a large number of amorphous polymers. He has indeed found that the volume of activation for secondary relaxation is almost always less than 10 ml $mole^{-1}$, while for the main relaxation it generally exceeds 100 ml $mole^{-1}$ near the glass transition temperature. For glycerol, the only molecular glass whose pressure dependence of the secondary relaxation is known to have been studied, the volume of activation for the secondary relaxation is 4 ml $mole^{-1}$; for the main relaxation it is 80 ml $mole^{-1}$ and increases with decreasing temperature and increasing pressure. Williams has indeed interpreted his results on polymers in terms of intra- and inter-molecular potential energy barriers.

DIMARZIO: I just wanted to point out that some time ago Charles M. Guttman and I used an Ising model to treat the kind of thing you've been talking about. We took a one-molecule-thick layer of paraffin molecules and we allowed the paraffin molecules to rotate about their long axis, which lies perpendicular to the lamella. The rotation angles correspond to spin in an Ising model and so you can do the problem exactly because you can do the two-dimensional Ising model exactly. We realized we could couple volume changes into the model because when the molecules rotated they would result in an expansion of the lattice and the coupling of volume into the system made the transition first order rather than lambda-like. That's rather interesting because it's exactly the kind of behavior you have in these plastic crystals.

SIMHA: I have two questions for Dr. Heijboer. First, you have indicated that the β relaxation, as observed by dynamic methods, does not shift with the length of the sidechain in the poly(methacrylate) series. On the other hand, dilatometry does show a displacement. In the same series of experiments, it was noted that at a frequency of 1 Hz, the β and glass peaks could no longer be cleanly separated in the butyl methacrylates. Perhaps the thermal expansion experiments on the above series should be repeated?

The second point concerns intra- versus inter-molecular effects in locating secondary relaxation temperatures. Your detailed experiments on poly(cyclo methacrylate) systems indicate no effects due to changes in the molecular environment. On the other hand, the thermal expansion of the homopolymer clearly reveals these processes and at the proper location upon frequency correction. This is a somewhat unexpected result. Moreover, in other polymers, a pressure dependence of sub-glass relaxations is observed. All one can say then is that an interaction between intra- and inter-molecular effects must be invoked, in this specific instance at least. For example, a flipping of the cyclohexyl ring may tend to push the surroundings apart.

HEIJBOER: Since neither mechanical measurements at 10^{-3} Hz, where the β maximum is clearly separated from the glass transition (FIGURE 3), nor dielectric measurements (References 14 & 15 of my paper) reveal any effect of the length of the side chain on the temperature location of the β maximum of the methacrylates, I think the thermal expansion measurements should indeed be repeated.

As for the intra- versus inter-molecular interactions, the fact that the location of most of the secondary loss peaks obeys Equation 1 with $\nu_0 \simeq 10^{13}$, is in my opinion a strong argument in favor of a preponderant influence of intramolecular interaction, that is of the intramolecular barrier, on the location of the loss maximum. This is also borne out by the fact that many secondary loss peaks are not affected by annealing.

On the other hand, I agree that the flipping of the cyclohexyl ring shows up clearly in the thermal expansion. This probably means that there should also be a considerable contribution of intermolecular interaction. However, I do not see how this should be reconciled with the observation that changes in the molecular environment do not affect the cyclohexyl loss peak. We even do not know the detailed molecular mechanism of the interaction of mechanical stress with molecular motions, at least as far as secondary loss peaks are concerned.

It should be mentioned that the effect of pressure on sub-glass transitions is much smaller than its effect on glass transitions. This also indicates that intermolecular interactions are less important for sub-glass transitions than for glass transitions.

GOLDSTEIN: Dr. Heijboer, the question of the intra versus inter is obviously partly an argument about which particular aspect of the beat relaxation one is most interested in. It's quite obvious that there are both intermolecular and, when possible, intramolecular contributions, so part of it is just a difference in focus rather than a real difference in the origin of the effect.

I did want to make just a few comments about some of the evidence you have offered for an intramolecular effect. I can't argue against a lot of it; it is very convincing. I'm not going to say that I can disprove what you say or come up with some argument that will answer every point you made.

There was one particular bit of evidence you cited though that I do want to make a comment about. You made the point that when you enlarged the group involved in the β relaxation, if it was an intermolecular effect you would tend to slow the process down due to steric effects. I'd like to point out that when we substitute a larger group for a given side chain, we don't do this by taking a rigid glass and sticking in that large group, crowding it into a space that isn't big enough to fit it, but what we do is synthesize a new molecule, take it up to the liquid state where it can adjust itself to the structure in the liquid state, then we cool it down into the glassy state. Presumably a larger group simply in the course of going through this process creates around itself the kind of environment that's congenial for it, so it's a little misleading to say that if we enlarge the group we increase steric interactions.

A second point concerns the metal glasses. In various places I've made the point that although I believe the beta relaxation is a universal feature of amorphous packing, there is some evidence against my belief, and some of it had to do with metal glasses: I have mentioned that H. S. Chen had looked for a secondary relaxation in one glassy alloy and not found it in the right place for it.

There was other evidence by Eisenberg and Reich who've also looked for secondary relaxations in metal glasses, and they've found some that were very sensitive to the history of the sample. I want to mention that Chen, who was here yesterday and not here today, showed me some new results of his on the same glass that he had previously looked at. This time he had used a method of differential thermal analysis and he believes he has resolved a β relaxation in about the place the β should be. He has some explanation as to why it didn't show up in the mechanical measurements, which he didn't have time to explain to me, and I wouldn't therefore try to repeat his description of this.

One last point: I don't know whether Dr. Heijboer agrees with Dr. Struik's picture of the β relaxation as being a kind of precursor to the main glass transition. [Dr. Heijboer stated that he does not]. In other words you agree with me that *if* Struik's point were correct it *would* imply a strong intermolecular significance for the beta relaxation: we are in agreement on that.

Okay, I want to ask just one last question for my own information. In your slide showing how the mechanical stress biases things to produce the β relaxation you showed an unsymmetrical potential well: The two minima did not have the same level initially in the absence of stress. I wonder why you did that?

HEIJBOER: It might be that my verbal presentation about the effect of enlargement of a group sounded a little misleading. What I tried to make clear is that the idea generally expressed in the literature (e.g., Reference 42 of my paper), namely, that the motion of a larger group requires a larger activation energy than the motion of a smaller one, is certainly not always correct. I do not object to the idea that a larger group on being frozen in might reserve a larger free volume for its motion than a smaller one. However, when we compare poly(*tert*butyl methacrylate) (PtBuMA) with poly(methyl methacrylate) (PMMA), we see that the β maximum of PtBuMA is lower than that of PMMA. This means that the number of groups participating in the β process is smaller; however, those that participate do so with the same ease: the activation energies for the two β processes are the same.

You also made the interesting observation that an increase in pressure produces a decrease in height of the dielectric loss peak without shifting its position on the temperature axis. If an intermolecular barrier were the governing factor, I would expect a change of the temperature of the loss maximum or of the activation energy, not a decrease in height. On increasing pressure the motion of part of the groups is blocked by the decreasing free volume; those that can still move do so with the same ease. This means that the governing potential barrier is not affected and is therefore probably intramolecular in nature!

Concerning your last question, I showed an unsymmetrical potential well because this is the situation for a monosubstituted cyclohexyl ring, and it was compounds containing this ring that I studied in most detail. However, the argument is the same for a symmetrical potential well, the only difference being the temperature dependence of the relaxation strength.

THE ANOMALOUS THERMAL PROPERTIES OF GLASSES AT LOW TEMPERATURES*

R. O. Pohl

Department of Physics
Cornell University
Ithaca, New York 14853

G. L. Salinger

Department of Physics
Rensselaer Polytechnic Institute
Troy, New York 12181

In the past several years there has been an intensive effort to understand the properties of amorphous dielectrics below 1 K. At these low temperatures thermal phenomena should be dominated by the properties of long-wavelength elastic waves, which are well understood. Wavelengths λ of thermal vibrations can be found from $h\nu = kT$ and $\nu\lambda = v$, where v, the sound velocity, is a few thousand meters per second. Thus below 1 K, $\lambda \sim 1000$ Å. Since this is much larger than microscopic disorder there should be little difference between the thermal properties of amorphous and crystalline dielectrics. Experimentally there is great regularity in the behavior of a particular thermal property for all amorphous dielectrics; but this behavior is very different than that for crystalline dielectrics. For example, the specific heat c of amorphous dielectrics plotted as c/T versus T^2 is shown in FIGURE 1 below 0.7 K. In general the specific heat c can be fit to

$$c = c_1 T + c_3 T^3, \quad (1)$$

where $c_1 = 1 - 5 \times 10^{-6}$ J g^{-1}K^{-2} and c_3 is larger than is expected from acoustic measurements. The thermal conductivity Λ of a variety of amorphous dielectrics as a function of temperature[1,2] is shown on FIGURE 2. Below 1 K,

$$\Lambda = AT^{\delta}, \quad (2)$$

where $\delta = 1.9 \pm 0.1$ and $A = 3 \times 10^{-4}$ W cm^{-1} K^{-1} within a factor of 3 for all the materials. Around 10 K, there is a plateau where $\Lambda = 10^{-3}$ W cm^{-1} K^{-1} within a factor of 2 for all substances. This is in marked contrast to the behavior of crystalline dielectrics which follow a T^3 dependence below 1 K and the addition of a few parts per million of an impurity can decrease the thermal conductivity by orders of magnitude.[3]

Anomalous behavior has also been noted for amorphous dielectrics in measurements of acoustic attenuation[4] and velocity,[5] dielectric constant,[6] thermal expansion,[7] nuclear magnetic resonance[8] and optical properties.[9]

A number of models have been proposed to explain these results.[10] We will concentrate on one that invokes systems having very few levels.[11-13] The connection between these systems and the nature of the glassy state is not known.

*This work has been supported in part by the Energy Research and Development Administration under Contract No. AT(11-1) 3151, Technical Report No. COO 3151-66 and in part by the National Aeronautics and Space Administration. Grant No. NGL 33-018-003.

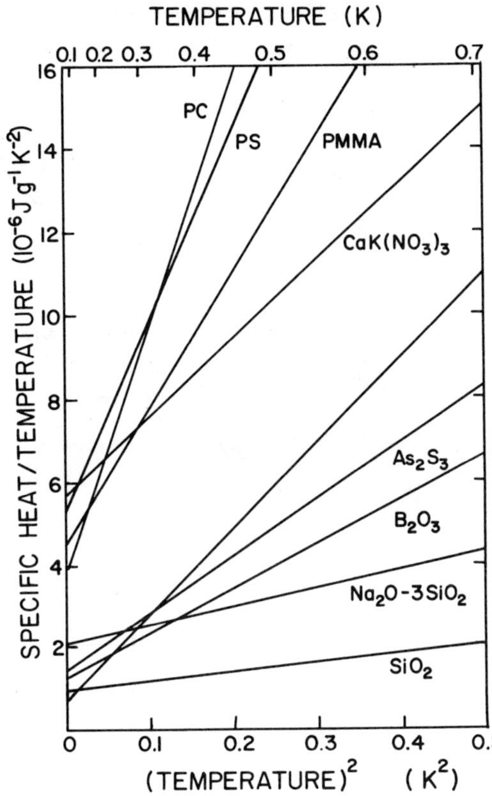

FIGURE 1. Specific heat of non-crystalline solids below 1 K plotted as c/T vs T^2. (After Stephens.[1])

In this paper we show that (a) specific heat measurements above 0.1 K indicate a distribution of local modes independent of energy; (b) ultrasonic attenuation measurements at low powers indicate that the local mode systems can have at most a few levels; (c) ultrasonic velocity measurements give information about phonon-local mode coupling parameters; (d) the measured thermal conductivity agrees with that calculated from the above information assuming that the energy independent distribution of modes observed in the specific heat is responsible for phonon scattering; (e) thermal expansion and far infrared experiments indicate a phonon assisted tunneling model; (f) several experiments, however, indicate that the modes observed in the specific heat measurements may not all scatter phonons.

Specific Heat

The specific heat of a solid is calculated from the temperature derivative of the internal energy which can be expressed as an integral of the product of the energy ϵ of the mode contributing, the number of such modes per unit energy $n(\epsilon)$, the probability that the mode is occupied $f(\epsilon/kT)$:

$$U = \int_0^{\epsilon_m} \epsilon\, n(\epsilon) f(\epsilon/kT)\, d\epsilon. \tag{3}$$

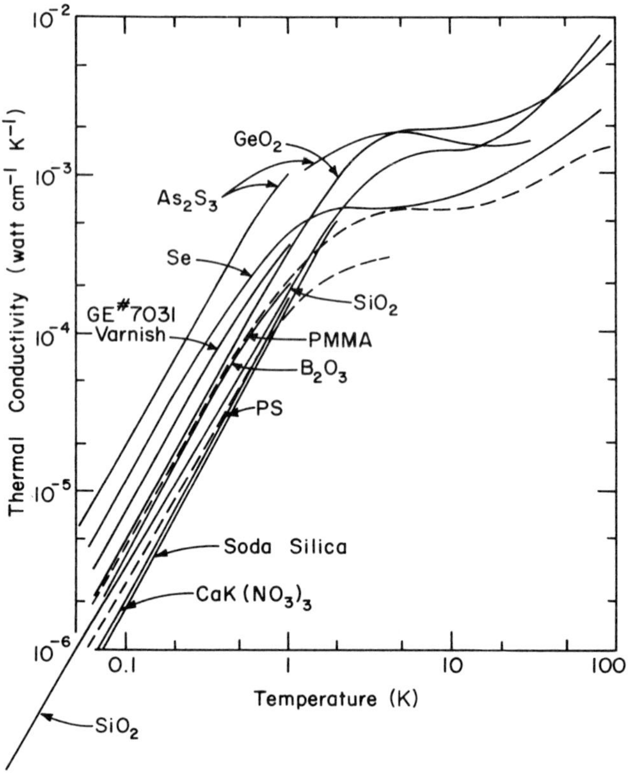

FIGURE 2. Thermal conductivity of noncrystalline solids. Note the extension of the SiO_2 data[2] to 0.025 K. (After Stephens.[1])

The upper limit of integration is usually determined by the condition that the sum of the density of states is the total number of those modes $\mathfrak{N}$ in the solid

$$\mathfrak{N} = \int_0^{\epsilon_m} n(\epsilon) d\epsilon. \tag{4}$$

However, since the distribution functions approach zero rapidly when $kT \ll \epsilon$, little error is made in replacing ϵ_m by infinity in Equation 3 when the low temperature behavior is of interest. Thus

$$U = (kT)^2 \int_0^{\infty} n(\epsilon)\, x f(x)\, \mathrm{d}x, \tag{5}$$

where $x = \epsilon/kT$. If

$$n(\epsilon) = \sum n_q \epsilon^q, \tag{6}$$

the low-temperature dependence of U depends on T^{2+q} and the specific heat is proportional to T^{1+q} since $c \propto \mathrm{d}U/\mathrm{d}T$.

The specific heats of solids below room temperature have been explained by the Debye theory[14] in which the theory for blackbody radiation developed by Planck is applied to elastic waves in homogeneous isotropic solids not necessarily crystals. The number of states per unit energy is proportional to ϵ^2 so that at low temperatures when the wavelength of the elastic wave is much longer than the microscopic disorder of the material, the specific heat c depends upon the absolute temperature cubed

$$\frac{c}{T^3} = c_{3,D} = \frac{16\pi^5 k^4}{5\hbar^3}\,\frac{1}{\rho v^3}, \tag{7}$$

where ρ is the mass density of the material and v is an average velocity of sound

$$\frac{1}{v^3} = \frac{1}{3}\left(\frac{1}{v_l^3} + \frac{2}{v_t^3}\right). \tag{8}$$

Here l and t refer to the longitudinal and transverse polarizations respectively. As shown, below 1 K, $\lambda > 1000$ Å; thus the specific heat of any material should be proportional to T^3 below 1 K, the magnitude depends upon the velocity of sound and the density of the material. We have avoided the common formulation using

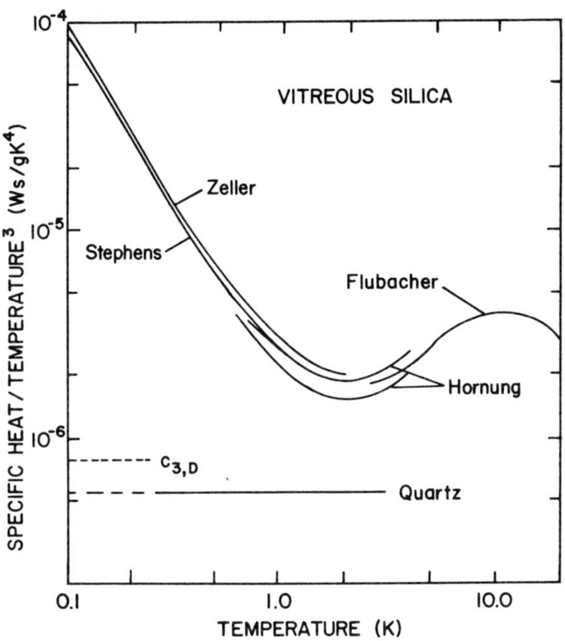

FIGURE 3. Specific heat of crystalline and vitreous SiO_2 plotted as c/T^3 vs T to show deviation from the Debye T^3 law. The line marked quartz was measured by Zeller and Pohl[16] and the dashed line represents the value of c/T^3 calculated from elastic measurements. The dashed line $c_{3,D}$ is the Debye contribution to the specific heat of vitreous silica calculated through Equation 7 (Reference 14). The curves represent specific heat measurements on different samples of vitreous silica, Stephens,[1] Zeller,[16] Flubacher,[17] and Hornung.[18]

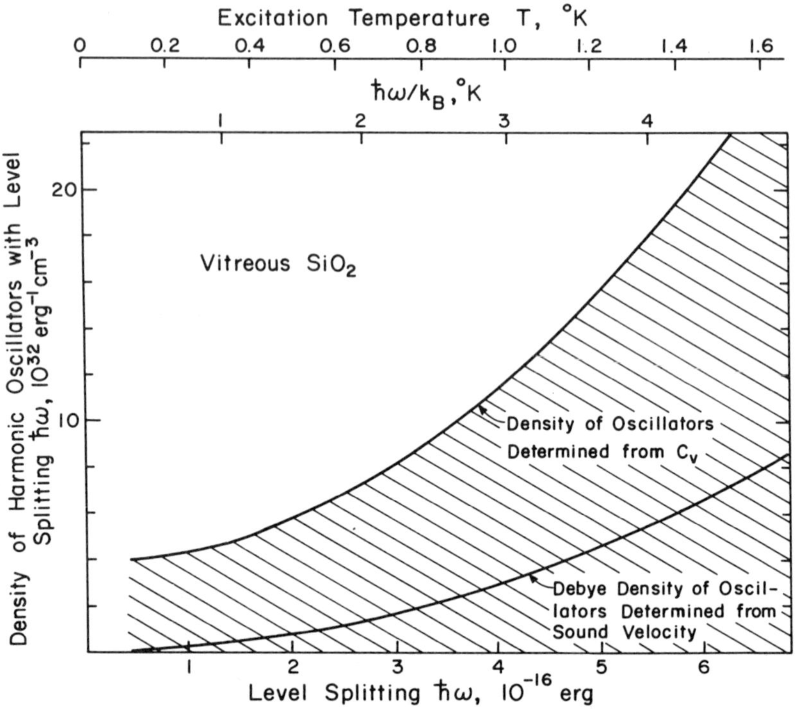

FIGURE 4. Density of states for SiO_2 glass. The experimental density of states, derived from specific heat measurements, was calculated under the assumption that the excess states are harmonic oscillators, as are phonons. If the systems consisted of two levels, their density of states would be twice as large. Systems with energy level spacing Δ are frozen out at $\Delta/kT = \frac{1}{3}$, so, for instance, all the states up to $\Delta/k = 1$ K are involved in the specific heat at $\frac{1}{3}$K. The top scale on this figure shows the temperature at which a system with energy level spacing Δ becomes thermally excited. (After Stephens.[1])

the Debye temperature θ because of ambiguities in defining θ for polyatomic noncrystalline solids.[15]

A plot of c/T^3 versus T is shown on FIGURE 3 for crystalline quartz. The results are typical for a large variety of crystalline materials, in which the calorimetrically measured specific heat is accurately determined by sound velocity measurements through Equation 7. For crystalline quartz[16] $c/T^3 = 5.5 \times 10^{-7}$ W s g^{-1} K^{-4} and $\bar{v} = 4.4 \times 10^5$ cm s^{-1}.

Data for the specific heat of vitreous silica,[17,18] also plotted on FIGURE 3, are typical for a great variety of amorphous solids. Above 1 K, c/T^3 has a hump that was attributed to discrete oscillations that could be identified from prominent peaks in the Raman spectrum.[17,18] More recently the specific heat of crystobalite,[19] a crystalline form of silica, was found to vary in the same way as vitreous silica. Neutron diffraction studies show a low frequency transverse acoustic mode.[20] In analogy with the more complex neutron diffraction and specific heat studies of GeO_2,[19] it is argued that the hump in c/T^3 above 1 K is due to a modification of the crystalline density of states. An indication of the universality of an increased density of low-frequency states in amorphous solids comes from electron tunneling experiments in amorphous metal films.[10] There is much interesting science to be learned in trying to explain the hump in c/T^3 above 1 K, and to correlate it with data on thermal expansion, internal friction, dielectric constants, nuclear magnetic resonance, and optical spectroscopy experiments. However, we turn our attention to the temperature range below 1 K.

Below 1 K the deviation of the specific heat from the Debye value increases until below 0.2 K the calorimetrically measured specific heat is more than an order of magnitude greater than the Debye prediction. As shown in FIGURE 1 these data are typical for all amorphous materials and can be described in Equation 1 with $c_3 > c_{3,D}$. Thus as shown in FIGURE 4 from Equation 6,

$$n(\epsilon) = n_0 + (n_2' + n_{2,D})\epsilon^2, \tag{9}$$

where $n_{2,D}$ is the Debye distribution of states. The coefficient n_0 implies that some number of states per unit energy is independent of energy. The value for n_0 depends upon the model chosen but seems to have a value in the range of 4–25 × 10^{32} $\text{erg}^{-1}\ \text{cm}^{-3}$ or about $10^{17}\ \text{cm}^{-3}$ up to 1.5 K.

The models to explain these effects fall into two classes. One depends on lack of long-range order mainly through variations in density.[10] These models are attractive because a crystalline solid should have a more uniform density than an amorphous one. However, the theories usually involve parameters that are not

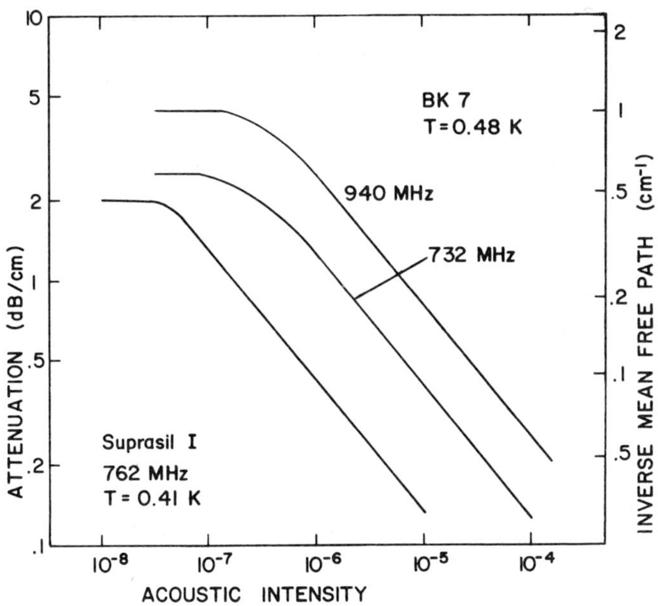

FIGURE 5. Ultrasonic attenuation of borosilicate and SiO_2 glass as a function of acoustic intensity. The inverse mean free path is that due to the two-level system only. At power levels below 10^{-7} W/cm^2 the inverse mean free path is constant and for the borosilicate glass glass varies as ω^2; i.e., $(940/732)^2 = 1.67 = 1/0.6$. At powers above 10^{-7} W/cm^2 the attenuation is proportional to the square root of the power in agreement with theory.[4] (After Arnold *et al.*[4])

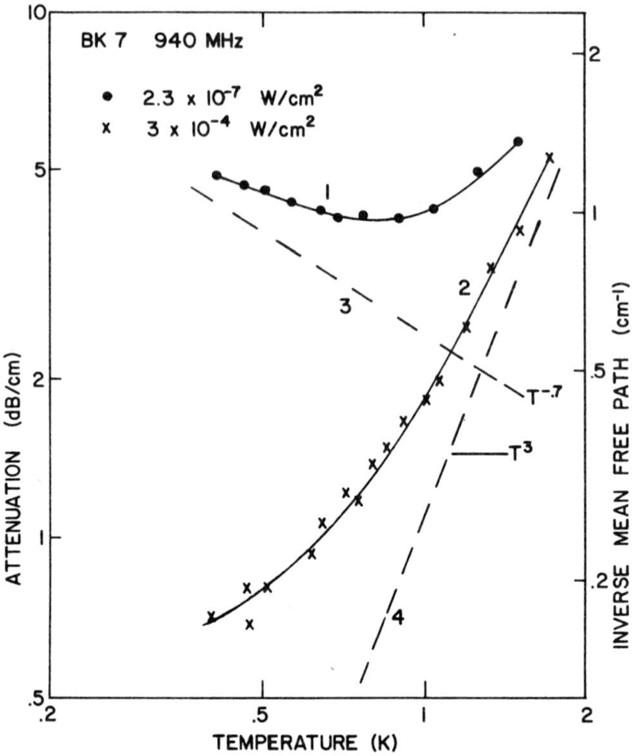

FIGURE 6. Temperature dependence of the ultrasonic attenuation of borosilicate glass at 940 MHz at two different powers. The full circles show the attenuation in the almost unsaturated region and the increase in this attenuation below 0.6 K is clearly seen. The triangles show the saturated attenuation approaching a constant value of 0.6 dB/cm^2. Curve 3 was obtained by subtracting curve 2 from curve 1. Curve 4 was obtained by subtracting 0.6 dB/cm^2 from curve 2. The T^3 dependence of curve 4 is due to relaxation of the two level systems as described in the text. (From Arnold *et al.*[4] By permission of the *Journal of Non-Crystalline Solids.*)

easily experimentally accessible. The other group of models invokes a distribution of localized modes.[10] Of these the one receiving the most attention is the phonon-assisted tunneling model.[11-13] In this model it is assumed that because of the morphology of the system a group of atoms may have more than one equilibrium position that does not necessarily significantly increase the internal energy of the system. At low temperature the atoms do not have enough energy to surmount the barriers between configurations and they tunnel from one configuration to the other with the small energy difference made up by lattice vibrations. In its simplest form one can ignore the tunneling aspect of the model and just assume a local density of modes having a few discrete levels. Evidence for this model comes from ultrasonic attenuation experiments.

Ultrasonic Experiments

The attenuation of gigahertz sound waves is plotted in FIGURE 5 as a function of power level parametrized by frequency.[4] At very low powers the attenuation is constant. As the power is increased over a few orders of magnitude the attenuation decreases and the mean free path increases by an order of magnitude. This decrease in attenuation can be explained[11-13] if the local modes are assumed to consist of very few levels so that at higher powers the populations of the levels can be equalized leading to no net energy removed from the ultrasonic wave. Thus the mean free path increases. This is the same process as saturating a nuclear magnetic resonance signal.

The calculation for the acoustic attenuation of phonons resonantly scattered by local mode systems is very similar to the calculation of resonance absorption in the case of dielectric or anelastic relaxation. In our case, at low powers the acoustic beam causes periodic deformations of the two-level system, which perturbs the energy of the system. (For ease a two-level system is considered rather than a multi-level system.) The periodic perturbation causes transitions as outlined in quantum mechanics[21]:

$$\tau^{-1} = \frac{2\pi}{\hbar} \mid H_{ij} \mid^2 \rho(\omega). \tag{10}$$

The matrix element is given by

$$H_{ij} = \left(\frac{\hbar\omega}{2\rho v^2}\right)^{1/2} M, \tag{11}$$

where M is the coupling energy between the phonon and the two-level system. The density of available states $\rho(\omega)$ for a two-level system is $n_0 \tanh \hbar\omega/2kT$. The inverse mean free path is $l^{-1} = (\tau v)^{-1}$ so that

$$l_\nu^{-1} = \frac{\pi n_0 M_\nu^2}{\rho v_\nu^3} \omega \tanh \frac{\hbar\omega}{2kT}, \tag{12}$$

where the subscript ν refers to the polarization of the sound wave. Even at these low temperatures for gigahertz ultrasonic experiments $\hbar\omega \ll kT$ so that $l^{-1} \propto \omega^2/T$. The ω^2 dependence is seen in FIGURE 5 and in FIGURE 6 we see that $l_\nu^{-1} \propto T^{-0.7}$ at low temperatures and only for power levels below 10^{-7} W/cm^2.

The above discussion assumes that the occupation number of the levels is independent of the sound wave amplitude and depends only upon thermal excitations. Those conditions obtain only at low power levels. At higher powers transitions to the upper state occur at a faster rate than decays to the lower state, effectively saturating the two-level system and leading to increased mean free paths.

There is, however, a competing relaxation mechanism.[11-13] The sound wave compresses part of the solid and expands other parts. The two-level systems attempt to maintain thermal equilibrium with their surroundings by exchanging energy irreversibly with the sound wave. This process does not saturate and in the low temperature limit the inverse mean free path is proportional to T^3 and independent of frequency. This explains the curves in FIGURE 6.

The same authors have measured the variation in longitudinally and transversely polarized sound velocity[5] as a function of frequency and temperature using

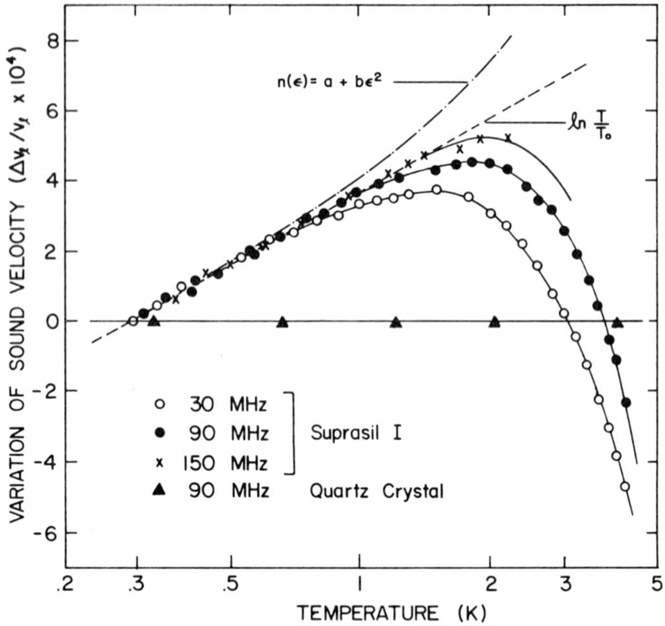

FIGURE 7. Relative variation of the longitudinal sound velocity $\Delta v_l/v_l$ plotted as a function of the temperature on a logarithmic scale. The straight line represents a variation proportional to ln T. The solid lines represent the theoretical prediction for the sum of the contribution of the resonant and the relaxation process, the latter dominating above 0.6 K. The dash-dot line represents the contribution of the resonant interaction alone assuming $n(\epsilon) = n_0 + n_2'\epsilon^2$. The filled triangles show the variation for crystalline silica. (From Piché *et al.*[5] By permission of *Physical Review Letters.*)

powers of 10^{-3} W/cm^2. Their results for $\Delta v/v \times 10^4$ are shown in FIGURE 7. Also shown is the behavior of a quartz crystal in which $\Delta v/v = 0$. Using the Kramers-Kronig relation the variation of the sound velocity can be related to the sound absorption α:

$$\left(\frac{\Delta v}{v}\right)_\nu = P\int_0^\infty d\omega' \, \frac{c}{\pi} \, \frac{\alpha(\omega' T) - \alpha(\omega' T_0)}{\omega^2 - \omega'^2}, \tag{13}$$

and

$$\alpha_\nu(\omega T) = \pi \, \frac{n_0 M_\nu^2}{\rho v_\nu^3} \, \omega \tanh \frac{\hbar\omega}{2kT}. \tag{14}$$

Therefore

$$\left(\frac{\Delta v}{v}\right)_\nu = \frac{n_0 M_\nu^2}{\rho v_\nu^2} \ln \frac{T}{T_0}, \tag{15}$$

where T_0 is a reference temperature. The decreasing part of the $\Delta v/v$ curve can be obtained from the relaxation measurements described above. The quantity $n_0 M_\nu^2$ is the coupling between the sound wave and the two-level systems, $n_0 M_l^2 \sim 2.6 \times$

10^8 erg cm^{-3} and $n_0 M_t^2 \sim 1.2 \times 10^8$ erg cm^{-3} for borosilicate glass. From specific heat experiments $n_0 = 8 \times 10^{-32}$ erg^{-1} cm^{-3}; therefore $M_l \sim 0.35$ eV and $M_t = 0.24$ eV. That is, longitudinal and transverse phonons couple equally well to the two-level systems. Results for silica are very similar. This large value of the deformation potential also means a large Gruneisen parameter.

The change in velocity of light in silica and borosilicate glasses was determined[6] through measurement of the temperature dependence of the dielectric constant by monitoring the shift in resonance frequency of a microwave cavity partially filled with the sample. The results are similar to the above with a bigger difference between borosilicate and SiO_2 glasses as shown on FIGURE 8. The relevant parameter is $n_0 p^2$, where p is the dipole moment. Using n_0 from specific heat experiments, p is about 0.3 D for SiO_2 and 0.66 D for borosilicate glass assuming the same value for n_0. It appears that different units are responsible for the motion in each of these materials. Since a Debye unit is 10^{-18} esu cm, 0.3 D corresponds to one electronic charge moving 0.06 Å. Thus the low value of the dipole moment precludes the motion of single atoms for which p would be higher.

Thermal Conductivity

In general the thermal conductivity can be expressed in the kinetic form by

$$K = \tfrac{1}{3}\int c(\omega)v(\omega)\ell(\omega)\,d\omega, \qquad \textbf{(16)}$$

where $c(\omega)$ is the specific heat per unit frequency range for those modes which have

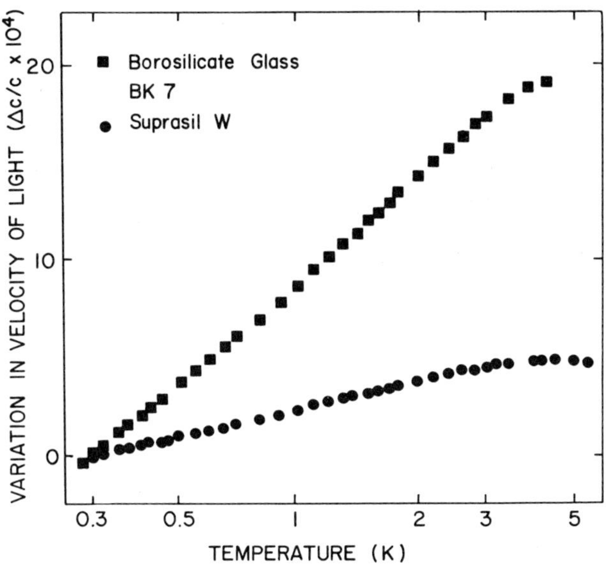

FIGURE 8. Relative variation of the velocity of light $\Delta c/c$ at 1.1 GHz in borosilicate and SiO_2 glass plotted versus temperature. The proportionality constant relating $\Delta c/c$ to ln T/T_0 is different for the two materials leading to different dipole mements. (From von Schickfus *et al.*[6] By permission of *Physical Review Letters*.)

a group velocity $v(\omega)$. Those of the modes that have a zero group velocity act as scattering centers and hence decrease $\ell(\omega)$. The two-level systems have no group velocity; thus we use the Debye expression for $c(\omega)$ and the mean free path as calculated from ultrasonic measurements.[19] At the low temperatures we only need the resonant scattering. In this case

$$\Lambda = \frac{\rho k^3 T^2}{6\pi^3\hbar^2}\left(\frac{v_l}{n_0 M_l^2} + 2\,\frac{v_t}{n M_t^2}\right)\int_0^\infty \frac{x^3 e^x(e^x + 1)}{(e^x - 1)^3}\,dx. \qquad \textbf{(17)}$$

All the quantities are known and the integral is just a number. At 0.2 K, $\Lambda = 1.1 \times 10^{-5}$ W/cm K and Zaitlin and Anderson[22] find 9×10^{-6} W/cm K for borosilicate glass. They also find that they can reproduce the entire thermal conductivity curve including the plateau at 10 K if they use the nonresonant scattering and let $n(\epsilon) = n_0 + n_2'\epsilon^2$ as required by the specific heat measurements. Their results for SiO_2 and borosilicate glass are quite good. For the polymer polymethyl methacrylate (PMMA) and for GeO_2 their results are not as encouraging.

Thus all these experiments, the specific heat, ultrasonic attenuation, sound velocity, dielectric constant, and thermal conductivity appear to be explained by a uniform distribution of two level systems.

Thermal Expansion

The original models for these systems ascribed the two levels to phonon-assisted tunneling between two configurations of groups of atoms having about the same energy.[11-13] The energy separation of the two levels was $\epsilon = (\Delta^2 + \Delta_0^2)^{1/2}$ where Δ_0 is the tunnel splitting for the symmetric case

$$\Delta_0 = h\Omega\sqrt{\sigma/\pi}\,e^{-\sigma} \qquad \textbf{(18)}$$

where $\sigma \propto d\sqrt{V}$ and $h\Omega \sim 10^{-2}$ eV, and ϵ is the energy difference between the ground states of the two wells. These quantities are defined in the inset of FIGURE 9. Up to now we have not needed any property of the tunneling to explain the results.

Recently White[7] has measured the linear thermal expansion α of SiO_2 down to 1.5 K and finds that $-\alpha/T^3$ increases dramatically at the lowest temperatures as shown in FIGURE 9. Similar preliminary measurements have been performed on PMMA and in that case $+\alpha/T^3$ increases at low temperature.[23] The thermal expansion is related to the specific heat by $\alpha = \gamma c\rho/3B$ where B is the bulk modulus, ρ is the density, and γ the Gruneisen parameter. γ is defined by

$$\gamma = -\frac{\partial \ln \omega}{\partial \ln V}. \qquad \textbf{(19)}$$

For SiO_2, γ is about -40 and for PMMA, γ is about $+40$ where $c = c_1 T$ only.

One can explain the large positive Gruneisen parameters for PMMA by noticing that as the temperature decreases the wells come closer together. Thus both V and d decrease slightly, but the tunneling frequency increases steeply because V and d appear in the exponent. The same explanation suffices for SiO_2 because when the temperature is lowered the SiO_2 lattice expands. Thus the wells get further apart and the tunneling frequency decreases and α/T^3 becomes more negative. Similar large expansion coefficients were found for OH^--doped NaCl in which it is known that the OH^- tunnels between equivalent potential minima in the Cl^-

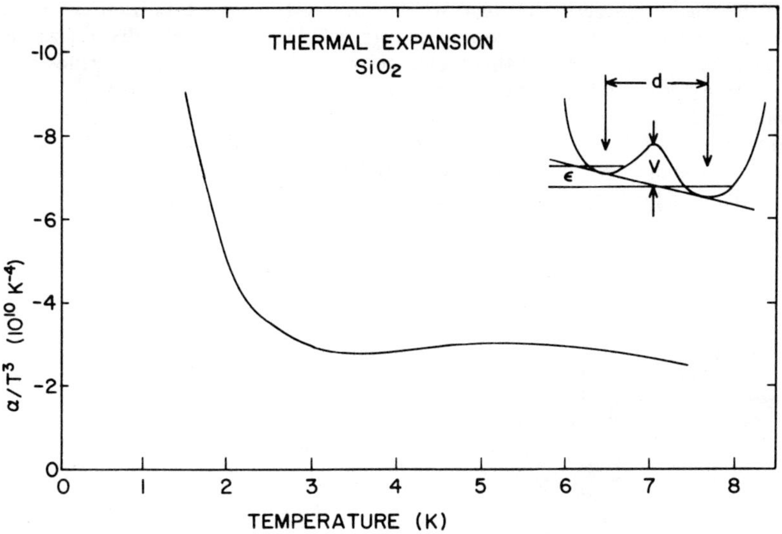

FIGURE 9. The thermal expansion α of vitreous silica plotted as α/T^3 vs T. Note that the thermal expansion of SiO_2 is negative over the entire region. The increase in the magnitude of α/T^3 may be due to phonon assisted tunneling the model for which is shown in the inset. A particle or group of particles may be in two states separated by a distance d and a barrier height V. The energy of the system in the two states differs by a small amount ϵ. At low temperatures the particles can get from one state to the other by tunneling through the barrier with the energy made up by the phonons.[11-13] (From White *et al.*[7] By permission of *Physical Review Letters*.)

vacancy.[24] However, in our case a two level system would suffice if the level spacing somehow depended upon the distance between wells.

Far-Infrared Studies

For several years, Sievers and his students have looked for evidence of the low energy states in far-infrared absorption. Recently, Mon and Chabal succeeded in measuring the optical absorption in four amorphous materials, GeO_2, PMMA, and two pieces of SiO_2 containing different amounts of water.[9] The data obtained at 4.2 K are shown in FIGURE 10. At first sight, the spectra show little similarity, and are strongly sample dependent, as evidenced in curves C and D for SiO_2. It turns out, however, that all spectra have a very characteristic temperature dependence in common, which is shown in FIGURE 11. Mon and Chabal measured the absorption between 1.2 and 4.2 K, for PMMA even between 0.54 K and 10 K. In their paper,[9] Mon *et al.* show that a straightforward description of this temperature and frequency dependence can be achieved with a level diagram as shown in FIGURE 12b. Each absorbing center consists of three states, two of which are closely spaced ($r\hbar\omega$, $r \sim 0.05$) relative to the spacing of the third state ($\hbar\omega$). The optical absorption is assumed to take place only between the states labeled 1 and 2. The temperature and frequency dependence results from the thermal population of the three states. At low frequencies (<6 cm^{-1}), an increase in temperature causes a decrease in absorption, since state 2 becomes increasingly more populated, while at higher frequencies, state 2 remains thermally depopulated. The increase in absorption in this frequency range results from a thermal population of state 1, out of which the absorption takes place.

The optical absorption and the model used to describe it shows a great deal of resemblance with that of alkali halide crystals doped with certain impurities known to tunnel between certain equivalent potential wells within the lattice site they occupy.[3] There the closely spaced states result from tunneling, while the wide

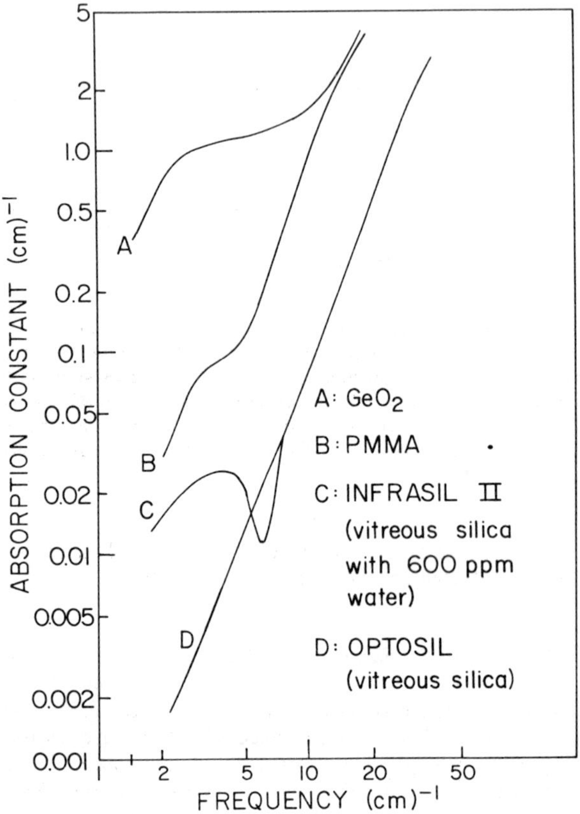

FIGURE 10. Absorption coefficient versus frequency for four different glasses at 4.2 K. (From Mon *et al.*[9] By permission of *Physical Review Letters*.)

spacing is caused by oscillator states. A spectroscopic study of the temperature dependence of absorption in several tunnel systems, e.g., KCl:Li, NaCl:OH, has been made by Kirby *et al.*[25] Guided by this similarity, Mon *et al.* argue that their observations in the amorphous materials result from similar tunneling and oscillator states, except that in the amorphous materials the splittings $\hbar\omega$ (and $r\hbar\omega$) are spread over a wide frequency range, possibly with a constant density of states $n(\epsilon)$ equal to that derived from the linear specific heat anomaly discussed earlier.

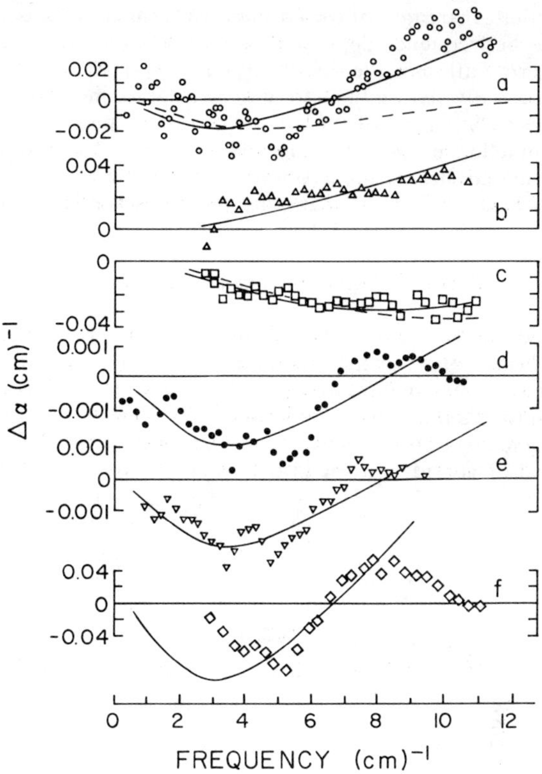

FIGURES 11. Changes in absorption coefficient with temperature versus frequency. The dots represent the experimental data, the dashed line the two-level model, and the solid line the three-level model. (a) PMMA: $\alpha(4.2\text{ K}) - \alpha(1.2\text{ k})$; $r = 1/20$. (b) PMMA: $\alpha(0.97\text{ K}) - \alpha(0.55\text{ K})$. (c) PMMA: $\alpha(8.68\text{ K}) - \alpha(4.25\text{ K})$. (d) SiO_2 (with 600 ppm H_2O): $\alpha(4.2\text{ K}) - \alpha(1.2\text{ K})$; $r = 1/40$. (e) SiO_2 (water free): $\alpha(4.2\text{ K}) - \alpha(1.2\text{ K})$; $r = 1/40$. (f) GeO_2: $\alpha(4.2\text{ K}) - \alpha(1.2\text{ K})$; $r = 1/20$. (From Mon *et al.*[9] By permission of *Physical Review Letters*.)

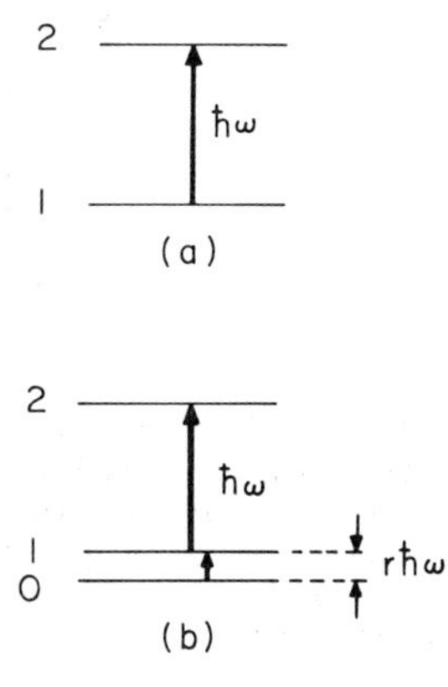

FIGURE 12. Two models of far-infrared absorption by the low energy states: (a) two-level, (b) three-level. The far-infrared transition is labeled $\hbar\omega$. (From Mon *et al.*[9] By permission of *Physical Review Letters*.)

Since the oscillator strength of the far infrared transition $\hbar\omega$ is not known, and since it may also be frequency dependent, the optical data cannot be used for an independent determination of the density of states $n(\epsilon)$. In amorphous substances $n(\epsilon)$ is therefore usually determined from specific heat measurements. FIGURE 4 shows an analysis by Stephens of the low-temperature specific heat of amorphous SiO_2.[1] In the tunneling model[11-13] proposed to explain the low energy states in glasses, it is postulated that the states observed in specific heat are also responsible for the phonon scattering. This we want to explore in some detail in the following.

Thermal Conductivity in an Electric Field

In an applied electric field E, tunneling defects in crystalline solids become polarized,[3] and hence, their energy splitting will change. Resonant scattering of phonons by these states will, consequently, move to a different frequency.[3] Stephens looked for a similar effect in glasses.[26] We have seen above that the thermal conductivity measurement, as well as the temperature and frequency dependence of the speed of sound and the real part of the dielectric constant (i.e., the

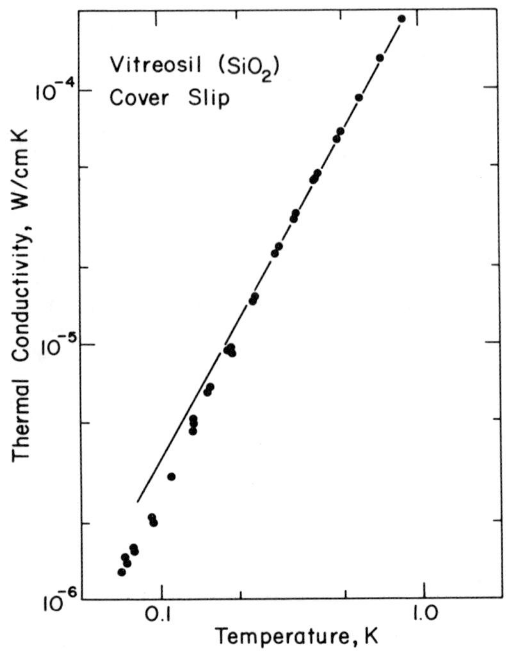

FIGURE 13. Thermal conductivity of the vitreosil high electric field sample in zero field. The vertical scale was determined by comparison to previous thermal conductivity measurements on the same material (solid line). The deviation below 0.2 K is due to the thermal resistance of an indium-glass interface, which was included in the measurement since the cold thermometer was soldered to the heat sink rather than separately to the glass. (After Stephens.[26])

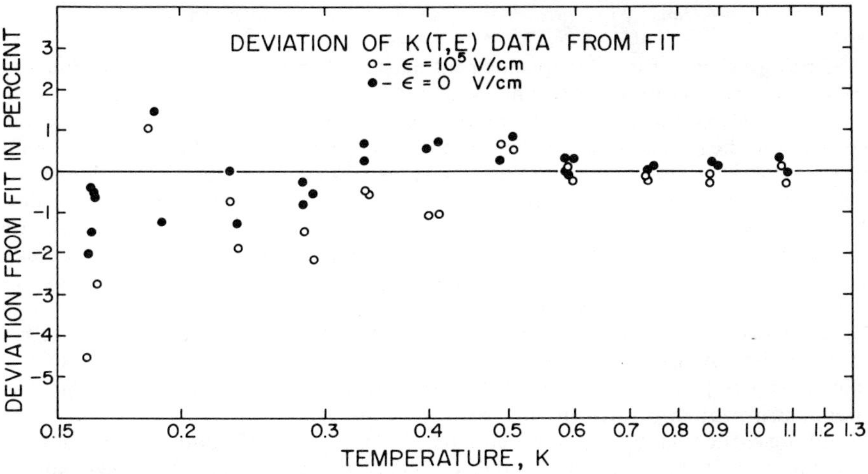

FIGURE 14. Thermal conductivity of the vitreosil high electric field sample plotted as the percentage deviation from a polynomial fit. The filled circles are the data for $E = 0$, the open circles are the data for $E = 10^5$ V/cm. (After Stephens.[26])

speed of electromagnetic waves in the medium) can be interpreted with the assumption of a constant density of states of the tunneling defects. The density of states derived from specific heat measurements, however, shows a nonlinear contribution (approximately proportional to ϵ^2) in the frequency range of interest for heat conduction below 1 K (FIGURE 4). Hence, Stephens argued as follows: If the density of states of tunneling defects is indeed constant, then an electric field will not alter the density of states $n(\epsilon, E)$ at a certain energy ϵ, since the number of states removed by the field E will equal that of the states whose frequency will be changed to ϵ by the field. Hence, regardless of the magnitude of the dipole moment of the tunneling defects, the thermal conductivity $\Lambda(T, E)$ should be field independent. Stephens measured $\Lambda(T, E)$ of a thin plate of silica with and without an applied field of 10^5 volt/cm (FIGURES 13 and 14). He analyzed the null effect observed in two ways: Using the dipole moment determined by Schickfus *et al.*,[6] he concluded that the density of the phonon scattering states had to be constant to within 6% over the range of frequencies carrying the bulk of the heat in the temperature range of his measurement (0.16 to 1.1 K, corresponding to the range of frequencies $\nu = \omega/2\pi = 10^{10}$ to 7×10^{10} sec^{-1}). In this range, the density of states obtained from specific heat (FIGURE 4) actually varies by a factor of two. Alternatively, Stephens could derive an upper limit for the dipole moment assuming that the density of the states which cause the phonon scattering was actually given by $n(\epsilon)$ determined from the specific heat. In that case, the density of states should vary with the applied field, and hence the absence of an effect of E on Λ could be used to determine an upper limit of the dipole moment of the tunneling states. Under this assumption, Stephens found an upper limit of the dipole moment in SiO_2 of 0.1 D = 0.02 eÅ (local field corrected), smaller than the value determined by Schickfus *et al.*[6] by a factor of three, and unreasonably small for tunneling atoms or even silicon oxide molecules.

Density of States from Specific Heat Measurements

The question whether the specific heat density of states $n(\epsilon)$ is equal to that responsible for the phonon scattering, as postulated in the tunneling model, was also studied by Goubau and Tait.[27] Since the tunneling frequency, and hence the coupling to the lattice should depend greatly on the barrier height, one of the first predictions of the tunneling model of glasses[11-13] was that the observed specific heat should be dependent on the time during which the measurement was performed. For short times, only the strongly coupled tunneling states can take up energy from the lattice, and hence the specific heat should appear smaller. Goubau and Tait were unable to detect such an effect even when the sample dimensions were chosen such that the heat could propagate through the sample in times of the order of 10^{-5} sec. FIGURE 15 shows the data obtained on polymethyl methacrylate. Although the tunneling model can probably be modified in such a way as to be brought into agreement with this result, the explanation of the discrepancy is probably much simpler, as well be discussed next.

In the earlier studies of the specific heat anomaly of amorphous dielectrics, no evidence was found that it was sample dependent. Hence, the theoretical model was designed with the assumption that the anomaly (as well as the thermal conductivity) is independent of the particular sample. A systematic study by Stephens, however, has turned up evidence that this conclusion was premature, at least as far as the specific heat anomaly is concerned.[28] FIGURE 16 shows the specific heat of

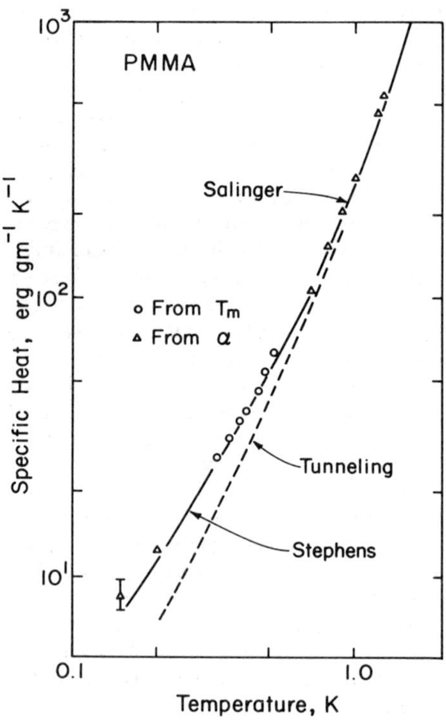

FIGURE 15. The specific heat of polymethyl methacrylate as measured on both long (5 sec) and short (50 μsec) time scales. The closed circles are short-time data determined from the thermal diffusivity α. The open circles are short-time data determined from the maximum amplitude, ΔT_m, of the heat-pulse signal at the bolometer. The dashed line is the tunneling-model prediction.[11-13] The solid line is the long-time data for PMMA from Stephens *et al.*[35]

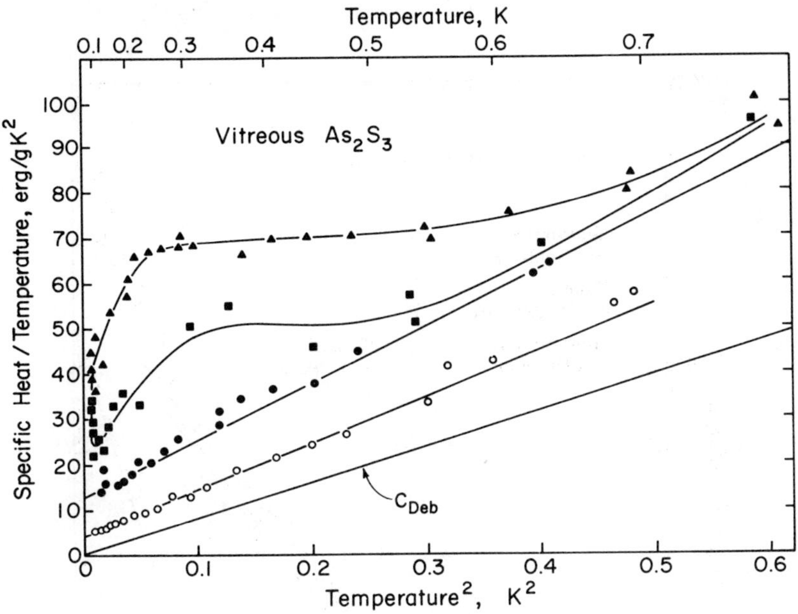

FIGURE 16. Specific heat of four As_2S_3 samples plotted as c/T vs T^2. The line marked C_{Deb} is the heat capacity predicted by the Debye model. The two upper curves are from samples which were produced at Cornell with successively more care to remove water of hydration. The next curve is from a sample that was supplied by A. J. Leadbetter. The lowest set of data is from a sample that was made by F. J. DiSalvo at Bell Labs. If one assumes that the differences between the upper three and lowest sets of data are due to the presence of two-level systems, one can calculate the density of these systems to be 68×10^{16} cm^{-3} for the upper curve, 26×10^{16} for the second one, and $\sim 10^{16}$ cm^{-3} for the third. Spark source mass spec analysis of the four measured samples showed the following impurity concentrations in the order given above: (1) 10^{19} to 10^{20} cm^{-3} Sb and 10^{17} to 10^{18} cm^{-3} Rb; (2) 10^{17} to 10^{18} cm^{-3} and 10^{16} to 10^{17} cm^{-3} Cd; (3) 10^{17} to 10^{18} cm^{-3} Ge; (4) nothing detectable. (After Stephens.[28])

amorphous As_2S_3. With increasing sample purity and/or perfection, a Schottky type anomaly disappears in As_2S_3, as does an anomaly beginning below 0.1 K, leaving an anomaly of the usual form (closed circles). Further care in producing the sample (chemical purity and/or physical perfection?), however, makes this anomaly shrink by more than a factor of two (open circles). The thermal conductivity of the latter two samples, however, differs by less than 20% (and even this difference is believed to be the result of the poor definition of the geometry of the sample[28]). Similar results were found for B_2O_3[2,8,29] and the ionic glass CaK $(NO_3)_3$[28]. In these glasses, a reduction of the anomalous specific heat results in zero change of the thermal conductivity. Consequently, the entire removable portion of the specific heat anomaly apparently does not scatter phonons. Whether all or at least part of the excitations causing the excess specific heat in the sample with the lowest specific heat scatter phonons, has to be left as an open question. Recently, the specific heat of amorphous solids was measured for the first time to temperatures well below 0.1 K.[2] The results obtained on several samples of SiO_2 are shown in

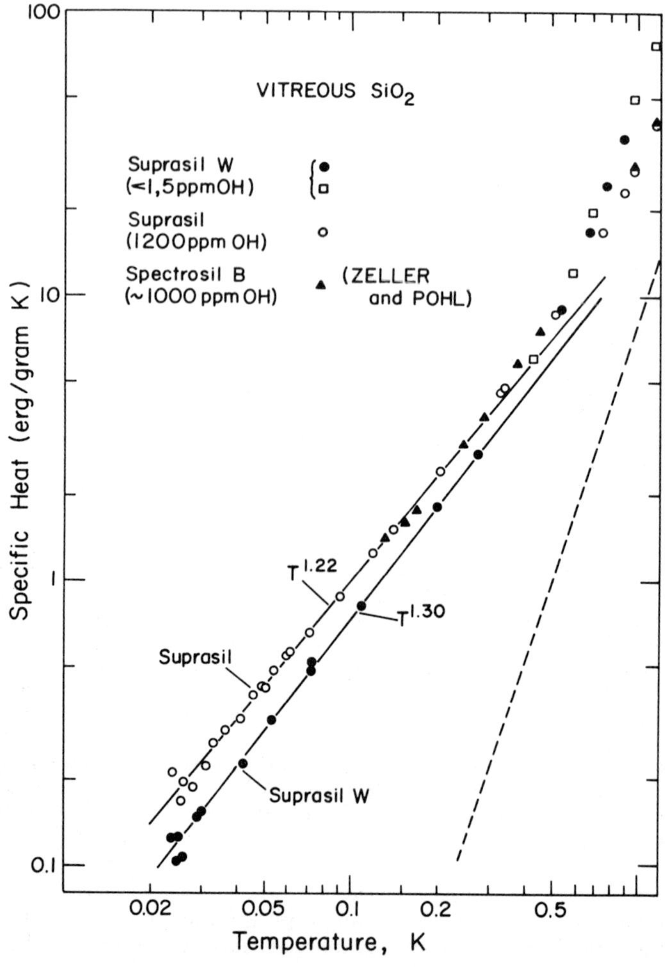

FIGURE 17. Specific heat of vitreous SiO_2 above 0.025 K, Suprasil and Spectrosil B have large OH^- concentrations, but small metal ion concentrations. Suprasil has 130 ppm chlorine and 100 ppm fluorine. Suprasil W has low OH^- and metal ion concentrations, but 230 ppm chlorine and 290 ppm fluorine (all numbers according to the manufacturer). Note that Spectrosil B and Suprasil have identical specific heats in the temperature range where both were measured ($T > 0.1$ K). Note also that SiO_2 with low OH^-, but high (~50 ppm) metal ion concentrations has been found to have lower specific heats than Spectrosil B above 0.5 K; this difference, however, vanishes below that temperature.[36] The dashed line marks the Debye specific heat of vitreous SiO_2, $C_{Deb} = 8\ T^3$ erg gm $^{-1}$ K $^{-4}$ based on $v_t = 3.75 \times 10^5$ cm/sec and $v_l = 5.80 \times 10^5$ cm/sec. (After Lasjaunias *et al.*[2])

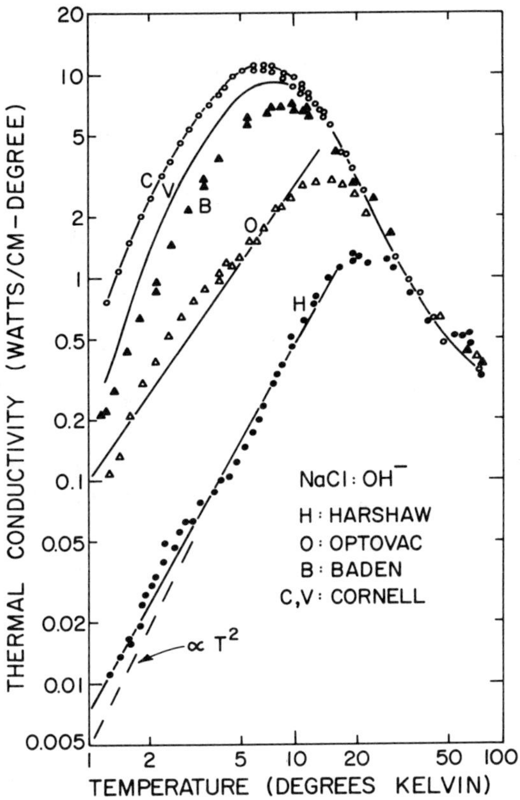

FIGURE 18. Thermal conductivity of commercial NaCl crystals from Harshaw and Optovac compared with a natural crystal of Baden halite and two Cornell-grown crystals. The dashed line varies as T^2. (After Klein.[30])

FIGURE 17. In addition to the sample dependence, the low-temperature data also show the limits to what is called the "linear specific heat anomaly," as inferred from the data obtained above 0.1 K (FIGURE 17, see the data by Zeller and Pohl[16]). It is important to realize, though, that the thermal conductivity of SiO_2 was found to be entirely sample independent.[2]

We are thus lead to the conclusion that at best only a fraction of the states seen in specific heat measurements are caused by the postulated tunneling states, and hence the specific heat results, which played such a major role in the formulation of the tunneling model,[11-13] have to be viewed with caution. On the other hand, we have at present no reason to believe that the thermal conductivity of amorphous solids is not truly intrinsic. It is most easily explained with the assumption of a highly constant density of states of scattering centers. [See the work on $\Lambda(T, E)$,[26] and both the ultrasonic and the dielectric work by the Grenoble group[4-6] lends strong support to the picture of a constant density of highly anharmonic states of low energy in all amorphous solids.] Finally, the far-infrared absorption measurements in Sievers's group[9] provide probably the most direct resemblance between

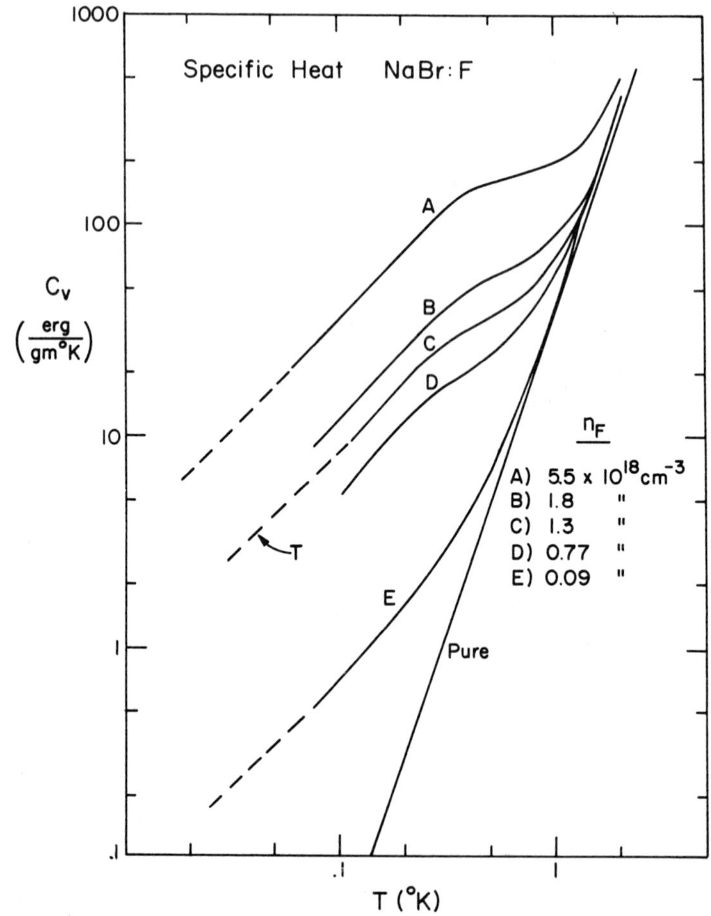

FIGURE 19. Specific heat of NaBr containing different amounts of NaF in solid solution. The dashed lines vary as T. (After Rollefson.[32])

these states and the tunneling-oscillator states studied extensively in crystalline solids containing certain defects. This raises the interesting question whether an "amorphous" thermal conductivity, and/or a linear specific heat anomaly can also exist in sufficiently disordered crystalline solids. FIGURE 18 shows the discovery of phonon scattering by tunneling defects in an alkalide halide host crystal, NaCl, by Klein.[30] The thermal conductivity decreases with increasing impurity concentration (identified since as the tunneling OH^- ion.[31]) The phonon scattering was explained by Sussmann[21] as resulting from resonance scattering by tunneling defects. Sussmann argued that the conductivity varied roughly as T^2 in the highly doped crystal, from which he concluded that the density of states $n(\epsilon)$ had to be constant, in a manner identical to that postulated later in glasses.[11-13] The specific heat of NaCl:OH has actually never been measured. In subsequent studies of more carefully doped NaCl:OH crystals it has been found, however, that $\Lambda(T)$ shows a far more pronounced structure than shown in FIGURE 18. From these findings it followed that the density of states of the tunneling defects in this material is really not very constant. Rather, all the OH^- ions in NaCl have fairly equal level schemes, similar to those of the other well-known tunneling defects,[3] e.g., KCl:CN or KCl:Li.

A linear specific heat anomaly in doped alkali halides has actually been observed in NaBr:F,[32] (FIGURE 19). Rollefson explained this with the tunneling theory developed by Sussmann, assuming a spread of asymmetric wells between which the F^- ion could tunnel. Rollefson found, however, that the thermal conductivity was not affected by these tunneling defects, indicating that their coupling to the lattice had to be much weaker than, for instance, that of OH^- in NaCl. Rollefson did observe that the anomalous specific heat varied linearly with the fluorine ion concentration in the crystal.

So much for the doped alkali halide crystals. These examples show that a behavior similar to that common to all amorphous solids can be found in crystals under certain conditions. Another interesting example for glasslike behavior has been discovered by Bilir[33] and by Slack *et al.*[34] in crystalline YB_{66}. The low-temperature thermal conductivity is almost exactly identical to that of silica, and the specific heat shows a linear anomaly at low temperatures of 2.6×10^{-6} J $g^{-1}K^{-2}$, which is similar to the value of 1.1×10^{-6} J $g^{-1}K^{-2}$ for SiO_2. Bilir has suggested that these phenomena are connected with low-energy tunneling states of the yttrium ion between almost equivalent potential wells.

Clearly, more work is needed in order to demonstrate under what conditions glasslike thermal behavior can be observed in disordered crystals, and, at Cornell, work is going on in this direction.

In conclusion, we want to reemphasize the point that we find most remarkable about the glassy anomalies: Why do all amorphous solids appear to have the same low-temperature thermal conductivity, both in temperature dependence and absolute magnitude? We believe that the understanding of this phenomenon will be crucial for the understanding of the origin of this anomaly.

References

1. STEPHENS, R. B. 1973. Phys. Rev. **B8:** 2896–2905.
2. LASJAUNIAS, J. C., A. RAVEX & M. VANDORPE. 1975. Solid State Commun. **17:** 1045–1049.
3. NARAYANAMURTI, V. & R. O. POHL. 1970. Rev. Mod. Phys. **42:** 201–236.
4. ARNOLD, W., S. HUNKLINGER, S. STEIN & K. DRANSFELD. 1974. J. Non-Cryst. Solids **14:** 192–200, and references cited therein.
5. PICHÉ, L., R. MAYNARD, S. HUNKLINGER & J. JÄCKLE. 1974. Phys. Rev. Lett. **32:** 1426–1429. The change in velocity of transverse modes was reported by HUNKLINGER, S. & L. PICHÉ. 1975. Solid State Commun. **17:** 1189–1192.
6. VON SCHICKFUS, M., S. HUNKLINGER & L. PICHÉ. 1975. Phys. Rev. Lett. **35:** 876–878.
7. WHITE, G. K. 1975. Phys. Rev. Lett. **34:** 204–205.
8. SZEFTEL, J. & H. ALLOUL. 1975. Phys. Rev. Lett. **34:** 657–660.
9. MON, K. K., Y. J. CHABAL & A. J. SIEVERS. 1975. Phys. Rev. Letts. **35:** 1352–1355.
10. MORGAN, G. J. & D. SMITH. 1974. J. Phys. **C7:** 649–664. Also WALTON, D. 1974. Solid State Commun. **14:** 335–339. See also the review by BÖTTGER, H. 1974. Phys. Stat. Sol. **B62:** 9–42.
11. ANDERSON, P. W., B. I. HALPERIN & C. M. VARMA. 1972. Phil. Mag. **25:** 1–9.
12. JÄCKLE, J. 1972. Z. Phys. **257:** 212–223.
13. PHILLIPS, W. A. 1972. J. Low Temp. Phys. **7:** 351–360.
14. See, for example, the solid state text book by KITTEL, C. 1971. Introduction to Solid State Physics. 4th edit.:215. John Wiley and Sons, Inc. New York, N.Y.

15. Anderson, O. L. 1959. J. Phys. Chem. Solids. **12:** 41–52.
16. Zeller, R. C. & R. O. Pohl. 1971. Phys. Rev. **B4:** 2029–2041.
17. Flubacher, P., A. J. Leadbetter, J. A. Morrison & B. D. Stoicheff. 1959. J. Phys. Chem. Solids **12:** 53–65.
18. Hornung, E. W., R. A. Fisher, G. E. Brodale & W. F. Giauque. 1969. J. Chem. Phys. **50:** 4878–4886.
19. Bilir, N. & W. A. Phillips. 1975. Phil. Mag. **32:** 113–122.
20. Leadbetter, A. J. 1969. J. Chem. Phys. **51:** 779–786.
21. Sussmann, J. A. 1964. Phys. Kondens Materie **2:** 146–160.
22. Zaitlin, M. P. & A. C. Anderson. 1975. Phys. Stat. Sol. **B71:** 323–327.
23. Lyon, K. & G. L. Salinger. Unpublished.
24. Case III, C. R. and C. A. Swenson. 1974. Phys. Rev. **B9:** 4506–4511.
25. Kirby, R. D., A. E. Hughes and A. J. Sievers. 1970. Phys. Rev. **B2:** 481–509.
26. Stephens, R. B. 1976. Phys. Rev. B. To be published.
27. Goubau, W. M. & R. H. Tait. 1975. Phys. Rev. Lett. **34:** 1220–1223.
28. Stephens, R. B. 1976. Phys. Rev. B **13:** 852.
29. Lasjaunias, J. C., D. Thoulouze & F. Pernod. 1974. Solid State Commun. **14:** 957–961.
30. Klein, M. V. 1961. Phys. Rev. **122:** 1393–1402.
31. Rosenbaum, R. L., C. K. Chau & M. V. Klein. 1969. Phys. Rev. **186:** 852–864.
32. Rollefson, R. J. 1972. Phys. Rev. **B5:** 3235–3253.
33. Bilir, N. Low Temperature Heat Capacities of Open-Structured Crystals. Ph.D. Thesis, Stanford University, Dept. of Materials Science and Engineering, May 1974. Unpublished.
34. Slack, G. A., D. W. Oliver & F. H. Horn. 1971. Phys. Rev. **B4:** 1714–1720, Also Slack, G. A., D. W. Oliver, G. D. Brower & J. D. Young. J. Phys. Chem. Solids. To be published.
35. Stephens, R. B., G. S. Cieloszyk & G. L. Salinger. 1972. Phys. Lett. **38A:** 215–217.
36. Stephens, R. B. 1974. Ph.D. Thesis. Cornell University. Unpublished.

CAN TUNNELING LEVELS EXPLAIN THE ANOMALOUS PROPERTIES OF GLASSES AT VERY LOW TEMPERATURE?

B. I. Halperin

Bell Laboratories
Murray Hill, New Jersey 07974

The previous two speakers have summarized some of the anomalous properties of glasses at very low temperatures.[1] As they have indicated, most or all of these anomalies can be explained at least *qualitatively* by the assumed presence of localized two level systems known as "tunneling levels".[2–7] However, it is not yet clear whether any reasonable statistical distribution of tunneling levels can explain *quantitatively* all of the various properties that have been observed. This talk will review some of the theoretical considerations underlying the possible role of tunneling levels.

Tunneling levels occur when an atom or group of atoms can exist in two nearby configurations that are local minima of the potential energy, separated by a barrier. The Hamiltonian for a pair of tunneling levels can be described by a two-by-two matrix[3,4]

$$H_0 = \tfrac{1}{2}\begin{pmatrix} \Delta & G \\ G & -\Delta \end{pmatrix}, \tag{1}$$

where $\Delta = E_1 - E_2$ is the difference in energies of the ground states in the two wells, neglecting overlap, and G is the matrix element arising from the overlap between the wave functions in the two wells. We may write

$$G = \hbar\omega_0 e^{-\lambda}, \tag{2}$$

where ω_0 has the order of magnitude of a typical phonon frequency, and λ is proportional to the product of the thickness of the barrier, the square root of the barrier height, and the square root of the mass of the tunneling group. On diagonalizing H_0 we find that the ground state Ψ_0, and the excited state Ψ_e, are linear combinations of the original states Ψ_1 and Ψ_2, representing the ground states in the two separate wells, with coefficients that depend on the ratio Δ/G. The energy difference between the ground and excited states is given by

$$E = (\Delta^2 + G^2)^{1/2}, \tag{3}$$

which is roughly equal to the larger of the two quantities, $|\Delta|$ and G. Note that when $\Delta = 0$, Ψ_0 and Ψ_1 are even and odd combinations of Ψ_1 and Ψ_2, and are not localized in either well.

The most important couplings between a pair of tunneling levels and the outside world occur via the long wavelength electric field and the long wavelength strain field of the glass. In the presence of an electric field, $\vec{E}$, we must add to H_0

a term

$$H_d = \tfrac{1}{2}\,\vec{E}\cdot\vec{d}\begin{pmatrix}1 & 0\\ 0 & -1\end{pmatrix}, \tag{4}$$

where the dipole moment $\vec{d}$ is equal to an effective charge e^*, times the displacement involved in moving from well 1 to well 2. In principle, there will also be off-diagonal terms in H_d, arising from the derivative of the matrix element G with respect to the electric field; however, such terms are expected to be quite small and negligible in practice. The most important coupling to the phonon field will occur via a term in the Hamiltonian of the form

$$H_p = \tfrac{1}{2}\begin{pmatrix}1 & 0\\ 0 & -1\end{pmatrix}\sum_{ij} \Lambda_{ij}\epsilon_{ij}, \tag{5}$$

where ϵ_{ij} is the macroscopic strain tensor at the site of the tunneling-level pair, and the matrix of coupling constants Λ_{ij} is a symmetric tensor. The matrix Λ_{ij} is characterized by three perpendicular eigenvectors, whose spatial orientation is random in a glass, and by three eigenvalues, which we shall denote γ_1, γ_2, γ_3. There will also be a small off-diagonal matrix element to H_p coming from the volume derivative of G, which may be important for the thermal expansion at low temperatures, but is probably unimportant otherwise.

The most likely type of transition between the ground and excited states occurs with emission or absorption of a phonon, to conserve energy, and is proportional to the square of the matrix element of H_p between the *ground* and *excited states*. It is easy to show that for a given value of Λ_{ij},[3,4]

$$\langle 0 \mid H_p \mid e \rangle \propto G/E. \tag{6}$$

For a given value of E, this is maximized when λ has its minimum value

$$\lambda_{min} \equiv \ln(\hbar\omega_0/E), \tag{7}$$

so that $G = E$ and $\Delta = 0$. For $\lambda > \lambda_{min}$, the matrix element falls off exponentially. Thus, as the barrier becomes larger, the relaxation rate decreases as $e^{-2\lambda}$. For λ sufficiently large, the relaxation rate of the excited state becomes so slow that equilibrium does not occur on the time scale τ of an experiment, and the level pair in question will not contribute to the experimentally measured specific heat. Roughly, for a level pair to contribute to the specific heat at temperature T, we must have $E \lesssim T$, and $\lambda_{min} < \lambda < \lambda_{max}$, where

$$\lambda_{max} = \tfrac{1}{2}\ln \Gamma_0\tau, \tag{8}$$

and Γ_0 is of order 10^{12} sec^{-1}. For $T \lesssim 1\ K$ and $\tau \approx 10^3$ sec, we have $\lambda_{min} \approx 5$ and $\lambda_{max} \approx 20$.

In order to estimate the specific heat or other properties of the system, we must first discuss the distribution $n(\Delta, G)$. The distribution of the variable Δ, (at fixed G) is relatively easy to discuss. Since there was no a priori distinction between the levels 1 and 2, it is clear that the distribution should be an even function of Δ. Furthermore, if we think of E_1 and E_2 as independent random variables, the root mean square value of Δ would have the same magnitude as fluctuations in E_1 and E_2, which we would estimate to be of the order of 0.1 eV or more. We would arrive at a similar estimate of Δ_{rms}, the root mean square value of Δ, if we assume that the difference $E_1 - E_2$ is due to strains in the glass, on the atomic scale. Thus for small Δ we may write

$$n(\Delta, G) = n(0, G) + 0(\Delta^2/\Delta_{rms}^2), \tag{9}$$

where the second term is completely negligible for Δ of order 1 K.

The distribution of G is more difficult to predict. In Reference 3 we made the guess that λ (and hence $\ln G$) would be more or less uniformly distributed, from small values to very large values. Indeed, we know that there must exist a very large number of nearly degenerate states that can be reached by surmounting a barrier of the order of a volt or so, since we know that the ground state of a glass has an entropy that is typically of the order of $1/2\, k_B$ per molecule. (The number of atoms that must be readjusted to reach a new stable state may be rather large, however, leading to a very large effective mass m^*, and a correspondingly large value of λ.) If one assumes a uniform distribution for λ, one finds that the specific heat C varies according to [3,4]

$$C \propto (\lambda_{max} - \lambda_{min})T. \tag{10}$$

The first factor depends only logarithmically on T and on the time τ, so that the specific heat would be nearly linear in temperature. It is now clear that the simple form of $n(\Delta, G)$ discussed above is not correct in detail. The high-frequency specific heat measurements of Goubau and Tait[8] show much less dependence on τ than would be predicted from this assumption. Indeed, if one assumed a uniform distribution of λ, out to values much beyond 20, one would be led to an immediate contradiction with earlier experiments. It would be very difficult to keep a thermally isolated sample of glass below, say, a few tenths of a degree, because the amount of energy released by levels with $E \gtrsim 1$ K, and lifetimes between one hour and several days, would very rapidly cause the sample to heat up. Thus it seems necessary to assume a distribution in which λ is restricted to values small compared to 20. (Of course, we may also have λ large compared to 30, but such levels will have no effects at low temperature.)

By assuming an enhanced density of states with λ in the vicinity of 5 (i.e., with $G \approx 1$ K) we will find specific heat which grows more rapidly than linearly with T, for $T \sim 1$ K, and we may thereby attribute the enhanced T^3 term in the specific heat to an appropriately chosen distribution of $\ln G$. Hopefully, we may still retain the assumption that Δ is uniformly distributed in the range of interest.

It is interesting to note that according to our assumptions, the presence of an electric field $\vec{E}$ should have very little effect on the specific heat, thermal conductivity, or other properties. In effect, the electric field will shift the value of Δ (cf. Equations 1 & 4), by an amount which is random, because of the random orientation of $\vec{d}$. Since Δ is already uniformly distributed, the distribution of energies should be almost unaffected by electric fields. This may account for the negative results reported by Stephens[9] for the electric field dependence of the thermal conductivity.

Physical properties other than the specific heat depend on various aspects of the distribution of levels. Let $n(\Delta, G, \vec{d}, \Lambda_{ij})$ be the density of levels with given values of the specified parameters. We may define an expectation value $\langle A \rangle_E$ for some variable A, as

$$\langle A \rangle_E \equiv \frac{\int A n(\Delta, G, \vec{d}, \Lambda_{ij})\delta[E - (\Delta^2 + G^2)^{1/2}]}{n(E)}, \tag{11}$$

where

$$n(E) \equiv \int n(\Delta, G, \vec{d}, \lambda_{ij})\, \delta[E - (\Delta^2 + G^2)^{1/2}], \tag{12}$$

is the density of levels at energy E, and where the integral is over $\Delta, G, \vec{d}$, and Λ_{ij}, with G greater than some convenient lower cutoff ($\lambda < \lambda_{\max}$). It can be readily shown that the microwave absorption measurements, such as those carried out in vitreous silica by von Schickfus *et al.*[9] should measure the product of the density of levels and the expectation value of the dipole matrix element

$$< |d|^2 G^2/E^2 >_E,$$

for $E = \hbar\omega$, where ω is the microwave frequency. On the other hand, the dielectric relaxation at low frequencies is most sensitive to the density of levels with $E \approx k_B T$ and relaxation rates comparable to the measuring frequency, weighted by $|d|^2\Delta^2/E^2$.

The mean free paths for phonons at low temperatures are believed to be limited by resonant scattering by the localized two-level systems. The scattering rate is proportional to the difference in the initial occupations of the ground and excited states of the level pairs, and hence decreases with increasing temperature, proportional to[4] coth $(\hbar\omega/2k_B T)$.

The mean free paths for longitudinal and transverse phonons are determined respectively by[3,4] $n(E)$ times

$$M_l^2 \equiv <\gamma_l^2 G^2/E^2>_E, \tag{13}$$

$$M_t^2 \equiv <\gamma_t^2 G^2/E^2>_E, \tag{14}$$

where γ_l and γ_t are the coupling constants averaged over the orientation of the level pair, given by

$$\gamma_l^2 = \tfrac{2}{15}(\gamma_1^2 + \gamma_2^2 + \gamma_3^2) + \tfrac{1}{15}(\gamma_1 + \gamma_2 + \gamma_3)^2, \tag{15}$$

$$\gamma_t^2 = \tfrac{1}{10}(\gamma_1^2 + \gamma_2^2 + \gamma_3^2) - \tfrac{1}{30}(\gamma_1 + \gamma_2 + \gamma_3)^2. \tag{16}$$

The thermal conductivity is primarily determined by the mean free path for transverse phonons. As was pointed out in the previous talk,[1] recent experiments by Lasjaunias *et al.*,[11] have found specific heats which varied from sample to sample, while the thermal conductivity remained constant. This suggests that several distinct kinds of tunneling levels must be present. The type of level whose concentration varies from sample to sample must have relatively small elastic coupling constants, so that it should make a relatively small contribution to the phonon scattering.

The mean free path of either transverse or longitudinal phonons may be measured by a conventional ultrasonic attenuation experiment at sufficiently low incident power. However, the fraction of level pairs in resonance with a phonon of any given frequency is quite small, and saturation effects set in at very low power levels, where the energy absorbed would not be sufficient to raise the temperature of the sample as a whole by an appreciable amount.[3] Measurements of ultrasonic velocities[12] and attenuation[13–15] at low temperatures, as a function of frequency, temperature, intensity, and pulse duration, and studies of the nonlinear interactions in a sequence of pulses, should give us a wealth of information about the distribution of levels and coupling constants. Much data has already been obtained for the case of fused silica,[12–15] and the results have been at least partially explained. More theoretical and experimental work is necessary in this field however.

A number of physical effects come into play in determining the behavior of the ultrasonic attenuation. For example, at low power, the number of levels which can be excited by a phonon of a given frequency will depend on the frequency breadths of the levels. These, in turn may depend in a complicated way on the interactions between different level pairs.[16] At higher power levels, "power broadening" of the levels may be important.[13] For short pulses, the spread in frequency of the phonon pulse, itself, may be important. The lifetime of the excited levels is of importance for pulses of long duration. At high power levels, resonant absorption ceases to be important, and ultrasonic attenuation occurs via a nonsaturating relaxation process,[3–5] in which the participating level pairs have $E \lesssim 2k_BT$, rather than E close to the incident phonon frequency. The wide distribution of the coupling matrix elements (Equation 6) expected in practice, will probably have a marked effect on the nonlinear ultrasonic attenuation, but calculations so far have not taken this into account.

I should like to remark, in closing, that although a number of possible explanations other than tunneling levels have been proposed for the low temperature anomalies in glasses,[2,7,17–26] none of these explanations seems very plausible to me. Since long wavelength phonons should be well described by continuum elastic theory, it is clear that some kind of additional low energy excitation is necessary to explain the specific heat and other anomalies. If these are vibrational levels, they must be produced by a very large deviation of the associated elastic constants from their average values, and this would only seem to be probable if the vibrational modes in question are localized on an atomic scale. We may note that it is not sufficient to set some local elastic constants equal to zero, to produce a mode of energy $\lesssim 1$ K. It would also be necessary to assume that the various anharmonic force constants are anomalously small, since the zero-point motion of the atoms will bring these into play. In fact, the most likely way to produce a low-lying excitation is to have a local elastic constant that is *negative*, and employ a positive quartic anharmonicity to restore stability. Such a situation, of course, leads to a double-well potential, and the low-lying level is nothing but the tunneling level that we have been discussing all along.

I may also remark that placing weakened force constants along sets of lines, as in dislocations[26] or microcrystallite edges,[22,25] will not substantially affect these considerations. In order to produce a specific heat large compared to the phonon contribution, the lines of defects must be much closer together than the wavelength of thermal phonons. The vibrational properties of an isolated line are therefore irrelevant—unless the force constants in the vicinity of the line are so radically altered that one has a set of low energy excitations strongly localized on the line, and practically decoupled from the rest of the lattice. In this case the anharmonic force constants will again be important and one has essentially a line of tunneling states.

In principle, low-lying excitations may be electronic in nature,[18,19] rather than arising from the lattice. For example, we may consider the possibility of an electron tunneling between several localized states. In such a case, however, one would normally expect a large electric dipole moment associated with transitions between the two states and one would expect to see a significant dielectric relaxation, which has not been found. The dipole mements obtained from microwave absorption[9] also seem too small for an electronic explanation.

It is also possible to produce low-lying excitations from interacting spins.

Various experiments have indicated that the number of free spins in insulating glasses is normally very small, however.[27–30] The lack of spins is also an argument against a simple electronic explanation of the specific heat.

One must also recognize the possibility that the short phonon mean free paths arise from a mechanism unrelated to the excess specific heat. Scattering of phonons by inhomogeneities in the elastic constants or densities, on the length scale of 10^3 Å, might account for the low thermal conductivity,[24] but would not be consistent with the observed dependence of ultrasonic attenuation on incident power.

Summary

Although tunneling-level-pairs can qualitatively explain most of the anomalous properties of glasses at very low temperatures, it is not yet clear whether any reasonable statistical distribution can quantitatively account for all the data. I have reviewed here some of the theoretical considerations.

Acknowledgments

The author is grateful for helpful conversations with B. Golding, C. M. Varma, P. W. Anderson, R. Pohl, and G. Salinger.

References

1. Pohl, R. O. & G. Salinger. 1976 Ann. N.Y. Acad. Sci. This volume.
2. Zeller, R. C. & R. O. Pohl. 1971. Phys. Rev. **B4:** 2029.
3. Phillips, W. A. 1972. J. Low Temp. Phys. **7:** 351.
4. Anderson, P. W., B. I. Halperin & C. M. Varma. 1972. Phil. Mag. **25:** 1.
5. Jäckle, J. 1972. Z. Phys. **257:** 212.
6. Rollefson, R. J. 1970. Ph.D. thesis, Cornell Materials Science Center. Report No. 1382.
7. Stephens, R. B. 1971. Unpublished report.
8. Goubau, W. M. & R. A. Tait. 1975. Phys. Rev. Lett. **34:** 1220.
9. Von Schickfus, M., S. Hunklinger & J. Jäckle. 1975. Phys. Rev. Lett. **35:** 876.
10. Stephens, R. B. 1975. Preprint.
11. Lasjaunias, J. C., A. Ravex, M. Vandorpe & S. Hunklinger. 1975. Solid State Commun. **17:** 1045.
12. Piché, L., R. Maynard, S. Hunklinger & J. Jäckle. 1974. Phys. Rev. Lett. **32:** 1426.
13. Golding, B., J. E. Graebner, B. I. Halperin & R. J. Schutz. 1973. Phys. Rev. Lett. **30:** 223.
14. Arnold, W., S. Hunklinger, S. Stein & K. Dransfeld. 1974. J. Noncryst. Solids **14:** 192.
15. Golding, B., J. E. Graebner & R. J. Schutz. 1976. Phys Rev. **B14.** In press.
16. Joffrin, J & A. Levelut. 1975. J. Phys. (Paris) **36:** 811.
17. Fulde, P. & H. Wagner. 1971. Phys. Rev. Lett. **27:** 1280.
18. Kaplan, T. A., S. D. Mahanti & W. M. Hartmann. 1971. Phys. Rev. Lett. **27:** 1796.
19. Redfield, D. 1971. Phys. Rev. Lett. **27:** 730.
20. Rosenstock, H. B. 1972. J. Noncryst. Solids **7:** 123.
21. Takeno, S. & M. Goda, 1972. Prog. Theor. Phys. **48:** 1468.
22. Baltes, H. P. 1973. Solid State Commun. **13:** 225.
23. Walton, D. 1974. Solid State Commun. **14:** 335.

24. MORGAN, G. J. & D. SMITH. 1974. J. Phys. **C7:** 649.
25. USHA & L. S. KOTHARI, 1974. Solid State Commun. **15:** 579.
26. LU, M.-S. 1975. Ph.D. thesis, Cornell Materials Science Center. Report No. 2501.
27. HORNUNG, E. W., R. A. FISHER, G. E. BRODALE & W. F. GIAQUE. 1969. J. Chem. Phys. **50:** 4878.
28. GUBSER, D. U. & P. C. TAYLOR. 1972. Phys. Lett. **40A:** 3.
29. DISALVO, F. J., J. TAUC & J. V. WASZCZAK. 1972. Bull. Amer. Phys. Soc. **17:** 344.
30. DISALVO, F. J., A. MENTH, J. V. WASZCZAK & J. TAUC. 1972. Phys. Rev. **B6:** 4574.

DISCUSSION

A. Leadbetter, *Moderator*

University of Exeter
Exeter, England

A. BIENENSTOCK (*Stanford University, Stanford, Calif.*): Dr. Halperin, You got the matrix elements from the shift of the velocity and N_0 from the specific heat. That gave you enough, I thought, to get the ultrasonic attenuation, but I don't recall your telling us how the ultrasonic attenuation so obtained agreed with experiments.

HALPERIN: In fused silica, the phonon mean-free path extracted from the ultrasonic attenuation at very low power levels, where there is no saturation effect, seems to agree rather well with the mean free path extracted from thermal conductivity measurements. The shift in sound velocity in turn has been successfully related to the attenuation via a Kramers-Kronig type of relation, but this involves extrapolations outside the range of directly meaasured mean-free paths. All of these quantities depend only on the *product* of the density of states and the average of the square of the matrix element. The density of states and matrix elements enter separately in the nonlinear acoustic attenuation experiments, but here the interpretation is more complicated, and has not been fully worked out.

MOYNIHAN: Dr. Pohl, were any other characterization measurements done on these different arsenic sulfide samples you looked at? Such as the ir spectra or possibly running the heat capacity on a differential scanning calorimeter to see the difference in thermal history? Did you make any additional effort to characterize these samples in terms of hydrogen, oxide, or hydroxyl impurities?

POHL: Yes, Stephens looked for instance for OH water absorption in the B_2O_3 and found nothing that resembles a correlation between OH concentrations and the specific heat.

MOYNIHAN: How about the arsenic sulfide?

POHL: The same problem. I think we should discuss this in somewhat more detail, but there is no correlation that we have been able to detect at this point. Clearly there must be something but we have not found it.

MOYNIHAN: One may also look at the thermal history of the materials—fictive temperature, if you want. This might be a difference.

POHL: Have there been systematic studies? The answer is no.

LEADBETTER: There have been studies on silica with different thermal histories, and the specific heats are somewhat different, but at higher temperatures.

MOSS: A question arose about possible experiments as I was listening to Dr. Halperin and Dr. Pohl. I wondered if there would be a way of perturbing, in a given material, the distribution of these states merely by taking a rapidly quenched glass and a fully relaxed glass and measuring the specific heat on both of them at low temperatures? Would not one expect to see a difference?

POHL: I would really like to put this in the form of a question to this group, what do you think is the best way of affecting a glass? I mean Dr. Moynihan already touched on this point and I want to ask this question, what do you think is the proper thing to do?

MOSS: I would certainly think that the distribution of levels that was discussed here would be much different in a rapidly quenched glass and in a fully relaxed glass; the barrier heights might be larger and so on.

HALPERIN: A priori, I do not know whether rapid quenching would increase or decrease the density of levels at low energy.

POHL: What rate of quenching and so on would one suggest to do?

MACEDO: If you go back and you calculate fluctuations with those two temperatures, you find that, since you can change the equilibrium temperature of the glass or the liquid by let's say 5% the variation in fluctuations will be rather insignificant, I think.

LEADBETTER: We don't take any convincing that there *may* be tunneling states: You are led inexorably to this conclusion as soon as you think about it. It's also clear that they can be used very well to rationalize many properties. It's also clear that there are very considerable difficulties left. Halperin himself has suggested some specific experiments where we can go forward. What people have sought for for many years is, what is the critical point of the system? Where do these effects appear and where don't they appear? In other words, what kind of defects have we got? It's okay to talk about two-level systems but what the hell is it that's moving? And we run into difficulties here with the dipole moments for example. Now has anyone got any contributions in this area? This is one thing I think we should discuss. The other is that if we can perturb this two level model in some way to take into account the difficulties, then has anyone got any suggestions for what's needed in addition to those Halperin has made?

Thirdly, maybe we have to throw the whole damn thing away and maybe there's a quite different approach that we can use. Now can we structure the discussion somewhat along these lines?

D. WALTON (*McMaster University, Hamilton, Ont.*): Dr. Halperin, I think your experiment has been reported by R. B. Bohn (1974. J. Appl. Phys. **45:** 2133). He measured the specific heat at low temperatures for a glass ceramic in the glassy state and then he heated it up and let it become a ceramic. I'm completely ignorant about the details of how one does this but apparently in this state it is probably partly crystalline. When it becomes a ceramic the linear term in the specific heat went up by as much as a factor of three.

HALPERIN: Was that a polycrystal?

WALTON: No, it was a glass and then it's partially crystallized when it becomes a ceramic.

LEADBETTER: Yes, I have done a similar experiment as has Pohl, and it is found that devitrified glasses may have a similar approximately linear anomalous specific heat to the parent glass. [Shows slide.] This is calcium magnesium silcate. The devitrified glass is more than 90% crystalline, but still has a cement matrix of amorphous material.

BIENENSTOCK: Almost all the glasses upon which I've heard reports of an anomalous specific heat at low temperatures are ones within which the atoms had low coordination numbers. Have there been experiments say on glassy metals in which all the coordination numbers are relatively high? Or amorphous germanium or silicon in which the atoms are very tightly linked?

LEADBETTER: The answer is no I think.

SALINGER: There have been measurements of specific heat of glassy metals at low temperatures. I think the argument is how big is the C_3 term, the coefficient of T^3? And I don't think it's even been settled whether there is a big C_3 term or not.

BIENENSTOCK: I understand now that in the metals you'd have a problem with the metalloid atoms, but in amorphous germanium you have everything very tightly linked and it's not clear that you have the same flexibility as in the other systems.

M. LIPSICAS (*Yeshiva University, New York, N.Y.*): Dr. Pohl, I'm not an expert on glass, and I'm not an expert on low temperatures but I'm surprised that you don't mention the fact that in specific heat measurements there was a big change around 1968, when George Seidel and one of his students started AC specific heat measurements. This was the idea that the Russians had suggested about 10 years before and since then there have been a lot of measurements of AC specific heat and it seems to me that if you're interested in tunneling situations you should measure specific heat as a function of the frequency. There's no difficulty whatsoever in doing it, and in fact, the experiment that you described, I must say, is very crude in today's terms because one can use, for instance, light-emitting diodes to put the heat in, and if you do not have enough absorption you can coat your sample with a little bit, a very small amount, of metal just to get enough absorption; you can vary the area over which you illuminate, which already changes both the amount of material used and the speed of response, etc. You have all sorts of possibilities; you have very sensitive detectors, which have rapid response these days; so, as far as the state of the art is concerned, there's no question whatsoever that you can do this. In fact, as far as germanium is concerned, work was done at Stanford and Bell Labs using the AC techniques (Greene, King, Zubeck & Hauser. 1972. Phys. Rev. **B6:** 3297) already four years ago.

LEADBETTER: At what temperature?

LIPSICAS: Not below 1.2°K.

LEADBETTER: Okay.

LIPSICAS: No, what I'm saying is that as far as the *technique* is concerned they used exactly these techniques of AC specific heat and I disagree with you as far as the difficulties are concerned. I think these days getting down to 20 millidegrees, as far as the low temperature physicist is concerned, is no great effort because you can use a dilution refrigerator (now available commercially), etc. I agree with you that it's much more difficult than working at higher temperatures, in principle, but I think people are already set up to do this. If Wheatly can go down to one millidegree, 20 millidegrees is well within the state of the art today.

LEADBETTER: Okay, I'm sure one of our low temperature experts could answer that. Bobby, are you going to answer this?

POHL: I think my answer to this is that the grass is always greener on the other side of the fence. (Laughter.)

BIENENSTOCK: One system you might think about is $CuAsSe_2$ in which as far as we can determine, the lowest coordination number is three; that is, about half the seleniums are three-fold coordinated; the rest seem to be four-fold coordinated. I think that the higher the coordination number, the fewer the degrees of freedom.

BRAWER: Dr. Pohl, in your arsenic sulphide glasses what's the mean free path of your phonons down at say a hundred millidegrees or 50 millidegrees?

POHL: The answer is really quite general: it's of the order of a hundred phonon wave lengths from about roughly one degree on down in all glasses.

BRAWER: It's about a hundred phonon wave lengths? How does this compare to the size of the sample you're using in your measurements?

POHL: Much smaller, unless one measures samples about 50 microns thick. In such samples, Stephens did indeed find a contribution to the phonon scattering resulting from properly roughened surfaces.

BRAWER: Something like this wouldn't explain the constancy of the thermal conductivity in your arsenic sulphide.

POHL: The conductivities reported in this talk were measured on samples about 5 millimeters thick. In these samples the mean free path is the result of bulk scattering alone.

WEINBERG: I would like to address my question either to Dr. Pohl or to anyone else in the audience who may care to respond. Is it at all possible to try to approach this question from a somewhat different point of view? Could one for example start with a crystalline structure, where one does not have a heat capacity anomaly, and try to distort it in some way to induce a heat capacity anomaly? In this manner one could, perhaps, ascertain specific structural changes which lead directly to the heat capacity anomaly.

My second question, which is somewhat related to my previous question, is the following. Can one go over to a somewhat simpler system? For example, should one expect a heat capacity anomaly in the type of system that Dr. Johari was talking about today? In the case of plastic crystals one can induce a glass transition, and one has more of a handle on things since positional structural order is maintained and only orientational disorder persists.

LEADBETTER: May I comment on the second question because I think that's an excellent suggestion: People have thought of this but whether anybody is planning to do it I don't know. Thank you for reinforcing it. I'll answer your first question too, by asking you one back. Tell us how to distort a crystal in a controlled manner?

MOSS: With neutron radiation.

LEADBETTER: Sure you can and it's partially been done some years ago by Westrum although I don't think it was ever published, but you know you get a lot of mess when you irradiate something.

MOSS: One may take magnesium oxide and irradiate it to a point where the diffraction peaks disappear and are replaced by diffuse scattering peaks. The crystal is really filled with dislocation loops, well characterized by diffuse scattering that has been measured. One may then take such a sample, which is an insulator, and run its specific heat at low temperatures.

POHL: I would like to answer the question by asking you another one. How long does it take until the radioactivity in the sample has decayed to the point that you can actually measure at 0.1 degree Kelvin without getting the self-heating problem?

MOSS: I know certainly that people have done very extensive x-ray studies of neutron-irradiated MgO and BeO.

POHL: One sample of silica was irradiated some 10 years ago by Birch and White in Sydney and they measured the specific heat at low temperatures. Because of self-heating in the silicon dioxide they were able to go to only about $2\frac{1}{2}$ degree Kelvin. The specific heat anomaly was reduced at higher temperatures. At the low temperatures ($< 3°K$) the specific heat was unaltered, as far as one could tell from these measurements. We have just recently received this sample from Dr. Birch, and intend to measure it at low temperatures. Instead of neutron irradiation, Stephens has used low-temperature plastic deformation on a lead crystal. Within the experimental error he was unable to see any difference on the specific heat between the undeformed and the deformed sample. There are several other cases that I could describe. One of the materials Si Moss is particularly interested in is the omega-beta phase transition in zirconium-niobium. If you have the right concentration, then the omega phase exists in very small domains. In that material Dr. Liu at Cornell has been able to indeed observe not only a thermal conductivity as in glasses but also specific heat anomaly. More importantly, upon anealling (aging it is called in that business), when these omega phases become less mobile, the linear anomaly decreased and the thermal conductivity increased. So this could be a rather interesting model substance for a glass, although if you ask me what is moving around in this material at low temperatures, the answer is that we can only guess that it is the motion of individual atoms within the omega phase.

WALTON: I want to report an experiment concerned with Brillouin scattering from vitreous silica; it was done by my colleague Howard Jackson. At 2.4°K he found that the lifetime of a longitudinal phonon in vitreous silica was roughly 7 megacycles, but more importantly on the way down to 2.4 degrees Kelvin the lifetime of the phonon always increased.

JOHARI: I would like to point out that a negative coefficient of thermal expansion has been observed in hexagonal ice below 80°K. An explanation in this case has been offered in terms of excitation of intermolecular bending vibrations.

RELATION OF CRYSTALLIZATION BEHAVIOR TO STRUCTURE IN AMORPHOUS SYSTEMS

D. Turnbull

Harvard University
Division of Engineering and Applied Physics
Cambridge, Massachusetts 02138

While the thermodynamic characteristics of the melt → glass transition and of the glass suggested a microcrystallite model of glass structure, the high resistance of pure melts and glasses to crystal nucleation seemed to indicate that the crystallization must require some essential reconstruction of the short-range order (SRO). Diffraction studies show that the number and spacing of nearest neighbors, as defined by the Wigner-Seitz (Vornoi) construction, are, generally, little changed by crystallization. However even under these conditions, the angular distributions of the nearest neighbors, i.e., the topology of the SRO, can be quite different in the amorphous and crystallized states. For example, crystallization of a directionally bonded random network requires topological reconstruction of the SRO. Apparently, an analogous reconstruction of the SRO topology would have to attend the crystallization of a nondirectionally bonded system in the Bernal dense random-packed (DRP) structure. The high resistance of pure metal melts and of glass-forming alloy melts to crystal nucleation may reflect that the topology of the SRO in these melts is DRP-like. Using the DRP model for the melt, Spaepen and Meyer have calculated an upper limiting value for the crystal melt tension in monatomic systems, which is consistent with the available experimental results on metals.

The concepts and arguments presented here have been surveyed, with literature citations, and developed in a number of papers[1–5] by the author and his associates.

References

1. BAGLEY, B. G., H. S. CHEN & D. TURNBULL. 1968. Mat. Res. Bull. **3:** 159.
2. TURNBULL, D. 1969. Contemp. Phys. **10:** 473.
3. TURNBULL, D. 1974. J. Phys. **35** (Colloque-4): C4.1–4.9.
4. TURNBULL, D. 1975. J. Electron. Mater. **4:** 771.
5. SPAEPEN, F. & D. TURNBULL. 1976. Proceedings 2nd International Conference on Rapidly Quenched Metals. B. C. Giessen & N. J. Grant, Eds. In press.

STABILITY AND LOCAL ORDER IN SIMPLE AMORPHOUS PACKINGS

Michael Hoare

Department of Physics
Bedford College
Regent's Park
London NW1 4NS, England

INTRODUCTION

The study of simple sphere packings has been a recurring theme in the theory of amorphous structure, the importance of which was recognized long before the discovery of monatomic, metallic glasses gave it more immediate relevance. Indeed a preoccupation with the geometry of simple packings can be traced back to the earliest Democritean tradition and is quite prominent in the speculative atomism of Boscovitch, Davy, and others almost a century and a half before modern crystallography and the first thought of structure determination. In our own time it has taken on aspects that go far beyond the physicochemical problems that concern us at this meeting: one may cite little-known applications to the structure of the atomic nucleus[1,2] and of viruses[3] and to the mechanics of fluidized beds.[4] Even more remarkable connections exist with the theory of general relativity (through the Regge calculus[5]) and the statistical theory of linguistics.[6]

By far the most elaborate study of disordered atomic packings remains that of Bernal[7-9] and his followers[10,11] though some earlier, very thorough work on locally-ordered, noncrystallographic packings was done by Boerdijk[12] and Frank and Kasper.[13] The relevance of Bernal's work to the theory of the glass transition was immediately realized by Cohen and Turnbull,[14] not without some scepticism from more traditional glass theorists.[15] Bernal's theory, as he freely admitted, is descriptive rather than explanatory and scarcely distinguishes between the liquid and glassy states, both being included in the well-known characterization, "... homogeneous, coherent, essentially irregular assemblages of molecules containing no crystalline regions, nor, in their low-temperature form, holes large enough to admit another molecule..." There is an essential, though quite proper, vagueness in all the above terms, of which the first, asserting *homogeneity*, is perhaps crucial. In his wider context it is clear that Bernal meant this to imply an effective absence of spatial correlation between molecules at distances greater than the dimensions of his five "canonical polyhedra," i.e., virtually from the second-neighbor distance outwards. How seriously are we to take this in approaching a theory of the real glassy state?

Bernal's theory and the language in which he frames it are both heavily influenced by the extremely ingenious experiments that he carried out on the packing of ball bearings—though it could be argued that, whether or not we have actually played with such three-dimensional models, the tendency to think in terms of touching hard spheres, or, equally misleadingly, the rigid-looking ball and spoke diagrams of most crystallography texts, is almost irresistable. Nevertheless it can be overcome and, as I hope to demonstrate, must be if we are to explain anything so complex as the glass transition. If we need to have a picture in mind it should at least be nearer to that of packing caviar or frog spawn, an exercise which, even if only performed mentally, is a valuable corrective to "hard-sphere thinking." Fortunately perhaps, the computer has made such operations unnecessary as well as aiding enormously in the analysis of the results. It is this type of model building that I shall be describing here and which I shall suggest can lead to a clarification of what may be the essential character of the glass transition. Although I shall deal mainly with the mechanics of soft-packed structures with two-body central forces, certain properties will emerge that would seem to be shared with systems of nonspherical units and those having angle-dependent potentials.

Soft versus Hard Packings

As I have indicated, it is now possible, given a fair amount of computing time and some programming ingenuity, to simulate the packing of real atoms under a given interaction potential—in other words to prepare assemblies of soft, sticky, partially penetrable spheres in (in principle) any number of dimensions. Not only is it relatively easy to design and build such structures, but also they may be "relaxed" in the computer to confirm their stability and locate the precise position of a particular potential energy minimum in configuration space and the value of its associated binding energy. In this way we may attach a definite numerical measure of the "efficiency" of a packing independently of macroscopic measures such as the "density" and "surface area."[16-20] A variety of dynamic experiments may also be carried out; one may perform the vibrational analysis of small motions about a given potential minimum[18-22] or follow the natural motion of a finite system at given total energy by full solution of the equations of motion.[23,24] One may also investigate "unnatural motions" under the influence of fictitious applied forces and with sudden or gradual adiabatic cooling induced by withdrawal of kinetic energy. Monte Carlo methods for performing ensemble averages are likewise possible[25]—in short one may make all manner of excursions in either phase space or configuration space, either systematically, or at random, or following natural motion. All this is possible with assemblies of up to some 1000 atoms, that is, with systems of the same order of size as the original Bernal model, either in the isolated "cluster" state or with periodic boundary conditions. But one conspicuous thing *cannot* be done—the determination of an unequivocal ***absolute minimum*** for the potential energy over all configuration space. No method short of a systematic search in all $3N - 6$ dimensions has yet been devised, and none is likely to be.

The computer is no less valuable in producing visual renderings of interesting structures that may be viewed from any angle (or even from "inside") as well as through stereo projections, ciné film and other special techniques. We have indeed come a long way since Morrell and Hildebrand's heroic attempt to model a real liquid using gelatin balls.[26]

The transition from "hard" to "soft" packings involves more than just a move in the direction of atomic reality for, as well as posing the problems of mechanical and thermodynamic stability in mathematically acceptable form, it induces a total change of descriptive language. Hard-packed assemblies are unpleasant in many respects: Statically they give rise to "jammed" configurations and unnatural "clearance regions";[28] dynamically they can lead to unrealistic "rattling" correlations.[29] Mathematically these difficulties follow from the lack of differentiability of the potential—the lack therefore of principal radii of curvature in the potential-energy surface, the nonapplicability of the Principal of Virtual Work, the impossibility of a proper theory of stress accommodation.

Bernal maintained throughout that "... the key word in the structure of liquids is ... *impenetrability*." And others have more or less tacitly assumed that the slope of the potential curve for atoms in "contact" [*sic*] is so steep as to render unimportant any subtle effects due to attraction of atoms at greater than the pair distance. Whereas this approximation is probably in order for determining the structure of the normal liquid above its melting point, I believe it to be seriously in error at temperatures in the neighborhood of the glass transition and, moreover, to have played a major part in the misunderstanding of this phenomenon and its consequences. The reason for this is basically simple and, one would have thought, impossible to overlook. In the neighborhood of the neutral position for a particular interatomic "bond" in a solid structure, be it for a Lennard-Jones potential or the more likely Morse potential in a metal, the repulsive contribution is by no means as "hard" as it would be in a collision at thermal energies but shows a degree of compliance quite sufficient to permit relatively complicated adjustments in the coordination sphere of a particular atom. As our later calculations will show, the cooperative character of positional adjustments near an N-atom minimum configuration can lead to the formation of quite large and intricate centrally symmetric structures which would be totally impossible to build with hard spheres. In order to emphasize this point still further we have plotted the Lennard-Jones and softer Morse potential in an unusual manner in FIGURE 1, showing percentage compression relative to the minimum energy point against corresponding fraction of binding energy. The points marked on the Lennard-Jones curve in the figure indicate the degree of compression found in the minimum "bond lengths" present in particular structures we shall later describe, as well as the shortest interatomic distance in the Lennard-Jones face-centered cubic (fcc) lattice.

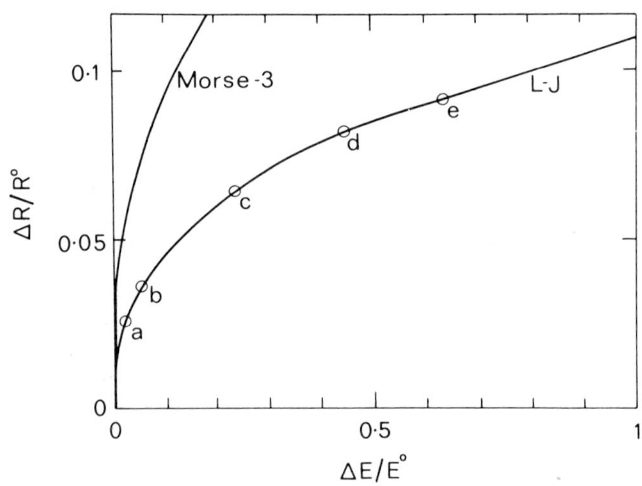

FIGURE 1. Potential curves for different 2-body force laws. Lower curve: the Lennard-Jones potential $V(R) = R^{-12} - 2R^{-6}$ in scaled units. Upper curve: Morse potential $V(R) = \exp[-6(R-1)] - 2\exp[-3(R-1)]$. The curves show only the compressive part of the potential well drawn as the fractional compression to the $V = 0$ point versus the corresponding fraction of binding energy. The points identify the *minimum* atomic spacing found in some of the minimal structures to be discussed. (a) fcc argon lattice. (b) 13-atom icosahedron (FIGURE 3c). (c) 55-atom isocahedron (FIGURE 6b). (d) 115-atom RID structure (FIGURE 5). (e) 471-atom structure (FIGURE 9).

Principles of Soft Packing

In practice we are considerably more limited in the study of soft packings than the previous section may have suggested. It would be most satisfying if we could compute the free energy of formation of a variety of alternative amorphous structures and compare the values for each over a range of temperature with each other and with that for the stable lattice. Although some calculations of the vibrational free energy of isolated clusters have been made, it is difficult to obtain reliable values outside the range of harmonic oscillations or for more than a few alternative structures. Nevertheless there are some indications that for solidlike structures the thermodynamic stability is determined by energetic rather than entropic conditions, at least for relatively cold, compact units in the size range up to a few hundred atoms. Apart from the computational difficulties involved, it is in any case natural to investigate first the potential energy characteristics of typical structures and attempt to draw qualitative conclusions so far as possible from these. A similar standpoint has been taken in a number of recent papers emphasizing the "potential energy" approach to the glass transition.[30–32]

Suppose we set out to discover those "interesting" regions of the configuration space of a moderately large number of particles (say $N = 100$) that can be expected to indicate configurations thermodynamically "metastable" in the sense used by Kautzmann.[33] More precisely these will be regions so separated by the topography of the potential energy surface that the phase point of the system will remain there for effectively infinite time when its momentum coordinates are projected out, in spite of a finite total energy. Such a system would, of course, be nonergodic and the region would, of necessity contain at least one potential-energy minimum. We suspect that the most interesting minima are those that are the lowest possible not corresponding to lattice-type order. In a finite system it is by no means to be expected that fragments recognizably latticelike occupy the position of lowest available potential energy, neither can it be assumed that the lowest minimum configuration could ever be achieved in any conceivable experiment. What methods of search are open to us? A considerable variety in fact. We may consider:

(a) Spontaneous assembly in a dynamic simulation.
(b) Applying some form of growth algorithm.
(c) Analogy with elements in known crystalline structures.
(d) Design.

Although we shall draw on evidence under all these headings the main emphasis in our own work has been on the last. The idea of *designing* packed structures suggests a subjective element that other model builders have gone to great lengths to avoid. Yet this is to neglect an important and entirely rigorous aspect of the problem: what we might call the *thermodynamic variation principle*. Quite simply, if we can discover, by whatever means, a structure A that can be shown to possess a lower free-energy of formation (or generally less potential energy) than some alternative B, then A is at a thermodynamic advantage over B whatever alternative structures C, D, E . . . it may be possible to find. If, in particular, it should emerge that A is noncrystallographic while B is a fragment of lattice, then we will have demonstrated a situation of some importance and the existence of a nucleation barrier. The fact that this type of experiment is of somewhat limited use in the prediction of known lattice structure need not deter us too much in applying it to the investigation of *local* structure and we have had some success in predicting the anomalous symmetries of very small metal particles in this way.[21]

Although a more difficult computational problem, the search for a minimal saddle point for the interconversion of two structures is subject to a similar variation principle. The discovery of a particular saddle point may, depending on the energies involved, eliminate all appreciably higher saddles from interest.

Packing Amorphons

Although our earliest explorations of potential energy surfaces were somewhat haphazard, we came to recognize certain guiding principles that supplement the variational principle discussed above. In summarizing these we can draw on the work of many other authors, many of whom worked without extensive computations and had no particular connection with the theory of glasses. A definite, though informal, logical pattern emerges somewhat as follows:

(a) We may cite the conjecture of Boerdijk[12] that the most efficient *local* packing structures are those which maximize the "tetrahedriality" of nearest-neighbor relationships.

(b) Given this, we find it almost inescapable that groups of 20 nearly regular tetrahedra will tend to associate such that 12 atoms form the vertices of a regular icosahedron with a 13th at its center. This train of thought has been followed by many authors independently (e.g., Werfelmeier,[1] Shternberg,[34] Pauling,[2] Franck,[35] Allpress and Sanders,[36] Sadoc, Dixmier, and Guinier,[37] Komoda,[38] and numerous others). Of these only Frank and Dixmier *et. al.* emphasized the likelihood of the icosahedron occurring in the extended phase, the other authors mentioned being mainly concerned with isolated clusters. Bernal, though acknowledging Franck's influence, always minimized the importance of the icosahedron, perhaps because, having a central atom, it does not qualify as a canonical polyhedron.

(c) Given the great stability of the 13-atom icosahedron, we have a short step to the recognition that soft-packed isocahedra are readily assembled, with only

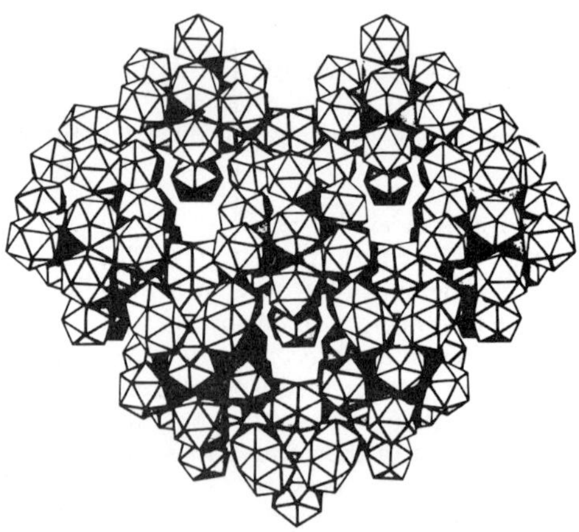

FIGURE 2. Icosahedral subunits of the unit cell of Cu_4Cd_3. The unit cell of 1124 atoms contains 568 icosahedra, 124 Friauf polyhedra (truncated tetrahedra) and some hundreds of smaller prismatic units. Each icosahedron has about half its vertices occupied by Cd and half by Cu. (From Samson.[40] By permission of W. H. Freeman and Company. Copyright 1968.)

slight distortion, into larger units in which they are joined face to face, point to point and interpenetrating in various ways. (This type of structure is well known in the crystallography of intermetallic compounds where, particularly in the work of Samson,[39,40] the analysis of such forms has reached a highly-developed art. FIGURE 2. reproduced from Samson's study of Cu_4Cd_3 shows the type of complexity possible in unit cells of over 1000 atoms.

(d) Recognizing that, whereas icosahedra can readily be assembled into all manner of ring and branched-chain structures, their composition into larger, compact, "polytetrahedral" units is severely limited by strain, we consider how "bridging units" may be introduced to relieve this. The 6-atom octahedron is particularly effective in this way and studies of intermetallic compounds (IMCs) amply demonstrate the complexity of local, noncrystallographic structures that can be formed in this way in mixed systems. Thus octahedra and tetrahedra can be combined in almost innumerable ways that tend to local symmetry and avoid the two special combinations giving the close-packed lattices.

(e) Accepting that the design of a systematic space-filling structure with densely-organized icosahedra is probably impossible,* one interesting alternative can be found for combining units of icosahedral symmetry (icosahedra, dodecahedra, rhombic tricontahedra) into centrally symmetric structures of considerable size. This is to use the framework of a *radial net*.[42] We shall explain this with examples in the following section.

The steps outlined above are effectively those by which we arrived at a number of remarkably compact, symmetrical, and in some cases strikingly beautiful *packing amorphons* which, in isolation, prove to be local minima for at least the Lennard-Jones and similar potentials. We choose this name in obvious extension of the term invented by Grigorovici[42,43] in his studies of the structure of amorphous bonded networks and in doing so deliberately invite the drawing of certain analogies between the two types of system.

In the next section I shall describe and exhibit a number of the more interesting packing amorphons and follow this with an account of some additional types of computer experiment of the mechanics of soft packings. Finally some conclusions from these will be drawn together into a tentative new account of the glass transition, which, I suggest, is viable for systems more complex than the atomic packings here described.

SOME LOCAL STRUCTURES

We shall make no attempt to catalogue systematically the many stable local structures that have been discovered in packings with a size range of a few to some hundreds of atoms. Those described below should serve to illustrate the kind of

*The question of whether some kind of systematic, noncrystalline, space-filling composition of icosahedra can be found has been posed by several authors.[13,14] In the strict sense—of arranging that every atom have regular 12-fold coordination—this is clearly impossible (as follows from the existence of a tetrahedral subgroup in the icosahedral symmetry). The possibility of finding some less regular open network cannot be ruled out so easily. We can, for example, build a Wurtzite lattice from rings of six icosahedra bridged by octahedra. Can this be disordered into a structure isomorphic with the Polk model? The answer seems to be no, for there are additional constraints to be met in the matching of triangular faces and these prevent the formation of the necessary five-membered rings. Yet perhaps something else analogous to the Polk model can be constructed by distortion of the icosahedral Wurtzite lattice. We leave this as a "dangling idea" in our logical scheme.

minimum locations that are available to and may attract the phase point of a finite system undergoing rapid cooling as it falls onto surfaces of progressively lower total energy. In them we can recognize certain common structural characteristics from which tentative predictions of dynamic behavior can be made and conclusions drawn about their possible statistical behavior should they occur as subunits of a more complex extended phase.

The next subsection recalls material that is reasonably well known; those that follow report experiments with soft-packings that have not previously been described.

Small Motifs

The smallest possible noncrystalline local structures were conjectured with the help of model building experiments[1,12,34] some time before it was possible to determine their precise geometry and binding energy by optimization of a potential function.[16,18] Prominent among these are the 7-atom pentagonal bipyramid (FIGURE 3a), the 8-atom stellated tetrahedron (Boerdijk[12]) and the 8-atom "dodecadeltahedron" (Werfelmeier[1]) (FIGURES 3b & 3e). The latter is interesting as perhaps the first intuition of a minimum configuration for a few atoms not all in "contact." We later confirmed its stability.[16] A measure of the relative stability of structures of the same number of atoms can be given by the binding energy E/N per atom present. The economy of the 13-atom icosahedral minimum (FIGURE 3c) ($E/N = 3.41$) is such that, though still unproved rigorously, it is almost inconceivable that this is not the absolute minimum available to 13 atoms with a potential soft enough to ensure the symmetry. Not only is this minimum very deep, but, unlike those of the smaller structures in the figure, it appears to be "protected" by relatively high saddle points in all directions. Two of the saddle points are known to be the cuboctahedral fcc structure (FIGURE 3d) and its hexagonal-close-packed (hcp) counterpart. ($E/N \simeq 2.91$). Both these have been shown to be mechanically unstable and to collapse spontaneously to the icosahedron.[17,18] The radial "bonds" of the icosahedron are always in compression; the surface bonds are in slight tension for the L-J potential but can be brought into compression by using a soft Morse potential.[17]

Intermediate Structures

It is convenient here to distinguish structures in the size range less than some 150 atoms corresponding roughly to the number needed to form up to a third concentric shell about a center. As illustrations we can consider the following:

(a) The soft-packed T26† structure, FIGURE 4a, was mentioned by Boerdijk.[12] Under the Lennard-Jones potential it has perfect tetrahedral symmetry and can be thought of as composed of four interpenetrating, slightly-distorted icosahedra ($E/N = 4.17$). It can be formed into a five-membered ring and thus into a variety of more complicated structures.

(b) The "deltahedron" DEL43 was described by Cundy[44] and arises by a covering of the surface of the 13-atom icosahedron with 20 octahedra (FIGURE 6a).

†The notations adopted here are not intended to be systematic and serve only for cross-reference within this article.

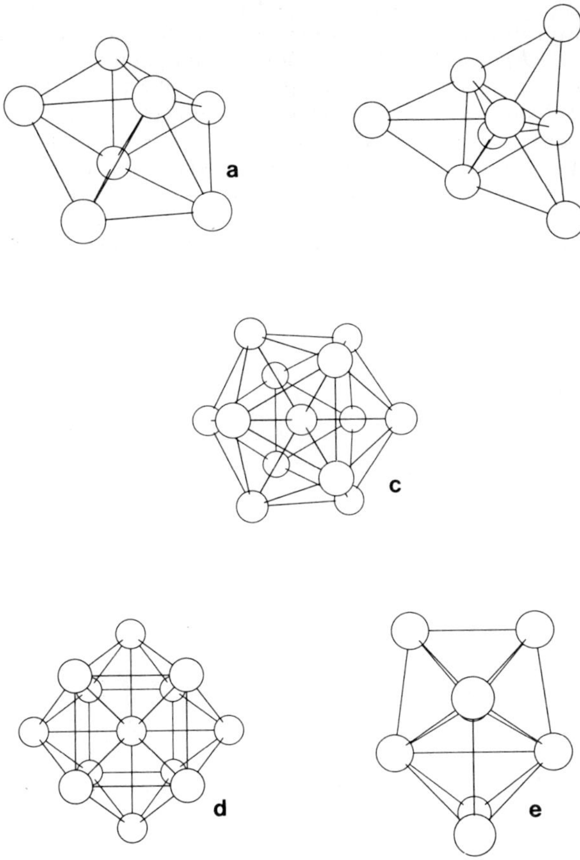

FIGURE 3. Small minimal structures for the Lennard-Jones potential. (a) Pentagonal biprism of 7 atoms. (b) Stellated tetrahedron of 8 atoms. (c) Icosahedron of 13 atoms. (d) Cuboctahedron of 13 atoms (unstable saddle point of fcc lattice symmetry). (e) Dodecadeltahedron of 8 atoms.

The Lennard-Jones minimum has perfect symmetry and an energy $E/N = 4.55$ units. Although devoid of crystallographic character, it posesses 20 tetrahedra and 40 half-octahedra.

(c) An alternative method of covering the icosahedron is to form the 33-atom dodecahedral structure (FIGURE 4b). With $E/N = 4.31$ this is not a particularly efficient minimum because the surface atoms are quite exposed. Pauling mentions this structure in his nuclear theory[2] assuming that both it and the rhombic triacontahedron (RTC) obtained from it by filling in the pentagonal facets will be regular and stable. Our experiments show that the symmetry of the RTC minimum is particularly sensitive to the character of the potential. Thus for the L-J potential it is irregular (FIGURE 4c), while for a Morse-3 potential it becomes perfectly symmetric (FIGURE 4d). These two configurations provide an excellent example of the crucial qualitative role which the shape of the potential can play in questions of local stability.

(d) On adding 72 further atoms to the DEL43 structure described earlier we obtain the beautiful structure RID115 shown in FIGURE 5. The surface of this is a *rhombicosidodecahedron* (RID, $E/N = 5.66$). The minimum configuration is perfectly regular under the Lennard-Jones potential with the surface bonds very slightly in compression ($d \simeq 0.998$). This figure illustrates perhaps better than any other so far what we mean by a "packing amorphon." By capping the twelve pentagonal facets we arrive at the closely related RID127 structure (FIGURE 7) in which some 60 surface bonds are slightly in tension. This structure can be assembled and dissected in many ways that serve to illustrate the complexity of its internal geometry. For example, it is, in effect, the "isocahedron of icosahedra," each of its 13-atom subunits bonded to neighbors by octahedral bridges. The five-

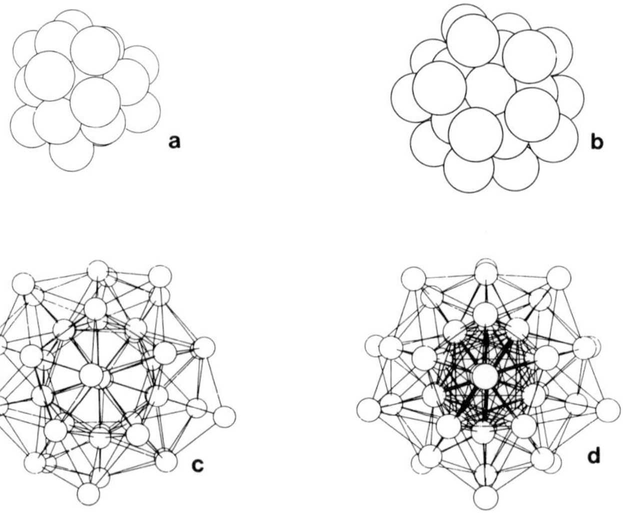

FIGURE 4. Intermediate structures. (a) 26-atom unit of tetrahedral symmetry. (b) Dodecahedron of 33 atoms. (c) Rhombic triacontahedron of 45 atoms at distorted Lennard-Jones minimum. (d) The same under the Morse ($\alpha = 3$) potential. Note the perfect symmetry of the last.

fold rings of icosahedra thus occurring, though not the whole structure, have been observed in IMC crystallography.[40] Alternatively one may dissect out a 55-atom "Mackay icosahedron," the "multiply twinned" structure having rudimentary close-packed faces of six atoms (FIGURE 6b).[45] Although this structure can grow further close-packed shells indefinitely, in the RID configuration this is prevented by positioning the third shell in "stacking fault" positions. We have here perhaps an indication of the nature of the free-energy barrier to crystallization.

Giant Amorphons

A fascinating property of icosahedral structures is the possibility of extending them hierarchically in the manner of the icosahedron of icosahedra illustrated above. In considering how much larger packing amorphons than this might be

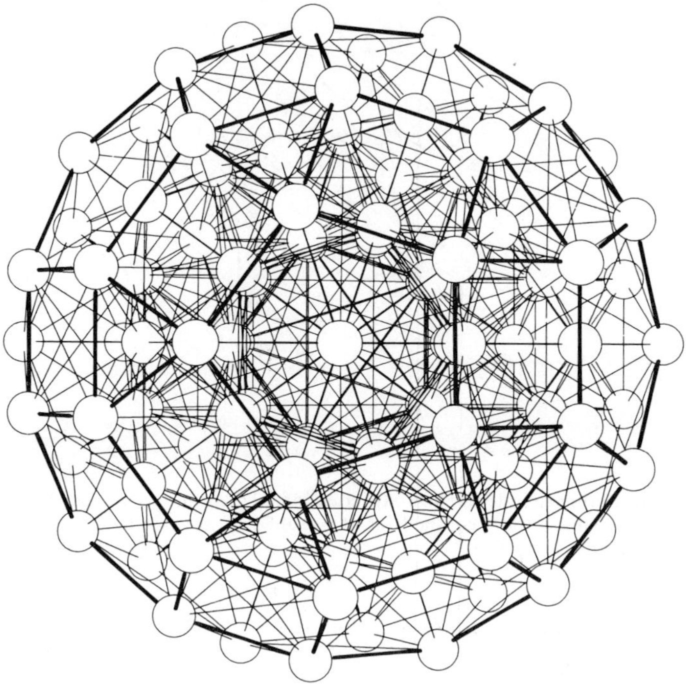

FIGURE 5. Rhombicosidodecahedral structure of 115 atoms at Lennard-Jones minimum. The surface "bonds" are very slightly in compression.

constructed, an obvious strategy is to compose 13 more complex units of icosahedral symmetry, or perhaps twelve such with a different central core. We tried this with various Lennard-Jones minimal structures of the required symmetry. Some, such as the D33 dodecahedral structure (FIGURE 4b) failed to give stable minima, but in one case, using Cundy's deltahedron DEL43, we were successful and obtained a very compact, centrally symmetric structure of 399 atoms made up of 13 of these units perfectly fitted together. This, illustrated in FIGURE 8b, gave $E/N = 6.22$. We now filled in the obvious concavities in the surface and obtained,

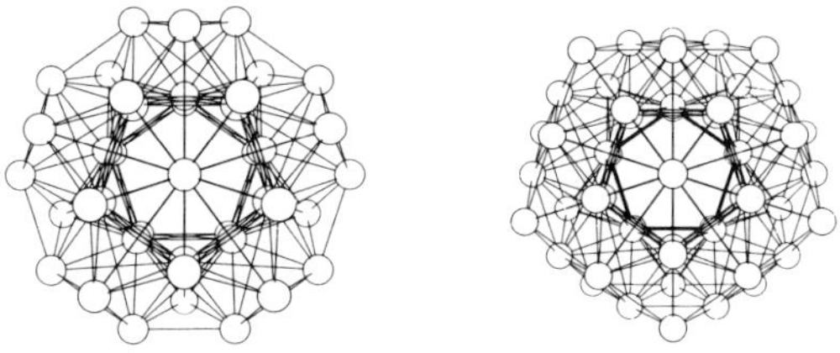

FIGURE 6. (Left) Icosidodecahedral structure of 43 atoms based on Cundy's deltahedron. A subunit of FIGURE 5. (Right) The Mackay "multiply twinned" 55-atom isocahedron. Also a subunit of FIGURE 5.

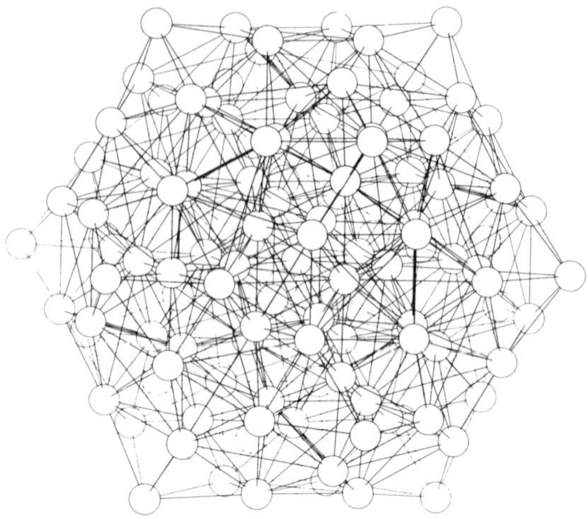

FIGURE 7. Rhombicosidodecahedral structure of 127 atoms grown from the 115-atom unit in FIGURE 5. This is the "icosahedron of icosahedra" containing 13 13-atom subunits bridged by octahedra.

somewhat to our surprise the curious structure FIGURE 9. This has a core made up as just described, but its surface is that of a rhombic tricontahedron. In that its surface facets have rudimentary close-packed planes, it is akin to the family of Mackay icosahedra, but, insofar as it grows out of 13 icosahedra rather than a single one, it can hardly be described as multiply twinned in the usual sense. The total number of atoms is 471 and its energy corresponds to $E/N = 6.47$.

We conclude this list of examples with a structure that illustrates that there is scarcely any obvious limit to the size of local structures that can be obtained by judicious combination of subunits of icosahedral or dodecahedral type. Geometrically, the key idea underlying the generation of hierarchical structures, such as the "icosahedron of icosahedra" discussed above, is the *radial net*. This type of spatial relationship is rarely discussed in crystallographic treatises, though a brief introduction to its main types will be found in Reference 41. Of the various three-dimensional radial nets that have been classified it is the so-called 5^6 dodecahedral net, which underlies almost all of our present constructions. The basic framework

FIGURE 8. (Left) The "5^6" radial net. (Right) Hierarchical structure of 399 atoms built as an icosahedron of the 43-atom subunits of FIGURE 6a.

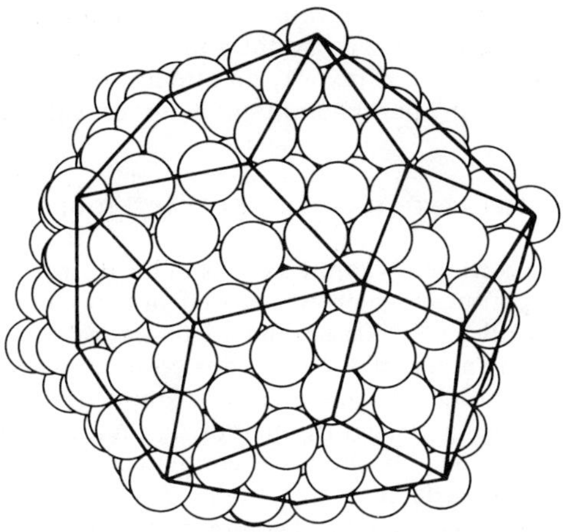

FIGURE 9. Rhombic triacontahedral structure derived by additions to FIGURE 8b. Contains 471 atoms.

of the 5^6 net is illustrated in FIGURE 8a, and can be envisaged in various ways. Its innermost unit can be seen as corresponding to the edges of the Voronoi polyhedra about the atoms of the 13-atom icosahedral structure, the next shell can be put into correspondence with the 13-atom subunits of the RID127 structure and so on, conceivably to a third and even higher level. This is, however, not the only strategy for building up very large structures based on the 5^6 radial net. Various units of tetrahedral symmetry can be placed at the vertices of the net forming thus the five-membered rings about the face of each dodecahedron. One such construction is illustrated in FIGURE 10, the basic unit being in this case the 26-atom T26 structure of FIGURE 4a. The hollow center of this can be filled very compactly with the Mackay 55-atom structure, FIGURE 6b, and the resulting whole, built into the next

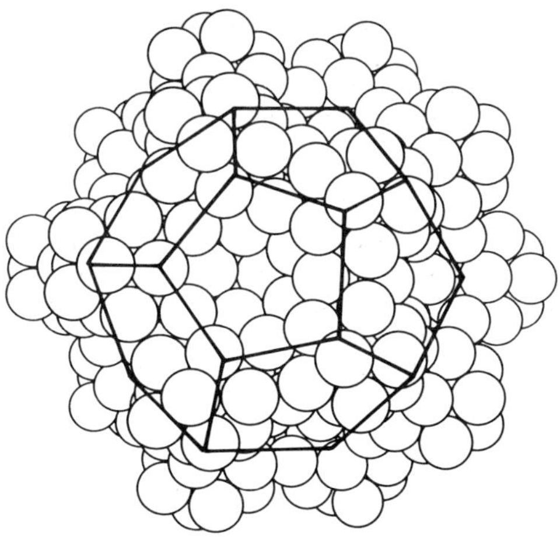

FIGURE 10. Dodecahedral 485-atom structure built of 26-atom subunits (FIGURE 4a). Envisaged as part of a "giant amorphon" based on the 5^6 dodecahedral net.

stage of the 5^6 net is an amorphon of, atomically speaking, enormous dimensions (In fact, 3965 atoms). I hasten to add that the above exercise is only an exploration of geometrical possibilities, not in any way an attempt to postulate the occurrence of such large structures in any particular material under realistic conditions.

Relaxation of the Bernal Model

Before going on to consider dynamic aspects of local structures, I shall mention a recent computer experiment which we carried out in collaboration with J. L. Finney of Birkbeck College.[46] This amounted to the relaxation of the original (1968) Bernal model, or rather of a 1000-atom core extracted from the original coordinates. The Lennard-Jones potential was applied to these and potential energy was minimized using an algorithm that discouraged violent motion over saddle points in the same neighborhood of configuration space. As we have described elsewhere in some detail,[47] the model did not undergo any dramatic changes of topology though certain local configurations did change, and there was an appreciable alteration in the computed radial distribution function (RDF). Figure 11 shows views of the central 100 atoms of the 999 treated before and after relaxation. There is no evidence of spontaneous crystallization and the RDF obtained shows an improvement in the direction of the profile observed in experimental alloy systems, particularly in correcting the previously anomalous asymmetric splitting of the split second peak. There is no visual or other evidence for the appearance of amorphons in the relaxed structure. This is not too surprising inasmuch as the original coordinates referred to a mass of "jammed" ball bearings, which would certainly need to pass over some quite remote saddle points to achieve this kind of local order.

Thus, in a somewhat too literal manner we have provided the answer to Turnbull's question of some years ago, "To what, if anything, does the Bernal model relax under a realistic potential?" without answering the more important one of, "To what kind of potential energy minima do simple atomic melts tend if cooled at the fastest rates possible under laboratory conditions?" All of which points to the fact that theoretical considerations of glassy structure must contain some reference to the conditions, even if hypothetical, of preparation and annealing of the sample.

Figure 12 shows the pair distribution function for the central 300 atoms of the unrelaxed Bernal model compared with the corresponding function for one of our larger optimized structures (the RTC471 structure of Figure 9). The two distributions are remarkably similar, except possibly for the fine-structure of the split second peak. The RDF for the optimized Bernal structure is, in fact, even closer to that for the RTC cluster of totally different geometry, which is, in turn, if anything, closest to experimental curves for amorphous alloys. These results illustrate how insensitive the radial distribution function is as an indicator or short-range amorphous structure and how limited are the conclusions that can be drawn from it. Further details of the optimization of the Bernal model will be found in the original paper.

The Dynamics of Local Structures

Before trying to bring the previous results to bear on the glass transition proper, I shall draw briefly on the results of some recent experiments on the dy-

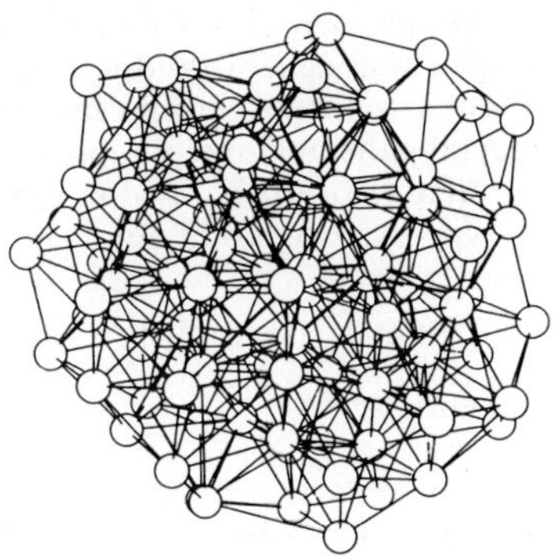

FIGURE 11. Central core of the Bernal model. (Left) As constructed by Bernal. (Right) After relaxation to a minimum in the Lennard-Jones potential. The object shown has 100 atoms and is extracted from the 999-atom central core of the "1968" Bernal model.

namics of isolated amorphous structures. Most of the Bedford College work on the dynamics of clusters[21,22] has been restricted to the vibrational analysis of structures in the harmonic approximation. We were able to demonstrate that, at temperatures conducive to effectively harmonic vibrations, the vibrational entropy

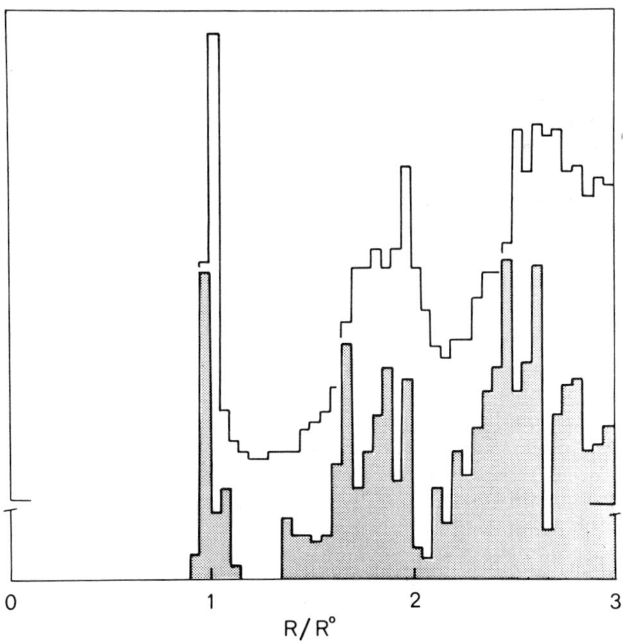

FIGURE 12. Pair distribution functions for the Bernal model (above) and that of a "packing amorphon" of similar size (below). The Bernal histogram is for 300 atoms taken from the central core of the *unrelaxed* "1968" model. The upper curve is for all atoms in the 471 atom RTC structure FIGURE 9.

does not seem to make a decisive contribution to the free energy of formation of small clusters in the range we have been discussing. These general findings have been borne out in the results of other workers.[47] To obtain further insight into the behavior or local structures at temperatures approaching the bulk melting point, it is necessary to go to a full "molecular dynamic" simulation of the natural motions and this has been carried out now for rare-gas type systems by a number of groups.[23-25,49-52]

Simulation of a Glassy Condensation

Recently a group at the Faculté des Sciences d'Orsay in Paris performed a computer simulation that involved the artificial quenching of a variety of isolated Lennard-Jones clusters from an initial randomly prepared liquid like state. The object of the exercise was to determine likely structures for homogeneously nucleated clusters of argon atoms, which they have succeeded in generating in supersonic jets and analyzing by electron diffraction.[48,49] The method followed was to arrange a continuous abstraction of kinetic energy until it was seen that the atoms in the cluster were localized and performing effectively harmonic vibrations. The mean atomic positions were then determined and RDFs and scattering curves were computed for comparison with experiment. The configurations obtained invariably showed evidence of noncrystalline order with enhancement of tetrahedral distances and the split second peak characteristic of atomic glasses. We later obtained sets of coordinates from the Orsay group and produced computer illustrations of the equilibrium configurations generated. There appeared throughout a strong tendency to motifs of five-fold symmetry and in one remarkable case we obtained the object illustrated in FIGURE 13. Although it is very difficult to distinguish in a "packed-sphere" diagram, the "ball and spoke" rendering clearly shows the presence of a RID115 nucleus (FIGURE 5) with some 14 other atoms distributed unsystematically about the surface facets. The generation of this structure from entirely random initial conditions to some extent justifies our special pleading in the previous section when we considered the actual Bernal model to be too tightly jammed to be able to relax to amorphonlike configurations.

The "Melting Transition" for Local Structures

Quite recently a number of independent authors have carried out extensive computer simulations of the dynamics of small, solid like Lennard-Jones clusters composed at known equilibrium positions.[23,48,53] The method has usually been to "warm" a solid cluster in equilibrium by gradual addition of kinetic energy and follow its motions as vibrations become anharmonic and delocalized motion sets in. One of the main clusters studied has been the $N = 55$ "Mackay icosahedron" (FIGURE 6b), which, though of multiple-twinned type, actually forms a subunit of some of the larger clusters studied here. As to be expected, the clusters become totally liquidlike at temperatures well below the bulk melting point; less predictable is the relative sharpness of the "melting transition," which takes place over a surprisingly narrow interval of energy. In the most comprehensive study so far, Briant and Burton[51] find a melting transition temperature of 35°K for the 13-atom L-J icosahedron rising to about 40°K in the region 50 to 100 atoms. (cf. bulk m.p. 84°K) Actually appreciable superheating and supercooling are observed, the

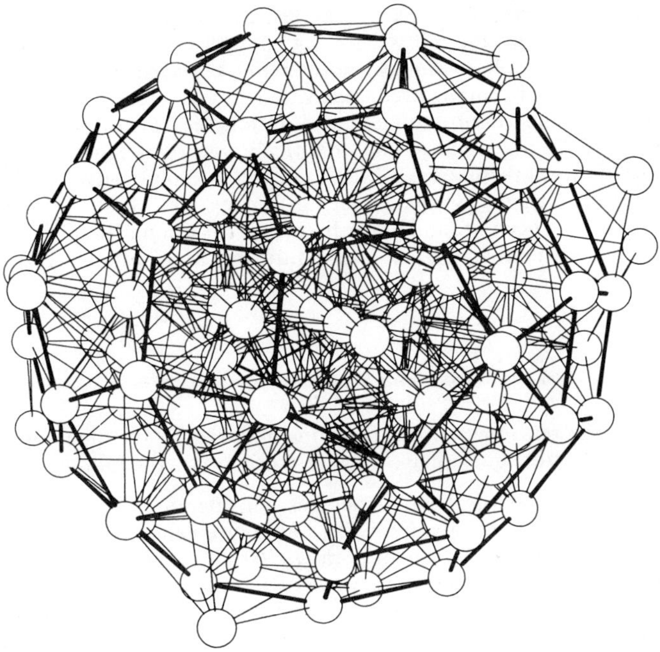

FIGURE 13. Structure generated spontaneously by "cooling" from computer-simulated liquid state. Note the presence of a 115-atom RID nucleus (FIGURE 5). We are indebted to J. Farges for supplying the coordinates of this model and for permission to reproduce it here.

quoted transition temperatures being obtained by a Maxwell construction. There is slight, though definite surface melting of the larger clusters at temperatures just below those required for the transition. We are investigating the feasibility of similar computations on our own, somewhat larger structures.

It will be noticed that I have refrained from drawing any conclusions from the better-known molecular dynamics simulations of liquid argon carried out at the Argonne Laboratory[58] and at Orsay.[59] This is because the presence of periodic boundary conditions in all these calculations cannot fail to destroy any vestiges of local order having a range approaching that for the structures we have exhibited here. We would estimate that a periodic "cell" containing some 10^5 atoms would be necessary before the conventional type of M-D calculation could hope to give rise to inhomogeneities of the kind we have predicted.

A Geometric Theory of the Glass Transition?

To a relative newcomer to the theory of the glassy state the multiplicity of models in the literature and the complexity of language in which they are formulated are alike bewildering. Altogether one hesitates to add a further dimension of argument to a subject that already seems to demand exegesis as much as logical analysis. The dangers of stressing geometrical explanation in what must be at root a dynamical *N*-body problem are clear and present in many branches of the glass literature. Just as the crystallographer is the last person likely to produce a theory of phase transitions so we may, if we are not careful, end up simply admiring the architecture of the amorphous state without in any way accounting for its existence of revealing anything of genuine predictive value.

Nevertheless I shall venture the conclusion that the key to the explanation of the glass transition is a geometric one of which an account can be given in terms relatively free of the mathematical subtleties in the interplay between phase space, configuration space and the simple 3-space of the system. Most of the ingredients for this prove to have been around in the literature for a long time though never, I think, properly articulated and, in one confusing area, almost certainly misapplied.

Local Order and Self-Limiting Structure

To establish the relevance of our previous material to the structure of a real atomically packed amorphous phase we would need to do the following:

(a) Demonstrate that the local structures considered are both mechanically stable in isolation and thermodynamically stable in a canonical ensemble at temperatures in the expected glass-transition range. *Or else* that there exist nucleation barriers with very long relaxation times preserving them against change to alternative forms, including the crystal nuclei. Further that the few structures discovered are truly representative of the many possible alternatives, perhaps less regular but sharing the same general size and structural characteristics.

(b) Show that their structural and dynamic properties are recognizably equivalent, or even enhanced, when they are composed of the mixed atomic species usual in amorphous alloys, and when they are embedded in, and mechanically coupled to, a surrounding matrix of indefinite structure.

(c) Adduce evidence that such structures are not merely stable under conditions of glass formation, but actually preferred among the alternatives available to a deeply supercooled liquid.

To these we might reasonably add the hope that any explanation relating to a glass transition in packed spheres might, in essence, be capable of extension to other types of glass-forming material.

In that we have only produced limited evidence under the first of these headings, we can only claim a tentative validity for what follows. Nevertheless if we are prepared to suspend doubts as to whether the experiments on isolated clusters are truly indicative of the behavior of the bulk phase, then the following *hypothetical* picture of the supercooled, amorphous packing emerges.

(a) The postulate of *homogeneity* in the terms insisted on by both Bernal and the "free-volume" school of glass theory[53–55] is questionable. In contrast there is a pronounced tendency at sufficiently low temperature to the formation of local amorphons with pentagonal and icosahedral elements of symmetry. These are at a thermodynamic advantage over *local* lattice structures of small dimensions and thus are protected from crystallization by the free-energy barriers to reconstructive transformation.

(b) Because of essential space-filling deficits these units are limited in size and possess surfaces with a degree of tensile strain. Nevertheless they can easily reach sizes of several hundreds of atoms—far larger than Franck's 13-atom icosahedra and large enough to give rise to relatively strained interstitial regions if they impinge on each other.

(c) The dynamic behavior of isolated clusters is to some extent mimicked by amorphons embedded in a solid matrix. In particular they show a relatively sharp melting transition at temperatures appreciable below the bulk melting point in the course of which disorganization begins at the surface and affects their inner shells least easily. Those local regions that cohere at a particular temperature possess considerable mechanical rigidity (more in fact than microcrystallites) and have no low saddle points for the transmission of shear.

If we entertain the possibility of this kind of inhomogeneity setting in, in the absence of crystallization, at some temperature well into the supercooled liquid region, what measurable properties can we expect it to confer on the substance? We know from various simulations[37] that the presence of amorphons of icosahedral type can be expected to "improve" the model RDF from that of the Bernal packing, expecially in the region of the second-peak splitting, though the RDF cannot be said to be a sensitive indicator of structural differences between different amorphous structures. We know from an increasing body of experimental information that anomalous dielectric, heat-capacity, thermal-conductivity, and other behavior invites the assumption of an ill-defined inhomogeneity, perhaps at the 100 to 1000-atom level. In short it is clear that a properly substantiated inhomogeneous model of the amorphous phase would be a welcome explanatory factor rather than an embarassment to most experimentalists.

However, it is in the explanation of the glass transition itself rather than the elucidation of other consequential effects that the role of the amorphon may prove to be crucial. If it is thc case that the growth of such regions is *self-limiting* and coupled with a tendency to form within a mobile and relatively disordered surface region (both these properties deriving from the same geometrical attributes), then an explanation rather than a description of the glass transition is at hand. We have only to envisage the number density of amorphons in the supercooled liquid rising (with only disproportionate tendency to increase in size) to see that a point can be reached where they impinge and, with relatively slight further decrease of temperature, congeal together throughout the mass. At this point a more or less catastrophic increase in viscosity would be observed depending to an extent on the slight degree of slippage and stress relief still possible at the boundaries of the "solid" regions.

I would pause here to assert that an explanation based on the above rather picturesque sequence of events would retain its credibility if we relaxed considerably the requirement of well-defined, centrally symmetric amorphons. It would be enough that there be a statistical tendency to the formation of structural motifs, irregular and perhaps transient, though on average recognizably in possession of the characteristics outlined above. The simple picture of a "congealing point" would then be somewhat blurred, with the mechanism of stress relief taking on something of the nature of a percolation problem with respect to the diminishing liquidlike connections running through the material. This need only entail a slight broadening of the transition range.

Tammann Revisited

To those acquainted with some of the early accounts of the glass transition several of the points made above will have a familiar ring. In fact, in overall *de-*

scriptive terms much of what I have said is almost a paraphrase of Tammann's classical explanation of the rigidifying (Erstarrung) of a glassy material near its transition temperature.[60] Tammann, it will be recalled, likened the onset of viscosity increase to the parallel phenomenon in clays whose platelike particles jam rigidly together when the interstitial water separating them falls to a critical proportion. This, along with more molecular descriptions by Simon[61] is perhaps the origin of a characteristic train of thought among European glass and viscosity theorists, many of whom, in distinct contrast to what one might call the "J. Chem. Phys." school, have emphasized the role of "microcrystallites," "paracrystallinity," "vitrons," and the like as structural entities. (See especially Eckstein,[62] Porai-Kosic,[63] Hosemann,[64] McLaughlin and Ubbelohde[65]). These theories, for the most part inherit the weakness in Tammann's original model, which is that no convincing microscopic reason is given for the appearance of rather stable, rigid, regularly sized and independent structural units in the temperature range of interest. Worse than this, several of the above authors have insisted that remnants of ordered regions persist above the normal melting point and contribute to viscosity anomalies in the mobile liquid range. These on the whole poorly substantiated and occasionally far-fetched claims have undoubtedly diverted attention from the virtues of Tammann's picture and its requirement of dynamic and structural inhomogeneity *in the neighborhood of* T_g.

The missing ingredient that, I suggest, transforms Tammann's description into a viable and predictive model is that of *self-limiting growth* based on noncrystallographic symmetries. This too is a relatively old idea, having been postulated by Frank[35] as the source of the nucleation barrier in "ordinary" supercooling and advocated by McLaughlin and Ubbelohde[65] in an attempt to explain prefreezing viscosity anomalies. The full importance of this concept in explaining the glass transition itself, not to mention its considerably greater plausibility (at T_g rather than T_f), seems not to have been sufficiently appreciated. At the same time, while the idea of amorphons arose in considerations of bonded networks, its application appears to have been restricted to structural interpretations and the prediction of the RDF.

There remains one respect in which the ideas we have arrived at through packing studies amount to more than the sum of these earlier perceptions. This is in the assertion that the amorphons responsible for the "congealing" transition in Tammann's sense might, even in monatomic systems, be considerably larger than Frank and others forsaw. Once the dominant structural motifs in the neighborhood of T_g extend to an average of some three- to four-coordination shells, a number of quite new possibilities are opened up: (a) The congealed matrix below T_g will possess small but definite regions of strained "connective tissue" between the more organized amorphons. (b) The latter may be large enough for there to be an element of differential melting at their surface, this contributing to a sudden onset of slippage and mobility with rising temperature. (c) The larger the regions of local order, the more reasonable to consider them as relatively uncoupled dynamically. All these factors combine to invite the explanation of calorimetric and kinetic anomalies along lines that have been hinted at in this meeting and elsewhere.

Conclusions

In the previous section I have not resisted the presumption that the elaboration of Tammann's picture to include self-limiting amorphons need not be limited to the soft-packed monatomic glasses modeled in our computer experiments. On considering each of the main classes of glass-forming substances (with the possible exception of ionic glasses) it is not difficult to find geometrical characteristics that might induce the formation of the required locally ordered centers. Some of these are listed in TABLE 1. Even in the case of polymers, there is the basis of an analogy, with the formation of micellar regions whose growth is frustrated not by packing deficits but rather by chain entanglements. As before, a statistical tendency to growth-limited local structure rather than conformity to a definite repeated pattern may well suffice to produce a glass transition.

Must a theory such as I have outlined stop short of the real test of its predictive value: the estimation of actual values of T_g? Perhaps the crucial question at the present stage is that of whether a viable theory of the glass-transition is possible, which obviates the necessity to face the full statistical mechanics of phase transitions—which reduces, in other words, the N-body problem to a few-body problem in an essential way, not merely as a convenient mathematical approximation. The picture we have outlined suggests that this may not be a forlorn hope and that thereby the glass transition can be both explained and shown, once and for all, not to be a "phase transition" as we normally understand this term. The key steps in

TABLE 1

GLASS-FORMING SUBSTANCES AND POSSIBLE LOCALLY ORDERED CENTERS

System	Local Geometry ?
Metals, rare gases	Packing amorphons
Silicates	Tilton structures
Ge, Si	Grigorovici amorphons
H_2O, EtOH	Clathrate structures
Carbohydrates	Spheroidal packing, Clathrate motifs
Polymers	Chain-hindered and micellar growth, "Spherulitic" structure
Ionic glasses	?

this program would be the recognition of the dominant units of local order, if any, in a substance and the determination of their "melting transition temperature" when driven by a relatively undifferentiated surrounding matrix. This is easier said than done. But suppose that an argon glass could be prepared and shown to be stable up to a transition temperature. It would not surprise me, in fact I might be willing to bet, that T_g would be in the region of 40°K—not because this is about the right proportion of T_f in comparison with other substances, but because it is the probable melting transition temperature for a three- to four-shell packing amorphon driven by a weakly-coupled heat bath.

A more detailed account of this work and its thermodynamic implications is in preparation.[66]

SUMMARY

In this paper I have described some recent experiments in the design and testing of stable soft-packed structures and considered their implication for the theory of the glass transition. Taken in conjunction with a variety of independent evidence, these results cast considerable doubt on the postulate of homogeneity in simple packings under a realistic interaction potential and suggest that relatively large, noncrystalline motifs with a tendency to local symmetry may be a prominent feature of "relaxed" glassy structures. It is suggested that three related consequences of the mechanics of such "packing amorphons" are essential to the nature of the glass transition. Their tendency to five-fold and icosahedral symmetry creates a free-energy barrier to nucleation and introduces a crucial property of local self-limiting growth. This latter property together with the known tendency to differential surface melting in such structures combines to create precisely the kind of medium-range texture and "congealing" described, though not justified, in Tammann's early account of the glass transition. This general explanation would appear to be capable of extension to more general types of glass-forming system.

Acknowledgment

The entire computer programming and graphical processing in this paper was carried out by John Andrew Barker, who is coauthor of Reference 66. We are indebted to the Science Research Council, London for financial support throughout the period of this project. Richard Hoare provided valuable assistance with model building.

References

1. Werfelmeier, W. 1937. Z. Physik. **107:** 332.
2. Pauling, L. 1965. Science **150:** 297.
3. Horne, R. W. & P. Wildy, 1961. Virology **15:** 348.
4. Higuti, I. 1960. Ann. Inst. Stat. Math. **12:** 257.
5. Wheeler, J. A. 1973. *In* Gravitation. J. A. Wheeler and C. M. Misner, Eds. W. H. Freeman. San Francisco.
6. Gani, J. 1975. Adv. Appl. Prob. **7:** 232.
7. Bernal, J. D. 1960. Nature. **185:** 68.
8. Bernal, J. D. 1964. Proc. R. Soc. London **280A:** 299.
9. Bernal, J. D. 1965. *In* Liquids: Structure, Properties, Solid Interactions. T. J. Hughel, Ed.:25. Elsevier. Amsterdam.
10. Finney, J. L. 1970. Proc. R. Soc. London **A319:** 479.
11. Collins, R. 1964. Proc. Phys. Soc. **83:** 553. *Ibid.* **86:** 199.
12. Boerdijk, A. H. 1952. Phillips Res. Rep. **7:** 303.
13. Frank, F. C. & J. S. Kasper. 1958. Acta Crystallogr. **11:** 184.
14. Cohen, M. H. & D. Turnbull. 1964. Nature **189:** 131. *Ibid.* **203:** 964.
15. Prins, J. A. 1965. *In* The Physics of Non-crystalline Solids. J. A. Prins, Ed.: 5. North Holland. Amsterdam.
16. Hoare, M. R. & P. Pal. Adv. Phys. **20:** 161.
17. Hoare, M. R. & P. Pal. 1971. Nature **230:** 5. 1972. *Ibid.* **236:** 35.
18. Burton, J. J. 1970. J. Chem. Phys. **52:** 345. 1973. *Ibid.* **56:** 3133.
19. Burton, J. J. 1973. J. Chem. Soc. Faraday II **69:** 540.
20. Bonissent & B. Mutaftschiev. 1973. J. Chem. Phys. **58:** 3727.
21. Hoare, M. R. & P. Pal. 1972. J. Cryst. Growth **17:** 77.
22. Hoare, M. R. & P. Pal. 1975. Adv. Phys. **24:** 646.
23. Kristensen, W. D., E. J. Jensen & R. M. J. Cotterill. 1974. J. Chem. Phys. **60:** 4161.
24. Briant, C. L. & J. J. Burton. 1975. J. Chem. Phys. **63:** 2045.

25. ETTERS, R. D. & J. KAELBERER. 1975. Phys. Rev. **A11:** 1068.
26. MORRELL, W. E. & J. H. HILDEBRAND. 1936. J. Chem. Phys. **4:** 224.
27. BARKER, J. A. & H. N. GLADNEY. 1975. J. Chem. Phys. **63:** 3870.
28. FUKANO, Y. & C. M. WAYMAN. 1969. J. Appl. Phys. **40:** 1656.
29. ALDER, B. 1972. J. Chem. Phys. **56:** 987.
30. GOLDSTEIN, M. 1969. J. Chem. Phys. **51:** 3728.
31. GOLDSTEIN, M. 1963. J. Chem. Phys. **39:** 3369.
32. ANGELL, C. A. & K. J. RAO. 1972. J. Chem. Phys. **57:** 470.
33. KAUTZMANN, W. 1948. Chem. Rev. **43:** 219.
34. SHTERNBERG, A. A. 1968. Rost. Kristallov. **5a:** 179. (Engl. Trans.: 1969. Growth of Crystals **8:** 256. Consultants Bureau, New York.)
35. FRANK, F. C. 1952. Proc. R. Soc. London. **A215:** 43.
36. ALLPRESS, J. G. & J. V. SANDERS. 1970. Aust. J. Phys. **23:** 23.
37. SADOC, J. F., J. DIXMIER & A. GUINIER. 1973. J. Non-Cryst. Solids. **12:** 46.
38. KOMODA, T. 1968. Japan. J. Appl. Phys. **7:** 27.
39. SAMSON, S. 1965. Acta Crystallogr. **19:** 401.
40. SAMSON, S. 1968. *In* Structural Chemistry and Molecular Biology. A Volume dedicated to Linus Pauling by His Students, Colleagues, and Friends. A. Rich & N. Davidson, Eds.: 487. W. H. Freeman & Co. San Francisco.
41. WELLS, A. F. 1970. Models in Structural Inorganic Chemistry. Appendix 3. Clarendon. Oxford.
42. GRIGOROVICI, R. 1968. Mat. Res. Bull. **3:** 13.
43. GRIGOROVICI, R. 1969. J. Non-Cryst. Solids. **1:** 371.
44. CUNDY, H. M. 1952. Math. Gaz. **36:** 263.
45. MACKAY, A. 1962. Acta Crystallogr. **15:** 916.
46. BARKER, J. ANDREW, J. L. FINNEY & M. R. HOARE. 1975. Nature **257:** 120.
47. MCGINTY, D. J. 1971. J. Chem. Phys. **55:** 580.
48. FARGES, J., B. RAOULT & G. TORCHET. 1973. J. Chem. Phys. **59:** 3454.
49. FARGES, J. Private communication, to be published.
50. BRIANT, C. L. & J. J. BURTON. 1973. Nature Phys. Sci. **243:** 100.
51. BRIANT, C. L. & J. J. BURTON. 1975. J. Chem. Phys. **63:** 3870.
52. BRIANT, C. L. & J. J. BURTON. To be published.
53. EYRING, H. 1936. J. Chem. Phys. **4:** 283.
54. TURNBULL, D. & M. H. COHEN. 1958. J. Chem. Phys. **29:** 1049.
55. TURNBULL, D. & M. H. COHEN. 1961. J. Chem. Phys. **34:** 120.
56. HUNKLINGER, S., P. PICHE, J. C. LASJAUNIAS & K. DRANSFELD. 1975. J. Phys. C, Solid State Physics **8:** L423.
57. GOLDSTEIN, M. Private communication. To be published.
58. RAHMAN, A. 1964. Phys. Rev. **136:** A405.
59. VERLET, L. 1967. Phys. Rev. **159:** 98.
60. TAMMANN, G. 1933. Der Glasszustand. Section IV, 12. Leopold Voss, Leipzig.
61. SIMON, F. 1930. Ergeb. Exakt. Naturwiss. **9:** 222.
62. ECKSTEIN, B. 1963. Glasstechn. Ber. **36:** 323. (See also Reference 15, p. 77.)
63. PORAI-KOSIC, E. A. 1959. Glastechn. Ber. **32:** 450. (See also Reference 15, p. 117.)
64. HOSEMANN, R. 1950. Z. Phys. **128:** 465. (See also Reference 15, p. 85.)
65. MCLAUGHLIN, E. & A. R. UBBELOHDE. 1958. Trans. Faraday Soc. **54:** 1804.
66. BARKER, J. ANDREW & M. R. HOARE. To be published.

RECURRING THEMES IN THE STRUCTURE OF GLASSY SOLIDS

G. S. Cargill III

IBM Thomas J. Watson Research Center
Yorktown Heights, New York 10598

INTRODUCTION

Understanding basic properties of amorphous materials requires realistic models for arrangements of atoms in these materials. Considerable progress has been made in formulating structural models and in comparing them with experimentally accessible structural data for many amorphous materials, including oxide glasses, amorphous silicon and germanium, and amorphous metallic alloys. Experimental data on atomic arrangements in amorphous SiO_2 (silica) were obtained by Warren *et al.*[1] in 1936; models for the atomic scale structure of SiO_2 have been proposed, criticized, and occasionally compared with experimentally accessible structural data since the 1930s. Interest in amorphous Si and Ge is of more recent origin; the first experimental data on atomic arrangements in amorphous Ge were published by Richter and Furst[2] in 1951; structural models and additional experimental data have been presented regularly during the last decade.[3,4] The first experimental structural data on amorphous metallic alloys that are stable at room temperature were published by Dixmier *et al.*[5,6] in 1963 and 1965. Many amorphous metal-metalloid alloys (e.g., Pd—Si, Ni—P, Fe—P—C, Co—P) containing approximately 20 at.% metalloid elements (Si, P, C. etc.) have now been examined by x-ray scattering, and models for atomic arrangements in these metallic glasses have been proposed, tested, and refined.[7]

The evolutions of models for atomic arrangements in these three types of amorphous solids will be reviewed in this paper. Particularly, recurring themes in the evolutions of models for atomic arrangements in (1) silica glass, in (2) amorphous Si and Ge, and in (3) metallic alloy glasses will be examined. Some contributors in these evolutions are listed in TABLE 1. In the latter sections of this review, some current views on the structure of metallic glasses will be summarized; recent results on anisotropies and long-range ordering in some model structures will also be described.

EVOLUTION OF STRUCTURAL MODELS

Continuous Random Models

The best developed models for atomic arrangements in all three of these classes of amorphous solids are the continuous random (CR) ones. Continuous random network (CRN) models for silica and for amorphous silicon and germanium, formed from tetrahedral units linked together to form continuous irregular three-dimensional networks, follow from the early proposals of Zachariasen.[8]

Silica Glass

Bell and Dean[9,10] have published detailed comparisons of their CRN model for SiO_2 with both x-ray and neutron radial distribution functions $\mathrm{RDF}(r) = 4\pi r^2 \rho(r)$,

TABLE 1

SOME CONTRIBUTORS IN EVOLUTIONS OF STRUCTURAL MODELS FOR VARIOUS AMORPHOUS SOLIDS

	SiO_2	Si & Ge	Metal-Metalloid Alloys, e.g. $Pd_{80}Si_{20}$
Microcrystalline models	Randall *et al.*[72] (1930) Valenkov and Porai-Koshits[25] (1937) Konnert *et al.*[26] (1973)	Howie *et al.*[27] (1973) Weinstein and Davis[28] (1973)	Graham *et al.*[29] (1965) Tyan and Toth[30] (1974)
Noncrystalline cluster models	Vitrons–pentagonal dodecahedra	Amorphons–pentagonal dodecahedra	Polytetrahedral and icosahedral clusters
	Tilton[31] (1957) Robinson[32] (1965)	Coleman and Thomas[33] (1967) Grigorovici and Manaila[34] (1968)	Farges *et al.*[35] (1975) Briant and Burton[36] (1975)
Continuous random models	Random networks	Random networks	Dense random packing of hard spheres
	Zachariasen[8] (1932) Warren *et al.*[1] (1936) Ordway[73] (1964) Bell and Dean[9] (1966) Evans and King[74] (1966)	Polk[12] (1971) Shevchik and Paul[75] (1972) Henderson and Herman[76] (1972) Steinhardt *et al.*[71] (1974) Evans *et al.*[70] (1974)	Finney[18] (1970) Cargill[20] (1970) Polk[57] (1970) Bennett[19] (1972) Sadoc *et al.*[48] (1973) Sadoc and Dixmier[59] (1975)

and this model has been used to interpret the vibrational properties of silica.[11] In this model, constructed from polystyrene spheres, representing silicon and oxygen atoms, and steel wires, representing Si—O covalent bonds, the Si—O—Si angles were distributed about 153°.[10]

Amorphous Ge and Si

Polk[12] was the first to construct a CRN model for amorphous Ge and Si. The comparisons of RDF(r) for this model and for other similarly constructed tetrahedral CRN models with experimental RDFs for amorphous Si and Ge provide considerable support for the model's validity.[12–14]

Metallic Alloy Glasses

Dense random packings of hard spheres (DRPHS)[15] may be thought of as the close-packed analogs of such CRN structures.[16,17] DRPHS structures have been produced by filling rubber blatters with ball bearings,[18] and similar structures have also been generated with various computer algorithms.[19] Radial distribution functions for such DRPHS structures have been compared with those obtained for amorphous metal-metalloid alloys (e.g., Ni—P, Pd—Si, Fe—P—C) containing approximately 80 at.% metalloid elements.[7,20] and for amorphous thin-film samples of some transition metals (e.g., Co, Fe) at low temperatures.[21,22] The DRPHS models reproduce characteristic features of the experimental distribution functions. CRN and DRPHS models have been used to calculate vibrational properties of amorphous Ge and Si[23] and of amorphous $Co_{80}P_{20}$,[24] respectively.

Homogeneity in Continuous Random Models

These continuous random models may be described as homogeneous, in contrast with microcrystalline and amorphous cluster models, which have also been proposed for some of these types of amorphous solids. In the CR models, the correlations between atomic positions appear to decay gradually with increasing interatomic separations, although short-range order (SRO) is strongly maintained in the CRN models and well-defined SRO is present in DRPHS models.

Microcrystalline Models

Microcrystalline models for amorphous solids[25] are heterogeneous in that highly ordered regions, microcrystals, are separated from one another by regions of much lower order, i.e., grain boundaries or extended regions of connective material. In these models, correlations between atomic positions decrease abruptly when the interatomic vector crosses the boundary between microcrystals. Although microcrystalline models have been proposed for amorphous SiO_2,[25,26] for Si and Ge,[27,28] and for metal-metalloid alloys,[29,30] no detailed prescriptions have been given for atomic arrangements in the grain boundary—connective material. At their present level of development, comparisons of experimental distribution functions (or interference functions) with those for microcrystalline models are much less convincing than are similar comparisons with continuous random models.

Noncrystallographic Cluster Models

Noncrystallographic cluster models constitute another type of heterogeneous description of atomic arrangements in amorphous solids. With these models, which have been proposed for SiO_2,[31,32] for Si and Ge,[33,34] and for amorphous metal-metalloid alloys,[35,36] noncrystallographic but highly ordered clusters of atoms play the same role as the microcrystals discussed above.

Silica and Amorphous Ge and Si

Tilton[31] and Robinson[32] have proposed "vitrons" based on pentagonal dodecahedra as structural building blocks for silica glass. Coleman and Thomas[33] and Grigorovici and Manaila[34] proposed "amorphons," also based on the pentagonal dodecahedron, as the major structural unit in amorphous Si and Ge. The amorphon corresponds to a vitron from which the oxygen atoms have been removed.

The latter authors[34] argued that small clusters of the pentagonal dodecahedral geometry are energetically favored over crystallographic configurations for the tetrahedrally coordinated Si or Ge because the number of surface dangling bonds per atom for such clusters is somewhat less than for a crystal containing the same number of atoms, and the tetrahedral angles between atoms in such clusters are only slightly distorted. Neither the vitron model for amorphous SiO_2 nor the amorphon model for amorphous Ge and Si, in their present states of development, has been as successful as the corresponding CRN models in reproducing experimental RDFs of SiO_2 or Si and Ge.

Metallic Alloy Glasses

Structural models for amorphous close packed materials (transition metal films and metal-metalloid alloys) have also been approached from the amorphous cluster point of view.[35,36] These heterogeneous models have been supported by observations that certain noncrystallographic clusters of small numbers of atoms with Lennard-Jones potentials have lower energies per atom than crystallographic clusters containing the same numbers of atoms.

In 1952 F. C. Frank[37] noted that a thirteen-atom cluster with twelve atoms at the face centers of a regular pentagonal dodecahedron centered on the thirteenth atom should have a lower internal energy, with pairwise Lennard-Jones interactions, than either of the crystallographic (fcc or hcp) arrangements, and he proposed that such noncrystallographic groupings would be very common in simple liquids. Hoare and Pal[38] have systematically enumerated minimum energy configurations for clusters of from three to sixty atoms under Lennard-Jones forces. They found three particularly compact noncrystallographic growth schemes, with tetrahedral, pentagonal, and icosahedral symmetries, which were appreciably more stable than fcc microcrystals having the same numbers of atoms. All of the lowest energy clusters obtained by Hoare and Pal[38] correspond to packing of approximately regular tetrahedra (atoms at tetrahedral vertices) face to face. Although high-density (low-energy) clusters can be produced by such tetrahedral packing, they cannot be extended indefinitely, because the tetrahedron is not quite a space-filling object. The fcc crystalline packing corresponds to packing tetrahedra *and* octahedra.

Farges *et al.*[35] have calculated distribution functions and interference functions for polytetrahedral clusters of 46 atoms and have found that they are similar to those obtained experimentally for small argon clusters, for amorphous thin films of Co, and to a lesser extent for an amorphous metal-metalloid alloy (Ni—P). They conclude that the arrangements of atoms in these materials are well represented by the polytetrahedral clusters. Briant and Burton[36] have also proposed that the 13-atom icosahedron is an important structural unit in amorphous close-packed materials. Structural models based rigorously on such highly ordered building blocks must apparently be hetrogeneous, with the polytetrahedral regions joined together by less ordered, lower-density and higher-energy regions.

Realistic Models—Useful Models

The above discussions suggest that we have a surfeit of models for atomic arrangements in these three classes of amorphous solids. Three separate criteria should be considered in evaluating the various competing models: (1) a model should be a realistic representation of atomic arrangements in the actual amorphous material, based on comparisons with experimentally accessible structural data; (2) it should be useful as the basis for predictive calculations of properties of the amorphous material; and (3) it should be susceptible to further refinement, as additional experimental structural data become available or as requirements of those actually using the models become more severe.

Realistic Models and Experimentally Accessible Structural Data

X-ray, electron, and neutron scattering measurements provide direct information on atomic arrangements in amorphous solids. Most amorphous solids are macroscopically isotropic. The scattering patterns, i.e., interference functions, then depend only on the scattering angle 2θ, or equivalently on the magnitude of the scattering vector $|\vec{K}| = K = 4\pi \sin \theta/\lambda$, where λ is the x-ray, electron, or neutron wavelength. Fourier sine transformation of the scattering measurements, i.e., of the interference function $I(K)$, yields the radial distribution function $\mathrm{RDF}(r) = 4\pi r^2 \rho(r)$ when the amorphous material consists of identical atoms. For a material composed of n different types of atoms, $\rho(r)$ can usually be interpreted as the weighted average of $n(n + 1)/2$ partial distribution functions $\rho_{ij}(r)$,

$$\rho(r) = \sum_{i,j}^{n} W_{ij}[\rho_{ij}(r)/c_j], \tag{1}$$

where W_{ij} are weighting factors that depend on concentrations c_i and c_j of atoms of types i and j and on the scattering strengths of these types of atoms.[1,7] Radial distribution functions for well-characterized models can be compared with those obtained experimentally, or interference functions calculated for the model structures can be compared with results of scattering measurements for amorphous materials.

Small-angle scattering (SAS) measurements provide information on chemical and structural homogeneity, just as the larger-angle scattering measurements characterize atomic scale structure. Small-angle scattering would be expected to result from materials with heterogeneous structures, e.g., those corresponding to microcrystalline or noncrystalline cluster models, if low density regions separate the microcrystals or clusters. However, the amount of SAS to be expected depends on the manner in which the microcrystals or clusters are arranged and joined together, and these aspects of such models have, up to now, received little attention.[39]

Densities of many amorphous solids have been measured; densities can also be calculated from well-characterized structural models. Comparisons of measured and calculated densities provide another component in accessing whether a model realistically represents atomic arrangements in a particular amorphous material.

Criteria for "Useful" Models

Realistic models for the three dimensional arrangements of atoms in amorphous solids are needed in developing and testing our understanding of the basic physical properties of these solids. Such tests usually involve computer calculations and require positional coordinates of large numbers of atoms. CRN and DRPHS models have been very useful as the starting point for such calculations.[11,23,24,40–43]

"Refinability" is another important criterion for the usefulness of structural models. CRN models for amorphous Ge and Si, constructed from tetrahedral units, have been refined by energy-minimization routines with realistic bond-bending and bond-stretching force constants. This refinement produced small changes in "atomic" positions without altering the topology of the structures.[44,45] DRPHS models, both computer-generated and physically constructed, have also been relaxed, using central force, pairwise interactions.[46,47] Such refinements have improved agreement between model and experimental distribution functions and have increased confidence that these are realistic models for atomic arrangements in the actual materials.

Another example of refinement of CR models involves use of two different sphere sizes in DRPHS modeling of atomic arrangements in metal-metalloid glasses, and incorporation of chemical ordering, e.g., allowing no metalloid-metalloid nearest neighbors, in computer-generated binary DRPHS models for these amorphous alloys.[48]

Current Views on the Structure of Metallic Glasses

In this section some current views on the structure of metallic glasses are summarized, here using the term "glass" to refer to amorphous metals and alloys produced in a variety of ways, e.g., evaporation, sputtering, electrical and chemical deposition, as well as quenching from the liquid state.[7,49] The metals and alloys are amorphous, or equivalently "noncrystalline," in the operational sense that their x-ray, electron, or neutron scattering patterns (diffuse, with a few broad, overlapping peaks) indicate that they do not possess well-defined, spatially periodic atomic arrangements, and these scattering patterns are inconsistent with those calculated for arrays of small crystals. The crystal structures employed in these comparisons are usually those of the material's equilibrium phases.[7]

Some Types of Amorphous Metals and Alloys

Most experimental work on amorphous metallic alloys in the last 10 years has involved materials prepared in amorphous form by rapid cooling from the melt. Duwez and his coworkers have developed techniques (splat cooling and hammer-and-anvil methods) for quenching small molten droplets at rates as high as 10^{6}°C/sec.[50] Methods have also been developed for rapidly quenching amorphous alloys in ribbon form.[51,52] Most amorphous metallic alloys produced by rapid quenching have been alloys of noble or transition metals with elements of groups IV or V (metalloids) containing between 15 and 30 at.% of the latter. Electrodeposition and chemical or electroless deposition have also been used to produce some amorphous alloys of the metal-metalloid type.[5,6,53,54]

Other amorphous metallic solids have been obtained by evaporation of metals in vacuum and condensation of their vapors on a substrate maintained at low temperature. Some nominally pure metals have been prepared by this technique. Amorphous films of Co and of Fe, with no intentional impurity additions, have been prepared by vacuum evaporation at 4°K and 10^{-8} Torr.[21,22] These films crystallize at approximately 50°K; their crystallization temperatures increase with increasing residual gas pressure during evaporation. Intentional addition of impurities, e.g., a few percent Si in Co, is known to increase greatly crystallization temperatures of such amorphous films.[55]

These amorphous metals and alloys are listed in TABLE 2. Other types of metallic alloy glasses have also been prepared and studied; some of these have been included in TABLE 2.

Structural Similarities

Detailed structural studies have been reported for most of these materials.[7] Interference functions for amorphous metal-metalloid alloys are very similar to one another, even among alloys produced by such diverse methods as rapid

TABLE 2

SOME TYPES OF AMORPHOUS METALS AND ALLOYS

Materials	Methods	Crystallization Temperatures
Metal-metalloid alloys		
Au—Si, Pd—Si, Fe—P—C, Mn—P—C Ni—Pd—P, Fe—Pd—P, Mn—Pd—P, Ni—Pt—P, . . .	Rapid quenching	300°–700°K
Ni—P, Co—P, Fe—P	Electrodeposition, vacuum evaporation	~600°K
Fe—Si, Co—Si, . . .	Vacuum evaporation (20°K)	60°–250°K
"Pure" elemental metals		
Co, Fe, Cr, Mn, Bi, Ga	Vacuum evaporation (4°K)	15°–100°K
Rare-earth–transition-metal alloys		
Tb—Fe, Gd—Fe, Gd—Co, . . .	R.F. and D.C. sputtering, vacuum evaporation	~700°K
Other alloy types		
Ag—Cu, Cu—Mg, Au—Fe, Pb—Sb, . . .	Vacuum evaporation	Wide range

quenching and electrodeposition. These interference functions have a sharp, well-defined first maximum, with a second maximum that is weaker and broader and has a shoulder on its large-angle side. Maxima and minima became rapidly weaker with increasing scattering angle. Interference functions for nominally pure amorphous thin films of transition metals Co, Fe, Cr, and Mn are also similar to those of the metal-metalloid alloys, except for the splitting of the second maximum in $I(K)$ for the transition metal films, as shown in FIGURE 1. Distribution functions $RDF(r)$ for the amorphous metal-metalloid alloys and for the amorphous transition metal films are also very similar, as shown by curves (a) and (b) of FIGURE 2. Both show the characteristic splitting of the second maximum, which is found for all of the metal-metalloid alloys with only one type of metal atom, and both have nearest neighbor maxima near the distance of closest approach (2.50 Å) in crystalline Co (fcc or hcp).

Detailed comparisons of measured scattering patterns of amorphous metal-metalloid alloys with those expected for small crystals of their equilibrium cry-

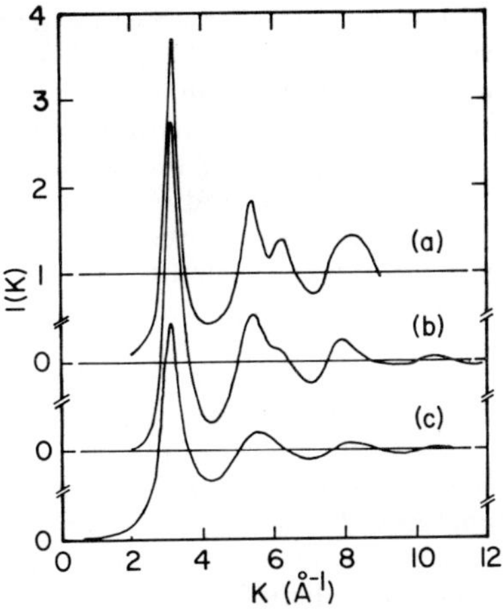

FIGURE 1. Interference functions for (a) amorphous Co (from Leung & Wright[22]), (b) amorphous $Co_{78}P_{22}$ (from Cargill & Cochrane[77]), and (c) liquid Co (from Waseda & Ohtani[78]).

stalline forms indicated that the amorphous alloys were not composed of small crystals, but possibilities of highly strained and defective crystals, perhaps with structures different from the equilibrium crystalline phases, have not been exhaustively tested.[5,6,56]

Dense Random Packing of Hard Spheres

RDFs for many amorphous metal-metalloid alloys are very similar to those obtained by Finney[18] and others for dense random packings of single-sized hard spheres, and this type of model is a very attractive alternative to microcrystalline models for these amorphous alloys.[20] X-ray distribution functions for the metal-metalloid alloys are dominated by contribution of metal-metal pairs because the metal atoms both are more numerous, typically comprising between 70 and 80 at.%, and have much larger x-ray scattering factors.

Polk[57,58] first proposed that the simple DRPHS model for these alloys be

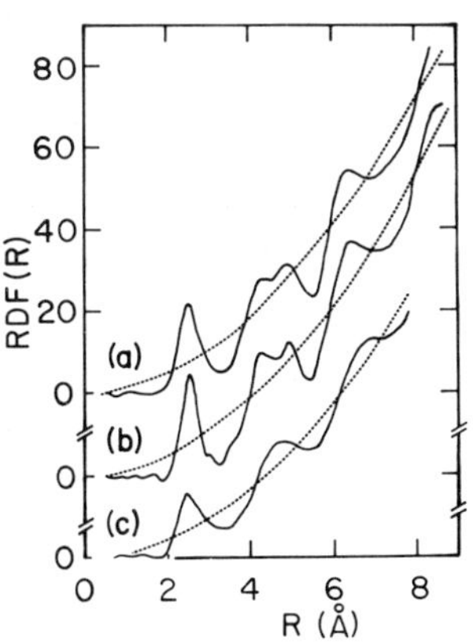

FIGURE 2. Radial distribution functions for (a) amorphous Co, with $K_{max} = 12$ Å^{-1} (from Leung & Wright[22]), (b) amorphous $Co_{78}P_{22}$, with $K_{max} = 16.9$ Å^{-1} (from Cargill & Cochrane[77]), and (c) liquid Co, with $K_{max} = 12.5$ Å^{-1} (from Schmitz-Pranghe & Kohlhaas[79]).

modified by allowing the metal atoms to occupy random packing structures somewhat less dense than those of Bernal[15] and Finney,[18] with metalloid atoms located in the larger holes inherent in such random packings. This insures that the metalloid atoms are surrounded by metal atoms, with metal-metalloid separations less than the sum of the corresponding Goldschmidt radii, i.e., configurations similar to those found in many transition metal phosphide, boride, silicide, and carbide crystal structures. This point of view is similar to that of Sadoc *et al.*[48] who proposed for the structure of these alloys a binary DRP model in which no small spheres, which represent metalloid atoms, are allowed to be near neighbors. These proposals for the role of metalloid atoms in these metallic glasses have been supported by recent measurements of partial distribution functions in an amorphous Co-P alloy by Sadoc and Dixmier.[59]

Two refinements of DRPHS type models for amorphous transition metal films have led to improved agreement between experimental and model distribution functions. These involve increasing the number of nearly perfect tetrahedra in computer-generated DRPHS structures[60] and relaxing DRPHS structures with respect to a realistic interatomic potential.[46,47]

Anisotropies and Long-Range Ordering in Continuous Random Model Structures

Continuous random models, e.g., dense random packing of hard spheres and tetrahedral continuous random networks, have been generally considered to be "ideally amorphous," with no significant regions of crystalline ordering, i.e., no periodically repeating structure, and with no overall structural anisotropy. Recent detailed studies of several CRN and DRPHS structures indicate that these models are less random and less isotropic than had been previously assumed.[61]

Direction-Dependent Scattering

For most amorphous materials, the scattering from a macroscopic volume is isotropic, i.e., independent of the orientation of the sample with respect to the scattering vector. However, it has recently become possible to observe anisotropy in electron scattering from small areas of amorphous films,[62] and to obtain images that report the difference in scattering from different microscopic regions.[63-65] Cochran[66] and others have shown that interpretation of such observations in terms of actual anisotropies or periodicities in the materials being examined is very difficult and involves careful considerations of instrumental factors as well as of atomic correlations. However, these observations have motivated several studies of anisotropic scattering properties of close-packed[61,67] and tetrahedrally coordinated[61,68] amorphous model structures.

The scattering intensity per atom, for a model structure of N identical scatterers, is given by

$$I(\vec{K}) = \frac{1}{N}\sum_{ij} \exp\,[i\vec{K}\cdot(\vec{r}_i - \vec{r}_j)]. \qquad \textbf{(2)}$$

The isotropic average scattering $\bar{I}(|K|)$, the average of $I(\vec{K})$ over all directions of the scattering vector $\vec{K}$, is given by

$$\bar{I}(|K|) = \frac{1}{N} \sum_{ij} \frac{\sin(|K| \, |r_i - r_j|)}{|K| \, |r_i - r_j|} . \tag{3}$$

In FIGURE 3 are shown $\bar{I}(|K|)$ for a spherical region of 996 central units of Finney's[18] 7934-unit DRPHS model and for the 519-unit CRN model of Polk.[12,69] In FIGURE 4, the behavior of the direction dependent intensity function $I(\vec{K})$ is shown, with $|K|$ corresponding to the first maximum of $\bar{I}(|K|)$ for both the DRPHS and CRN models. Points in the x,y plane correspond to the spherical angles θ and ϕ and the intensity is given by the height z of the "scattering net." For each model there are several directions for which the scattering tends to be quite large.

Random Reinforcement and Interference

Is the degree of anistropy in $I(\vec{K})$ for the DRPHS and CRN models greater than would be expected for *randomly occurring reinforcement and interference*? Even in a model where intrinsic correlations are relatively short ranged and, on

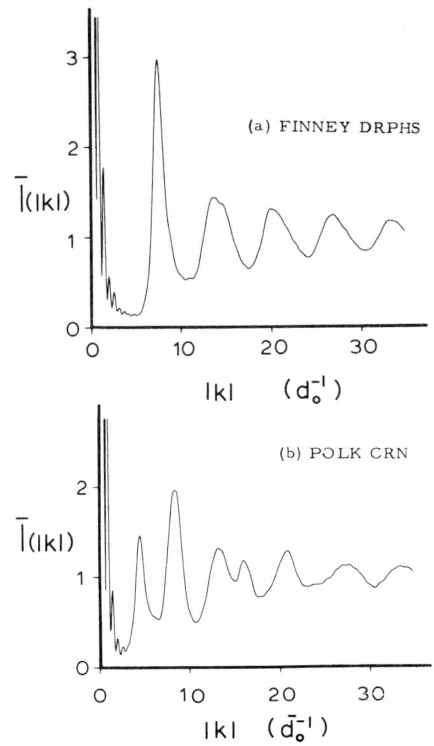

FIGURE 3. Directionally averaged interference function $\bar{I}(|K|)$ for (a) the 996 central units from a 7934-unit DRPHS model built by J. L. Finney[18] and (b) the 519-unit CRN model of D. E. Polk,[69] hand built and then relaxed with the aid of a computer. The scattering vector K is given for (a) in units of one divided by the hard sphere diameter d_0 and for (b) in units of one divided by the mean nearest neighbor distance $\bar{d}_0$. (After Alben *et al.*[61])

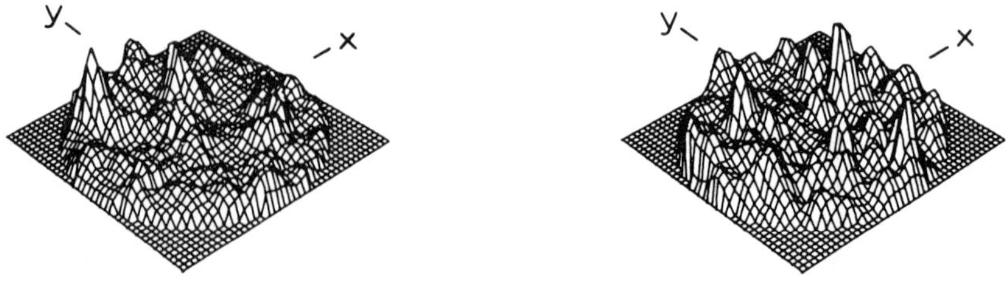

FIGURE 4. Dependence of the interference function $I(\vec{K})$ on the direction of $\vec{K}$: (a) for the 996 central units of the DRPHS model of Finney[18] with $|K| = 7.7\ d_0^{-1}$ and (b) for the 519-unit CRN model of Polk[69] with $|K| = 4.7\ \bar{d}_0^{-1}$. (After Alben *et al.*[61])

the average, isotropic in character, it must be expected that by chance the correlations will persist over a much longer range for some directions. This is illustrated in FIGURE 5 for the extreme case of a particular 519-atom cluster of scatterers randomly distributed within a sphere. The average density is the same as for the Polk CRN model, and $|K|$ corresponds to the first peak in $\bar{I}(|K|)$ for that model. For the random cluster there are no *intrinsic* correlations, i.e., no correlations associated with interactions among the atoms. Nontheless, for directions corresponding to the maxima seen in FIGURE 5, there must be periodic correlations in the projected atomic density.

These observations of apparent anisotropies in DRPHS, CRN, and truly random models can be compared with calculations for a cluster of characteristic dimension $\bar{R}$ of randomly placed scatters, in which the sum in Equation 2 is treated as a random walk in two dimensions. For this case, the expected range for the maximum value I_{max} of $I(\vec{K})$ for fixed $|K|$ depends just on $|K|$ and $\bar{R}$.[61]

Quantitive Comparisons

Values of $\bar{I}$, I_{max}, and $I_{max}/\bar{I}$ for the particular 519-atom random cluster, for the 519-atom Polk[69] CRN, and for the 996-atom Finney[18] DRPHS are given in TABLE 3. Also given is the range of $(I_{max}/\bar{I})_{random}$ obtained from the calculation described above for the $|K|$ and $\bar{R}$ values for each of the model structures. For

TABLE 3

CHARACTERISTICS OF THE SCATTERING ANISOTROPY FOR VARIOUS MODEL STRUCTURES. THE MAGNITUDE OF THE SCATTERING VECTOR CORRESPONDS TO THE FIRST DIFFRACTION RING*

	$\bar{I}$	I_{max}	$\frac{I_{max}}{\bar{I}}$	$\left(\frac{I_{max}}{\bar{I}}\right)_{random}$
519-Random†	0.92	7.3	7.9	6.6 ± 1.5
519-CRN	1.47	12.3	8.3	6.6 ± 1.5
996-DRP	2.93	38.9	13.3	7.6 ± 1.5
864-FCC	5.09	864.0	169.8	7.4 ± 1.5

*After Alben *et al.*[61]

†The scattering vector corresponds to the first diffraction ring of the CRN model.

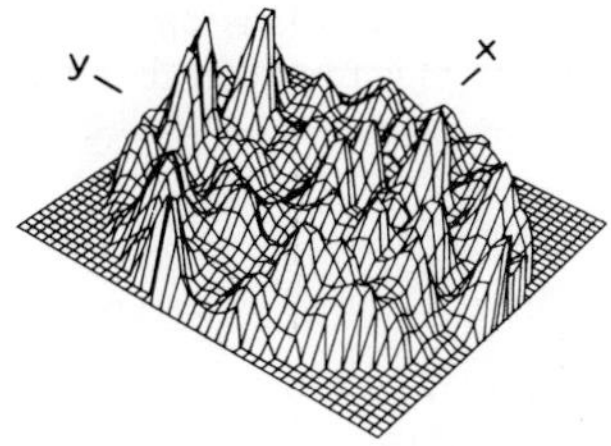

FIGURE 5. Dependence of the interference function $I(\vec{K})$ on the direction of $\vec{K}$ for $|K| = 4.7\ \bar{d}_0^{-1}$ for a spherical cluster of 519 randomly placed scatterers. Here $\bar{d}_0$ is the bond length in a diamond cubic structure crystal with the same density as this random model. (After Alben *et al.*[61])

further comparisons, values are also given for a 864-atom fcc crystal. $I_{max}/\bar{I}$ for the Polk CRN model is only 26% greater than that expected from randomly occurring reinforcement and interference, i.e., *by chance*. Similar results were obtained for other CRN models.[70,71] $I_{max}/\bar{I}$ for Finney's DRPHS model is 75% greater than expected by chance, but its anisotropy is far smaller than for a fcc crystal of similar size. Results for the Finney model are indicative of intrinsic order comparable to the model size.

Periodicities and Planes

The periodicities responsible for the $I(\vec{K})$ for the two strongest scattering directions for the DRPHS model are illustrated in FIGURE 5. This "projected density," in units of atoms per sphere diameter, is given by

$$P(z) = \int dx \int dy\, \rho(x, y, z), \qquad (4)$$

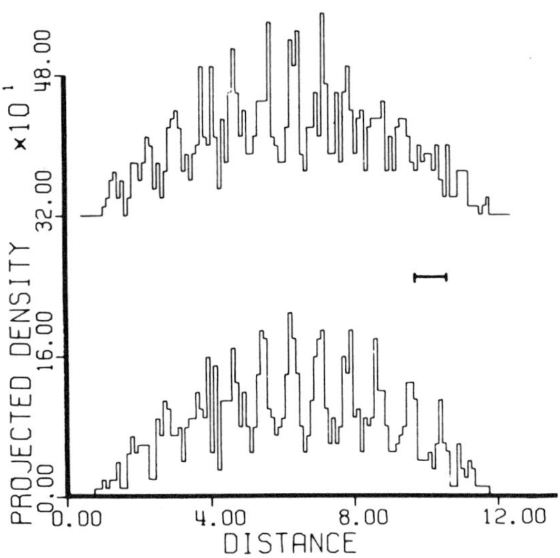

FIGURE 6. Projected density $P(z)$, in units of atoms per sphere diameter, as a function of distance, measured in sphere diameters, along two strong scattering directions for $|K| = 7.7\ d_0^{-1}$ for the 996 central units of the Finney[18] DRPHS model. The plane spacing corresponding to this $|K|$, $(2\pi/7.7)\ d_0 = 0.82\ d_0$ is indicated by the bars. Peaks in $P(z)$ correspond to planes of high density in the model. (After Alben *et al.*[61])

where the z axis is chosen to be parallel to the scattering direction of interest and $\rho(x, y, z)$ is the atomic density function

$$\rho(x, y, z) = \sum_{i=1}^{N} \delta(x - x_i)\, \delta(y - y_i)\, \delta(z - z_i), \qquad (5)$$

where x_i, y_i, and z_i are the coordinates of the ith atomic unit. Oscillations in the projected density $P(z)$ are seen to be a large fraction of the average density; in some cases these "planes" extend across the entire model. Similar results were obtained with Bennett's[19] computer-generated DRPHS structure.

One should not conclude from these results that the CRN or DRPHS structures are crystalline or microcrystalline. Rather, these observations indicate that the short-range order in these structures manifests itself over longer distances than had been anticipated, leading to multiaxial anisotropies and planar periodicities, which for some of the CRN models are not very different from anisotropies expected from randomly occurring reinforcement and interference in models consisting of random arrays of points.[61]

Conclusions

(1) Evaluations of structural models for various types of amorphous solids (SiO_2, Si and Ge, and amorphous metals and alloys) have followed similar paths, involving continuous random models, microcrystalline models, and non crystalline cluster models, as outlined in TABLE 1.

(2) Continuous random models, e.g., continuous random network (CRN) models for SiO_2 and for Ge and Si, and dense random hard sphere packing (DRPHS) models for amorphous metals and alloys, are now the most highly developed models for these materials; these more homogeneous models appear to be realistic and have been useful in extending theoretical methods to interpret some basic properties of these amorphous solids.

(3) Recent detailed examination[61] of several CRN and DRPHS models raise interesting questions concerning anisotropies and long-range ordering in these model structures.

References

1. Warren, B. E., H. Krutter & O. Morningstar. 1936. J. Amer. Ceram. Soc. **19:** 202.
2. Richter, H. & O. Furst. 1951. Z. Naturforschg. A **6:** 38.
3. Turnbull, D. & D. E. Polk. 1972. *In* Amorphous and Liquid Semiconductors. M. H. Cohen & G. Lucovsky, Eds.: 19. North-Holland Publishing Co. Amsterdam.
4. Bienenstock, A. 1974. *In* Amorphous and Liquid Semiconductors. J. Stuke & W. Brenig, Eds.: 49. Taylor & Francis. London.
5. Dixmier, J. & K. Doi. 1963. C. R. Acad. Sci. Ser. B **257:** 2451.
6. Dixmier, J., K. Doi & A. Guinier. 1965. *In* Physics of Non-Crystalline Solids. J. A. Prins, Ed.: 67. North-Holland Publishing Co. Amsterdam.
7. Cargill III, G. S. 1975. *In* Solid State Physics. F. Seitz, D. Turnbull & H. Ehrenreich, Eds. Vol. **30:** 227. Academic Press. New York, N.Y.
8. Zachariasen, W. H. 1932. J. Amer. Chem. Soc. **54:** 3841.
9. Bell, R. J. & P. Dean. 1966. Nature (London) **212:** 1354.
10. Bell, R. J. & P. Dean. 1972. Phil. Mag. **25:** 1381.

11. Bell, R. J. & P. Dean. 1970. Discuss. Faraday Soc. **50:** 55.
12. Polk, D. E. 1971. J. Non-Cryst. Solids **5:** 365.
13. Alben, R., P. Steinhardt & D. Weaire. 1974. *In* Tetrahedrally Bonded Amorphous Semiconductors. M. H. Brodsky, S. Kirkpatrick & D. Weaire, Eds.: 213. American Institute of Physics. New York, N.Y.
14. Graczyk, J. F. & P. Chaudhari. 1975. J. Non-Cryst. Solids **17:** 299.
15. Bernal, J. D. 1959. Nature (London) **183:** 141.
16. Chaudhari, P., J. F. Graczyk, D. Henderson & P. Steinhardt. 1975. Phil. Mag. **31:** 727.
17. Connell, C. A. N. 1975. Solid State Commun. **16:** 109.
18. Finney, J. L. 1970. Proc. R. Soc. A **319:** 479.
19. Bennett, C. H. 1972. J. Appl. Phys. **43:** 2727.
20. Cargill III, G. S. 1970. J. Appl. Phys. **41:** 2249.
21. Ichikawa, T. 1973. Phys. Status Solidi A **19:** 707.
22. Leung, P. K. & J. G. Wright. 1974. Phil. Mag. **30:** 185 and 995.
23. Alben, R., D. Weaire, J. E. Smith Jr. & M. H. Brodsky. 1975. Phys. Rev. B **11:** 2271.
24. Heimendahl, L. V. & M. F. Thorpe. 1975. J. Phys. F **5:** L87.
25. Valenkov, N. & E. Porai-Koshits. 1937. Z. Kristallogr. **95:** 195.
26. Konnert, J. H., J. Karle & G. A. Ferguson. 1973. Science **179:** 177.
27. Howie, A., O. L. Krivanek & M. L. Rudee. 1973. Phil. Mag. **27:** 235.
28. Weinstein, F. C. & E. A. Davis. 1973. J. Non-Cryst. Solids **13:** 153.
29. Graham, A. H., R. W. Lindsay & H. J. Read. 1965. J. Electrochem. Soc. **112:** 401.
30. Tyan, Y. S. & L. E. Toth. 1974. J. Elec. Mat. **3:** 791.
31. Tilton, L. W. 1957. J. Res. Nat. Bur. Stand. **59:** 139.
32. Robinson, H. A. 1965. J. Phys. Chem. Solids **26:** 209.
33. Coleman, M. V. & D. J. D. Thomas. 1967. Phys. Status Solidi **24:** K111.
34. Grigorovici, R. & R. Manaila. 1968. Thin Solid Films **1:** 343.
35. Farges, J., M. F. De Feraudy, B. Raoult & G. Torchet. 1975. J. Phys. (Paris) **36:** C2–13.
36. Briant, C. L. & J. J. Burton. To be published.
37. Frank, F. C. 1952. Proc. R. Soc. A **215:** 43.
38. Hoare, M. R. & P. Pal. 1971. Adv. Phys. **20:** 161.
39. Bienenstock, A. & B. G. Bagley. 1966. J. Appl. Phys. **37:** 4840.
40. Weaire, D., M. F. Ashby, J. Logan & M. J. Weins. 1971. Acta Met. **19:** 779.
41. Alben R. 1976. *In* Magnetism and Magnetic Materials—1975. J. J. Becker, G. H. Lander & J. J. Rhyne, Eds.: 136. American Institute of Physics. New York, N.Y.
42. Kelly, M. J. 1974. *In* Tetrahedrally Bonded Amorphous Semiconductors. M. H. Brodsky, S. Kirkpatrick & D. Weaire, Eds.: 174. American Institute of Physics. New York, N.Y.
43. Alben, R., D. Weaire & P. Steinhardt. 1973. J. Phys. C **6:** L384.
44. Steinhardt, P., R. Alben, M. G. Duffy & D. E. Polk. 1973. Phys. Rev. B **8:** 6021.
45. Boudreaux, D. S., D. E. Polk & M. G. Duffy. 1974. *In* Tetrahedrally Bonded Amorphous Semiconductors. M. H. Brodsky, S. Kirkpatrick & D. Weaire, Eds.: 206. American Institute of Physics. New York, N.Y.
46. Heimendahl, L. V. 1975. J. Phys. F **5:** L141.
47. Barker, J. A., M. R. Hoare & J. L. Finney. 1975. Nature (London) **257:** 120.
48. Sadoc, J. F., J. Dixmier & A. Guinier. 1973. J. Non-Cryst. Solids **12:** 46.
49. Cargill III, G. S. 1976. 2nd International Conference on Rapidly Quenched Metals, Boston, Mass., Nov. 1975. To be published.
50. Duwez, P. 1967. Trans. Amer. Soc. Metals **60:** 607.
51. Pond Jr., R. & R. Maddin. 1969. Trans. Met. Soc. AIME **245:** 2475.
52. Chen, H. S. & C. E. Miller. 1970. Rev. Sci. Instrum. **41:** 1237.
53. Bagley, B. G. & D. Turnbull. 1968. J. Appl. Phys. **39:** 5681.
54. Logan, J. & E. Sun. 1976. J. Non-Cryst. Solids **20:** 285.
55. Felsch, W. 1970. Z. Angew. Phys. **30:** 275.
56. Cargill III, G. S. 1970. J. Appl. Phys. **41:** 12.

57. POLK, D. E. 1970. Scripta Met. **4:** 117.
58. POLK, D. E. 1972. Acta Met. **20:** 485.
59. SADOC, J. F. & J. DIXMIER. 1976. Mater. Sci. Eng. **23:** 187.
60. ICHIKAWA, T. 1975. Phys. Status Solidi A **29:** 293.
61. ALBEN, R., G. S. CARGILL III & J. WENZEL. 1976. Phys. Rev. B. **13:** 835.
62. GRACZYK, J. F. & P. CHAUDHARI. 1973. Phys. Status Solidi B **58:** 163.
63. RUDEE, M. L. & A. HOWIE. 1972. Phil. Mag. **25:** 1001.
64. CHAUDHARI, P., J. F. GRACZYK & S. R. HERD. 1972. Phys. Status Solidi B **51:** 801.
65. HERD, S. R. & P. CHAUDHARI. 1974. Phys. Status Solidi A **26:** 627.
66. COCHRAN, W. 1974. *In* Tetrahedrally Bonded Amorphous Semiconductors. M. H. Brodsky, S. Kirkpatrick & D. Weaire, Eds.: 177. American Institute of Physics. New York, N.Y.
67. CHAUDHARI, P. & J. F. GRACZYK. 1974. Bull. Amer. Phys. Soc. **19:** 317; 1976. Phys Status Solidi B **75:** 593.
68. CHAUDHARI, P. & J. F. GRACZYK. 1974. *In* Amorphous and Liquid Semiconductors. J. Stuke & W. Brenig, Eds.: 59. North-Holland Publishing Co. Amsterdam.
69. POLK, D. E. & D. S. BOUDREAUX. 1973. Phys. Rev. Lett. **31:** 92.
70. EVANS, D. L., M. P. TETER & N. F. BORELLI. 1974. *In* Tetrahedrally Bonded Amorphous Semiconductors. M. H. Brodsky, S. Kirkpatrick & D. Weaire, Eds.: 218. American Institute of Physics. New York, N.Y.
71. STEINHARDT, P., R. ALBEN & D. WEAIRE. 1974. J. Non-Cryst. Solids **15:** 199.
72. RANDALL, J. F., H. R. ROOKSBY & B. S. COOPER. 1930. J. Soc. Glass Tech. **14:** 219.
73. ORDWAY, F. 1964. Science **143:** 800.
74. EVANS, D. L. & S. V. KING, 1966. Nature (London) **212:** 1353.
75. SHEVCHIK, N. J. & W. PAUL. 1972. *In* Amorphous and Liquid Semiconductors. M. H. Cohen & G. Lucovsky, Eds.: 381. North-Holland Publishing Co. Amsterdam.
76. HENDERSON, D. & F. HERMAN. *ibid.*: 359.
77. CARGILL, G. S. III & R. W. COCHRANE. 1974. J. Phys. (Paris) **35:** C4-269.
78. WASEDA, Y. & M. OHTANI. 1974. Phys. Status Solidi B **62:** 535.
79. SCHMITZ-PRANGHE, N. & R. KOHLHAAS. 1970. Z. Naturforsch. A **25:** 1752.

STRUCTURE OF THE AMORPHOUS STATE IN POLYMERS

Raymond F. Boyer

Midland Macromolecular Institute
Midland, Michigan 48640

Introduction

Interest in the detailed structure of amorphous polymers and copolymers, as well as in the amorphous state of crystalline polymers, is growing rapidly. In fact, this area is probably the last structural frontier for classical polymers now that the detailed nature of the crystalline state seems well defined for polymer single crystals, extended chain crystals, and the spherulitic nature of bulk crystallized polymers.[1]

Some measure of interest in the subject topic is afforded by noting recent symposia and special publications. For example, a full-day sumposium was sponsored by the American Chemical Society.[2,3] Several Plenary lectures and main lectures at the Madrid IUPAC Congress were concerned to varying degrees with this topic.[4] Eight articles in a recent issue of Kolloid Zeitschrift covered various specific aspects of the broad problem.[5] A definitive review by Robertson has just appeared.[6]

Arzhakov *et al.*[7] have summarized the current situation in the Soviet Union where so much effort has been expended in this field since Kargin *et al.*[8] first postulated the likelihood of local order in polymers. Yeh[9] has prepared a detailed review of world literature, with especial emphasis on Soviet literature. Flory has addressed this topic on several recent occasions, especially in support of the random coil structure.[10-12]

The author has offered three review articles: The first two[13,14] are concerned with understanding the empirical $\frac{2}{3}$ rule relating amorphous phase glass temperatures to crystalline phase melting points in semi-crystalline polymers; the third[15] is a commentary on the symposium of Reference 2. Because of the concurrent nature of this present paper and the material in Reference 15, I shall emphasize here mainly some newer views on the subject, together with necessary general background.

There are a small number of recurrent themes which will be stated here in the form of questions. Rigorous answers to these questions are not possible in our opinion at the present time; at most one can cite opinions and evidence from the literature.

(1) Since low-molecular-weight liquids possess short-range order and since amorphous polymers aae very viscous liquids, does the connectedness of polymer chains, and their high molecular weight cause more, less, or the same amount of order as in simple liquids?[16] This will be discussed in detail later with regard to *n*-alkanes and linear polyethylene.

(2) Is the amorphous state of polymers adequately represented as an ensemble of intermeshed random coils, with the unperturbed or theta dimension prevailing for any molecule in the ensemble? This view was first proposed by Flory who has recently summarized all available types of evidence in its favor.[10-12] Neutron-scattering data on polystyrene[17,18] and poly(methyl methacrylate)[19] as well as do-

main sizes in block copolymers[20] support this view. Any local order is presumably statistical in nature, occurring when neighboring chains happen to have similar directions in space over very short distances.

(3) Alternately, do packing considerations combined with intra- and interchain interactions force nonstatistical local order? Robertson[6] has concluded that there might be such local order over dimensions of 10 or at most a few tens of angstroms. Flory once stated[21] that any such local order was inconsistent with random coil dimensions, but has subsequently modified this point of view.[11]

(4) Do even more highly ordered regions exist, such as the folded chain model of Yeh[22] or the meander model of Pechhold[23] or the bundle model with internal folds of Arzhakov *et al.*?[7]

(5) Is some compromise possible, as proposed by Lindenmeyer[24,25] in which structured local order of the type in (4) is compatible with random coil dimensions? Neutron scattering data on atactic polystyrene (PS) by Wignall *et al.*[17] state that the chains are Gaussian with a persistence length between 5 and 15 Å and probably about 10 Å. This would appear to rule out the Yeh model[22] where he obtains measured dimensions of about 25 Å for atactic PS.

(6) Is it necessary to postulate a single model for all polymers, regardless of chemical structure; or for any given polymer at all temperatures? Should not the tendency for the random coil be enhanced by going to temperatures far above the glass temperature T_g of the polymer, and conversely, the tendency for local order increase as T_g is approached and packing conditions become more stringent? The notion seems to prevail that a discontinuity in structure should be expected on cooling down to T_g. But chain energetics and free volume are changing continuously as the temperature is lowered, with T_g simply representing a state where the available free volume no longer permits cooperative segmental motion within the time scale used to observe T_g.

We would expect that any tendency for local order would be minimized if backbone chains are flexible and intermolecular forces are low (elastomers above T_g); whereas high intermolecular forces (hydrogen bonding in the nylons) would promote a tendency for local order.

(7) Which model(s) can best explain certain bulk properties of amorphous glassy polymers such as crazing and/or shear band yielding?

(8) Which model(s) can best explain the reversible transformation from crystalline solid to the pressure random coil melt and vice versa? A detailed examination of this question appears later. It is also discussed from a different point of view in Reference 15.

(9) Finally, one must ask, "What is fact and what is artifact?" This question is especially pertinent to electron microscope observation as seasoned practitioners in this field recognize.[26] But it is also pertinent to scattering of light x-rays from bulk polymers where foreign particles and/or voids and/or minute crystals may give misleading results. This type of artifact has been discussed among others by Uhlmann and Teninger[27] and by Wendorff and Fischer.[28]

Definitions of Terms

One can list several different categories of amorphous polymers:

(1) Atactic, noncrystallizable polymers.
(2) Most random copolymers.

(3) Crystallizable polymers and copolymers in either of two states: the melt, the amorphous glass formed by rapid quenching from the melt.
(4) Polymer solutions.

Some noncrystallizable homopolymers are in fact stereo copolymers. Thus, normal atactic polystyrene has been described as arising from a random iso and syndiotactic placement of successive monomer units along the chain. Free radical polybutadiene may not be crystallizable because it is in fact a random copolymer of *cis*-1, 4, *trans*-1, 4, and 1,2-vinyl isomers.

Block copolymers in which both phases are amorphous are a special case of category 1 since the properties of the individual phases are similar to those of the parent polymers except near the interface between phases. Domain sizes vary as the square root of molecular weight of each phase, indicative of random coil dimensions for the polymer chains.[20]

Crystallizable polymers and copolymers pose a special problem because they may retain a detailed memory of their crystalline state even in the melt or quenched amorphous solid, and because they have a tendency to recrystallize—some of them very rapidly indeed.

Dilute solutions of polymers would appear to be the standard reference state for amorphicity, especially in a θ solvent where the polymer chain, by definition, exhibits unperturbed dimensions. However, crystallizable polymers may exhibit either or both of two types of order even in dilute solution:

(1) Intrachain order in the form of helicity[29] in solutions of isotactic PS and isotactic polypropylene.
(2) Interchain aggregation for polyethylene oxide[30] and ethylenepropylene copolymers.[31]
(3) Helicity and aggregation in syndiotactic polypropylene.[32]

Whereas one can define amorphous polymer types readily, a numerical definition, or even a precise qualitative definition of local order proves very elusive even for a given specific polymer. Petrie[37] could show schematics for order (or disorder) in smetic, nematic, and cholesteric liquid crystals. This capability is currently lacking for polymers. We shall try to define order in terms of the methods used to measure it.

First, one recognizes dynamic versus static order in polymers. Polymers at temperatures above T_g, as is common for elastomers, would exhibit dynamic local order centering around some average value. Even so, the highly viscous nature of polymer systems means a long time constant compared with that for low molecular weight systems. Below T_g any order which exists in the liquid state is frozen in.

Robertson[34] attempted a numerical definition of order in terms of the ratio d_a/d_c, where d_a is the density of a polymer in the completely amorphous state and d_c its density in the pure crystalline state. According to his model, randomly arrayed polymer chains should have a d_a/d_c of 0.625 whereas this ratio would approach unity for complete order. He showed that d_a/d_c is in the range of 0.90 to 0.95 for many polymers. We have examined a larger body of literature data than he used and found that d_a/d_c varies systematically with chemical structure.[35] The lowest value of d_a/d_c reported in the literature was 0.80. Robertson's calculations and interpretations have been criticized.[36]

Bothorel[37,38] has used depolarized Rayleigh scattering to measure order tendency in *n*-alkanes and related low-molecular weight materials. He uses the term correlation of molecular orientation (COM) to express local order with a parameter J. As will be seen in the next section, J increases linearly with chain length for the n-alkanes. In an alkane in the liquid state there is a distribution of configurations including some molecules in the all-*trans* form. These latter are more stable if paired with each other than if isolated. Hence, J seems to measure the percentage of chains existing as pairs.[38] For pure alkanes of $n > 5$, he estimates that 10%–15% of fully extended chains are present.

Patterson and Flory[39] have made depolarized Rayleigh scattering measurements on n-alkanes, and agree with Bothorel's results for the pure alkanes. In fact, they have gone to C_{36} at 140°C.[40]

Patterson and colleagues[41–44] have measured heats of dilution of linear alkanes, using as diluents shorter chain linear alkanes, branched alkanes, and spherical molecules such as CCl_4. After making all appropriate corrections, there is a residual effect, which these authors consider to be a measure of orientational order in the linear alkanes. This order parameter decreases with increasing temperature. Moreover, it correlates with a properly chosen function of Bothorel's J parameter, indicating that both methods are measuring the same intrinsic property of these linear alkanes.

Thus far neither the optical nor the thermodynamic methods have been extended beyond $C_{36}H_{74}$. There are obviously problems in doing so because of higher melting points, specimen purity, and so forth. Both methods agree that order increases with length of the n-alkane and is lessened by methyl side groups but neither method offers a visual image of the nature of the order, except that proposed by Bothorel[38] of association of fully extended molecules.

Stress optical coefficients (SOC) measured on cross-linked polymers in their rubbery (liquid) state affords some numerical measure of local order or correlation of molecular orientations. SOC is defined as the ratio between the strain-induced birefringence, Δn, and the stress f used to produce it.[45] According to classical rubber elasticity theory, SOC should be independent of swelling of the elastomer by diluent. In fact, SOC may decrease markedly, depending on the type of diluent. Such experiments are now interpreted to imply the existence of local order, or correlation of orientations, in the bulk polymer, with such orientation destroyed or reduced by diluent.[46,47]

Finally, we consider large angle x-ray scattering from amorphous polymer systems. Bjørnhaug *et al.*[48] have suggested some general procedures for estimating from radial distribution intensity curves the relative contributions of intra- and inter-chain effects for amorphous polymers. They estimate from molecular models the most common intrachain distances and calculate the expected scattering curve. The difference between this and the experimental scattering curve is ascribed to interchain distances. This method was applied only to a small number of polymers for which the interchain distances appeared reasonable in terms of chemical structure.

Corradini[49] had an even simpler scheme. He studied x-ray scattering from amorphous polyalphaolefins

$$[-CH_2—CH(CH_2)_nH-]$$

as a function of n, the length of the alkyl side group. He found an amorphous halo corresponding to a dimension which increased regularly with n. He interpreted this as an intermolecular dimension. He later described the situation as follows: Consider a segment of a given polymer chain; a segment of a neighboring chain has a probability $p(\parallel)$ of being parallel to the first chain for a short distance and a probability $p(\perp)$ of being perpendicular. He summarized his interpretation of the data, and his definition of local order, by the inequality: $p(\parallel) > p(\perp)$.[21]

Turner-Jones[50] subsequently verified the work of Corradini with an even more extensive series of poly-α-olefins. Again, she found a distance, 4.6 Å, that was independent of n, and a second distance that increased linearly with n, from about 10 Å for $n = 4$ to about 24 Å for $n = 16$. The relative intensity of the scattering peak assigned to the interchain distance decreased as more and more of the weight of the monomeric unit was in the side chain.

Corradini[49] noted the value of obtaining scattering curves for the same polymer at several levels of tacticity and hence crystallinity. The sharp lines of the crystalline specimen arise from known dimensions in the crystal lattice, i.e., the intermolecular distances are known. If an amorphous halo lies approximately at the same scattering angle 2θ as one of the crystalline peaks, it is plausible that an interchain distance is involved.

Krimm and Tobolsky[51] showed for PS that the 10 Å interchain peak increased in intensity as the specimen was oriented, thus providing support that it was not an intrachain peak.

Vainshtein[52] has suggested as a general rule that stiff polymer chains are more likely to form parallel bundles giving rise to an interchain scattering halo than would very flexible chains with their marked tendency to intertwine.

Thus, x-ray scattering from amorphous polymers gives a characteristic interchain distance with its implication that at least over short distances a few polymer chains are approximately parallel. Even here some caution is necessary since Corradini[53] calculates that even a random coil array can give similar interchain distances. What he does not know is the relative intensities to expect from the parallel and the coil arrays.

The Polyethylene Problem

Linear polyethylene (PE) is a long-chain linear alkane, —$(CH_2)_n$— where n may be typically 1000 to 10,000 or even greater. Neutron scattering data[54] on the melt and the crystalline solid PE is somewhat ambiguous because of a so-called clustering problem. Nevertheless, one is led to believe from this publication that random-coil behavior exists, especially in the melt, under ideal experimental conditions.

The liquid alkanes, say C_6 to C_{16}, might be considered as low molecular weight analogs of PE, or alternately stated, as PE oligomers. Various bodies of data exist to suggest the presence of local order in such alkanes and, moreover, order that increases with chain length n.

We have referred in the last section to the light-scattering studies of Bothorel[37,38] and of Patterson and Flory,[39,40] and also to the thermodynamic measurements of Patterson[41–44] as indicative of local order in n-alkanes.

TABLE 1 compiles data from several sources to indicate how Bothorel's parameter J seems to vary on going from C_{10} to C_{1000}. J appears to level off, but this is almost certainly a temperature effect rather than a molecular-weight effect.

Since heats of mixing and, hence, local order decreases vary rapidly between 25°C and 75°C for C_{16} and other n-alkanes,[42,43] one must assume that the value of J for C_{36} would be substantially higher at 25°C. Of course the C_{36} would crystallize first so that such a value cannot be measured. The alternate procedure of measuring J for C_{16} at 140°C would likely reduce it to zero. Alternately, the C_{36} might have been measured in solution at several concentrations and the data extrapolated to pure C_{36} at 25°C.

We conclude that at a fixed temperature, J would be increasing up to at least C_{36}. Bothorel's theory[38] predicts that optical anisotropy for the alkanes increases

TABLE 1

ORDER PARAMETERS FOR *n*-ALKANES AND POLYETHYLENE

Number of Carbon Atoms in *n*-Alkane*	J†	Temperature of Measurement	References
8	0.40	25°C	‡
10	0.82	25°C	‡
16	1.25	25°C	‡
36	1.11	140°C	§
1000¶	1.09**	140°C	§

*G. D. Patterson presents in Reference 3 data for the higher *n*-alkanes.
†*J* is Bothorel's parameter[37,42] for correlation of molecular orientations.
‡Table 5 of Reference 42. Data of Bothorel.
§Table 5 of Reference 11. Data of Patterson and Flory.
¶We assume this to be a lower limit for linear polyethylene.
**Obtained via an extrapolation technique that was not defined.

linearly with *n*. His measurements on solutions shows it still increasing linearly with *n* at C_{24}. Gent and Vickroy[55] found the optical anisotropy of PE to increase about 40% on going from 170°C to 120°C, indicating a very strong temperature effect.

Bothorel and Flory seem dramatically opposed in their interpretation of the implications for *n*-alkanes of optical anisotropy values. As already noted, Bothorel[38] believes that pairs of fully extended and completely aligned molecules can exist in the liquid. Flory[56] concludes that intermolecular correlative effects indicated by optical anisotropy do not necessarily denote parallelization of molecular chains. Bothorel suggests[38] that a tendency for alignment in the alkanes comes from London dispersion forces proportional to α_l^2/d^7 where α is the polarizibility in the chain direction and d is the intermolecular distance. The absence of side groups in the alkanes means that the d^7 term is uniquely small. This is consistent with the fact that measures of orientational order are much lower in branched alkanes than in linear alkanes.[42,43] Other polymer systems free of side groups and capable of close molecular approach are the polyalkylene oxides $[-(CH_2)_n—O-]_p$. Some of the fluorinated polymers, especially ones that assume a planar zigzag form, are also likely candidates.

Conversely, the fact that atactic poly(methyl methacrylate) (PMMA)[19] and polystyrene (PS)[17,18] show random coil behavior by neutron scattering may be a consequence of the bulky side groups and the large spacing between chains.

Additional neutron scattering experiments on PE are needed to see if the clustering problem[54] can be eliminated or whether it is a measure of molecular ordering in molten PE. Ching and Krimm[57] have a new ir study of mixed crystals of PE-H and PE-D. The tendency for desegregation, which they can measure, decreases as the ratio PE-H/PE-D increases. This is contrary to the "clustering" ratios reported in TABLE 1 of Schelten *et al.*[54]

The Reversible Transformation from Melt to Crystal

The reversible transformation shown below:

$$\text{Chain-folded Semi-crystalline solid} \quad \underset{T_m \pm \Delta T(^\circ K)}{\longleftrightarrow} \quad \text{Randomly coiled Disordered melt}$$

poses a number of physical and semantic questions pertinent to the subject of structure in amorphous polymers. I have discussed some of the physical aspects elsewhere (Section 7 of Reference 15), particularly as regards kinetic and driving forces for both directions of the transformation.

Here we wish to emphasize the semantic aspects, based so far as possible on physical facts, with the view of delineating some of the problems that arise in trying to define order in amorphous polymer systems.

We start in FIGURE 1 with the crystalline state C_1, which is envisaged as a bulk crystallized polymer containing mainly spherulites comprised of chain-folded crystals with twinning and with tie molecules. The specimen is semi-crystalline and, hence, contains amorphous regions. There may be fringed micellar crystals present. C_1 possesses three types of long-range order:

(1) The lattice spacings of the chain-folded crystals;
(2) The average long period of fold length of the crystals;
(3) The supermolecular organization of the numerous molecules in the spherulite. For general background on bulk crystallized polymers, see Reference 1.)

C_1 is now rapidly heated through the melting point. (We assume this process to be completely reversible for short time intervals in the melt.) The three types of long-range order disappear and one has the so-called amorphous melt. Now, Hosemann,[58] who has studied the highly defective crystal structure which sets in as T_M is approached closely, concluded that there is in the melt a considerable amount of order. According to schematic drawings of his,[58] this order indicates memory of order that existed in the crystal. Indeed, it is hard to avoid such a conclusion on simple kinetic grounds except for low-molecular-weight polymers.

The melted material can be held for various lengths of time above T_M (and, of course, the temperature may be increased). After a sufficiently long time, the random coil state, M_{RC}, is presumably achieved. This time will depend on temperature, molecular weight, chain stiffness, and other factors.

But there are, along the way, a series of melts, M_2, M_3, M_4, and so forth that

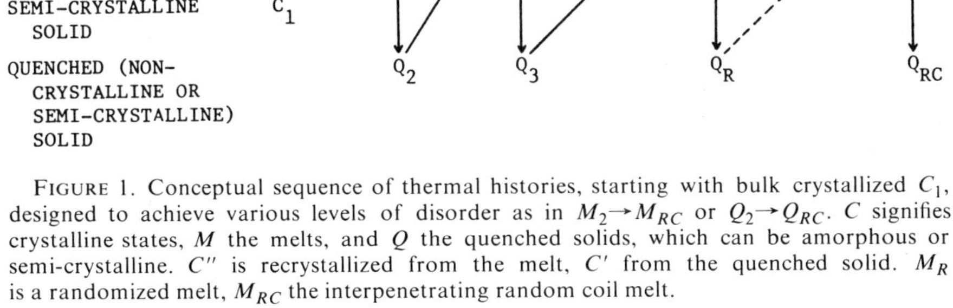

FIGURE 1. Conceptual sequence of thermal histories, starting with bulk crystallized C_1, designed to achieve various levels of disorder as in $M_2 \rightarrow M_{RC}$ or $Q_2 \rightarrow Q_{RC}$. C signifies crystalline states, M the melts, and Q the quenched solids, which can be amorphous or semi-crystalline. C'' is recrystallized from the melt, C' from the quenched solid. M_R is a randomized melt, M_{RC} the interpenetrating random coil melt.

are intermediate between M_1 and M_{RC} as regards memory of the crystalline state, C_1.

For example, Bunn[59] has shown x-ray scattering data from the melt of polybutene-1 which caused him to believe that short helices will persist in the melt. These were the 40_{11} helices found in the unstable crystal II type and not the 3_1 helices characteristic of stable type I crystals. The time at which the specimen was held in the melt was not stated. The important point is that some kind of local order consisting of short (length unspecified) helices within the chain and of the related interchain distance, exists in the melt.

Northolt *et al.*[60] have x-ray data showing the possibility of some type of order in the melt for nylons.

Zachmann has concluded from NMR studies[61,62] that the melt of polyethylene contains some kind of ordered structures. This opinion is based on line shapes compared with the shapes seen in dilute solutions. Even concentrated solutions of PE show evidence of order by this criterion. Zachmann[62] has been able to assign a lifetime of about 10^{-4} seconds for these ordered, or bundle structures, in the melt of PE.

M_R represents a kind of randomized state in which the memory structures of Hosemann have disappeared, and presumably even persistent nuclei are gone. We differentiate between M_R and M_{RC} since the latter is used in the sense of interpenetrating random coils as used in the introduction to discuss amorphous polymers. In view of the log time scale, the time for M_1 to M_R may be relatively short, that from M_R to M_{RC} relatively long.

Now any structure present in the melt is presumably frozen into the solid on quenching. Some polymers, notably PE and POM, are difficult to quench to the amorphous solid although even PE has finally been conquered.[63] It is not clear to us how much of this difficulty in achieving the quenched amorphous state results from structure present in the melt, or to very rapid kinetics of recrystallization. In any event, quenched solids with amorphous contents of 50% to 100% can commonly be obtained and may contain varying degrees of ordered structures in the amorphous regions.

There is then a hierarchy of structures, $M_1 \rightarrow M_{RC}$, which can exist in the melt and which can be frozen into the quenched amorphous solid. The latter should be ideal reference substances of known thermal history for use in structure studies on the amorphous state.

Finally, any one of the quenched states, Q_2 to Q_{RC}, or of the molten states, M_2 to M_{RC}, can be recrystallized. The structure of the recrystallized material will be different, as indicated by C_2' and C_2'', depending on the indicated thermal history.

The important question is: Having achieved the state M_{RC} or Q_{RC}, how long is required to return to the chain-folded starting material, similar to, but not necessarily identical to C_1 in all details? For low-molecular weight polymers there should be no problem. For very high molecular weights, the problems may be formidable. Low and high are used in relation to fold length: arbitrarily, MW $\equiv$ 1–3 fold lengths is low; MW $>$ 10–20 fold lengths is high. Effect of molecular weight on recrystallization kinetics and equilibrium crystallinity for polyethylene oxide fractions has been reported by Maclaine and Booth.[64]

The mental exercise pictured in FIGURE 1 is believed to be a valid one. It serves to emphasize the many levels of order that ultimately should be capable of definition and measurement before a full description of any amorphous state based on a particular thermal history can be defined.

The types of steps shown in FIGURE 1 have been carried out numerous times on many different polymers[65] but usually from the viewpoint of crystallization kinetics and morphology of the crystalline phase. The annealing of quenched nylon to develop a hydrogen-bonded noncrystalline structure[60] is an example of what might be affected.

No carryover from results on these crystallizable polymers to the structure of atactic polymers and copolymers is implied beyond that of developing experimental techniques applicable to both types of polymers.

Concluding Remarks

The main purpose of this review was to present an overview of a timely topic in the field of polymers. Divergence of opinions, a review of techniques commonly used for studying order, and an introduction to the semantic problems involved have been covered. Some of these topics have been treated in more detail elsewhere,[15] along with some topics not even mentioned herein.

We see no simple way to offer a satisfactory summary. For atactic PS and atactic PMMA, neutron scattering data from the bulk polymer shows random coil behavior. But is there local order—parallelism of chains over short distances but still distances greater than for an array of randomly coiled chains?

Finally, we note from Corradini[53] that three factors can affect the structure of the amorphous state:

(1) What the isolated chain wants to do in terms of its internal structure, i.e., act as a random coil.

(2) Packing considerations arising from space filling requirements. Here what orientational correlation is induced by packing appears in general not to interfere appreciably with random coil behavior, at least in atactic PS and PMMA.

(3) Only in the case of strong intermolecular forces such as the hydrogen bonding in nylons may there arise marked departures from random coil behavior.

To these we add strain-induced orientational order, which prevails to some extend during stress-strain and stress-optical coefficient measurements on vulcanized elastomers. These topics have been treated in detail in Section 3 of Reference 15.

References

1. KELLER, A. 1968. Reports on Progress in Physics. **31**(Part 2): 623ff.
2. Polymer Preprints. 1974. **15(2)**: 1–45, 324–343.
3. ALLEN, G. & E. S. PETRIE, Eds. 1976. J. Macromol. Sci. Physics. In press.
4. J. Polymer Science. 1975. **C-50:** 1–513. For invited lectures. Plenary lectures by Flory and Benoit covered material presented in References 11 and 18, respectively.
5. Kolloid Z. Z. Polym. 1973. **251(No. 11)**.
6. ROBERTSON, R. E. 1975. Annual Review of Materials Science. **5:** 73–97.
7. ARZHAKOV, S. A., N. F. BAKEEV & V. A. KABANOV. 1973. Vysokomol. Soeidin. **A-15:** 1154.
8. KARGIN, V. A., A. I. KITAIGORODSKII & G. L. SLONIMSKII. 1957. Kolloidn. Zh. **19:** 131.
9. YEH, G. S. Y. 1972. Critical Reviews of Macromol. Sci. **1:** 173–213.
10. FLORY, P. J. Opening lecture of Reference 2.
11. FLORY, P. J. 1973. Macromol. Chem. **8:** 1.

12. FLORY, P. J. 1975. Rub. Chem. Techn. **48:** 513. This is a reprint of Reference 11.
13. BOYER, R. F. 1973. Seventh Swinburne Award Address. Published by the Plastics Institute. London, SWI WOHL England. Also available from the author in reprint form.
14. BOYER, R. F. 1975. J. Poly. Sci. **C-50:** 189.
15. BOYER, R. F. To appear as part of Reference 3.
16. This question was posed by co-chairman Allen at the termination of the symposium of Reference 2. It also appears in his written ACS abstract.
17. WIGNALL, G. D., D. G. H. BALLARD & J. SCHELTEN. 1974. European Polym. J. **10:** 861.
18. BENOIT, H. 1974. Polym. Preprints **15(2):** 324.
19. SCHELTEN, J., W. A. KRUSE & R. G. KIRSTE. 1973. Kolloid Z. Z. Polym. **251(11):** 919.
20. MEIER, D. J. Midland Macromolecular Institute. Unpublished observations.
21. MILLIGAN, W. O., Ed. 1967. Proceedings of the Robert A. Welch Foundation Conferences on Chemical Research X Polymers. 163–167. Robert A. Welch Foundation, Houston, Tex.
22. YEH, G. S. Y. 1972. J. Macromol. Sci. **B-6:** 451.
23. PECHOLD, W., M. E. T. HAUBER & E. LISKA. 1973. Kolloid Z. Z. Polym. **251(11):** 818.
24. LINDENMEYER, P. H. 1973. J. Macromol. Sci. Physics. **B-8:** 361.
25. LINDENMEYER, P. H. 1975. J. Appl. Phys. **46:** 4235.
26. GEIL, P. H. 1974. Polym. Preprints **15(2):** 35. Illustrates numerous experimental parameters that must be varied to avoid artifacts.
27. UHLMANN, D. R. & A. L. RENNINGER. Polym. Preprints **15(2):** 28.
28. WENDORFF, J. H. & E. W. FISCHER. Kolloid Z. Z. Polym. **251(11):** 884.
29. KOBAYASHI, M., K. TSUMURA & H. TADOKORO. 1968. J. Polym. Sci. **A-2,6:** 1493.
30. CARPENTER, D. K., G. SANTIAGO & A. H. HUNT. 1974. J. Polym. Sci., Polym. Sym. **44:** 75.
31. BALDWIN, F. B. & G. VERSTRATE. 1972. Rubber Chem. Tech. **45:** 750.
32. STOFER, B. H. & H.-G. ELIAS. 1972. Makromol. Chem. **157:** 245.
33. PETRIE. S. E. B. Unpublished.
34. ROBERTSON, R. E. 1965. J. Phys. Chem. **69:** 1575.
35. Table II of Reference 15.
36. FISCHER, E. W. *et al.* Kolloid Z. Z. Polym. **251(11):** 8.
37. BOTHOREL & G. FOURCHE. 1973. J. Chem. Soc. Faraday II **69:** 441. This paper cites earlier publications by Bothorel and his collaborators.
38. BOTHOREL, P. 1968. J. Colloid Interface Sci. **27:** 529.
39. PATTERSON, G. O. & P. J. FLORY. 1972. Trans. Faraday Soc. **68:** 1098, 1111.
40. Reference 11, Table 5.
41. TANCREDE, P., M. D. CROUCHER & D. PATTERSON. 1974. Polym. Preprints **15(2):** 251.
42. LAM, V. T., P. PICKER, D. PATTERSON & P. TANCREDE. 1974. J. Chem. Soc. Faraday Trans. II. **70:** 1465.
43. CROUCHER, M. D. & D. PATTERSON. *Ibid.:* 1479.
44. DELMAS, G. & S. TURREL. *Ibid.:* 572.
45. TRELOAR, L. R. G. 1975. Physics of Rubber Elasticity. 3rd edition.
46. ISHIKAWA, T. & K. NAGAI. 1969. J. Polym. Sci. **A-2:** 7.
47. LIBERMAN, M. H., Y. ABE & P. J. FLORY. 1972. Macromolecules **5:** 550.
48. BJØRNHAUG, A., O. ELLEFSEN & B. A. TØNNESEN. 1954. J. Polym. Sci. **12:** 621.
49. CORRADINI, P. 1968. The Stereochemistry of Macromolecules. A. D. Ketley, Ed. **1:** 1. Dekker. New York, N.Y.
50. TURNER-JONES, A. 1964. Makromolecular Chem. **71:** 1, especially FIGURES 1 & 9.
51. KRIMM, S. & A. V. TOBOLSKY. 1951. Text. Res. J. **21:** 805.
52. VAINSHTEIN, B. K. 1966. Diffraction of X-Rays by Chain Molecules. Chap. VII: 338ff. Elsevier. New York, N.Y.
53. CORRADINI, P. Reference 4: 327ff.
54. SCHELTEN, J., G. D. WIGNALL & D. G. H. BALLARD. 1974. Polymer **15:** 682.
55. GENT, A. N. & V. V. VICKROY, JR. 1967. J. Polym. Sci. **A-2,5:** 47.
56. FLORY, P. J. Concluding remarks of Reference 11.

57. Ching, J. H. C. & S. Krimm. 1975. Macromolecules **8:** 894.
58. Hosemann, R. 1967. J. Polym. Sci. **C-20:** 1–17.
59. Bunn, C. W. 1974. Molecular Behaviour and the Development of Polymeric Materials. A. Ledwith & A. North, Eds. Chap. 10: 337. Chapman and Hall. London.
60. Northolt, G. M., B. J. Tabor & J. J. Vanaartsen. 1975. Prog. Colloid Polym. Sci. **57:** 225.
61. Zachmann, H. G. 1973. J. Polym. Sci. **C-43:**111.
62. Gölz, W. L. F. & H. G. Zachmann. 1971. Kolloid Z. Z. Polym. **247:** 814.
63. Zachmann, H. G. 1973. J. Polym. Sci. C-**43:** 111.
64. Zachmann, H. G. 1973. Kolloid Z. Z. Polym. **251:** 951.
65. Hendra, P. J., H. P. Jobic & K. Holland-Moritz. 1975. Polym. Lett., Ed. **13:** 365.
66. Maclaine, J. Q. G. & C. Booth. 1975. Polymer **16:** 680.
67. Miller, R. L. Midland Macromolecular Institute. Private communication.

DISCUSSION

A. Bienenstock, *Moderator*

Stanford University
Stanford, California 94305

RAVECHÉ: I'd like to ask Prof. Turnbull when he uses the term "topological rearrangement," can I assume by that in fact the radial distances are about right for the second and third nearest neighbors but the angular positioning has to change?

TURNBULL: Well, the angular positioning would even be different for the first nearest neighbors, and at least for the first nearest neighbors, and I suppose to some extent to the second nearest neighbors, the radial distances would be the same. Certainly for the first.

RAVECHÉ: We find in the computer simulations of fluids near freezing that the second nearest neighbor radial distances are about what they are in the crystal.

CARGILL: When you say the second nearest neighbors are at the same radial distance in the fcc crystal and in the amorphous or liquid regions of your diagram, I believe that you must really mean some sort of an interplaner spacing rather than the actual second neighbor spacing, which in an fcc crystal would be at $\sqrt{2}$ atom diameters and is associated with the octahedral hole configuration. This $\sqrt{2}$ distance should be absent in your model. This distance is in fact not seen for simple amorphous metals or liquids in actual experimental data.

J. BURTON (*Exxon*): I'd like to return to a question that Mike Hoare raised a moment ago about the role of the boundary conditions in these computer simulations. It was said that the small boundary, in this case I think it was the 256-atom simulation, did not prevent the forming of the ordered structure. Is that a correct understanding of what you said? You were able to get something that looked like the fcc material in the radial distribution constant and in the energy despite the boundary.

TURNBULL: That's correct.

BURTON: Now the problem is that the boundaries one uses in these simulations are cubic boundaries; they are boundaries where you have translational symmetry appropriate to fcc material. Such boundaries would not automatically force forming materials with that symmetry. However, if one were trying to nucleate a unit which was an ordered unit but which was incapable of being a space-filling unit with translational symmetry, the boundary on the small system would work very strongly against you. For instance if you were trying to make the kind of 13-atom icosahedron that Prof. Turnbull referred to a moment ago, which is the minimum energy structure for 13 atoms and which cannot grow into a space-filling structure with translational symmetry, then the boundaries might work against forming the structure. However, it does form if you have free boundaries. I think that in these simulations you have to be very careful to consider the difference between free boundaries and periodic boundaries.

TURNBULL: I agree that you have to be careful, but I think that's all that has to be said for them.

ANGELL: Perhaps in connection with this point somebody ought to mention that homogeneous nucleation has been observed as it occurs in sequential time in molecular dynamics calculations. I refer to studies of supercooled argon being performed by Rahman and McTague.

BIENENSTOCK: Prof. Angell is alluding to the difference between the *Monte Carlo* simulation technique where the progression of that simulation is not directly related to real time progression and also to the molecular dynamics simulation where the equations of motion are integrated numerically and are directly related to a real time progression. You can in fact relate that to the motion real time.

MILLER: Metallurgists have used the extremely rapid quenching technique "splat cooling" to form amorphous glasses from alloys and metals that ordinarily would crystallize. Could this technique be applied to organic liquids, such as the normal alkanes, to form completely amorphous glasses instead of crystalline materials?

TURNBULL: Well I'm afraid the methods rely very heavily on the high thermal conductivity of the material being quenched, and in order to have a similar result on the normal alkanes one would need to have a means of spreading the liquid into extremely thin films. In the case of the metals it's possible to get these cooling rates with thicknesses of the order of microns.

PATTERSON: There are people now who have been successful in making lots of amorphous materials including amorphous water. Rice's collaborators have succeeded in doing this by vapor deposition at low temperatures. For the lower alkanes it's entirely possible that if you vapor deposited the alkanes at 10 K you might get an amorphous alkane by that technique. So that's another technique you can use as well as quenching, splat cooling and quench rolling. I don't think anybody is willing to try to vapor deposit the higher alkanes. You just wouldn't get anything. The lower ones might work.

WEINBERG: As it has been mentioned in conventional cooling techniques in order to get a large degree of undercooling of most materials one has to remove these bulk heterogeneous impurities, I would like to ask Prof. Turnbull if anyone knows what these things are?

TURNBULL: In the case of crystallization of water I think there's a great deal of experience indicating what heterogeneities are effective. In the molten metals there's a scattered amount of information, not very extensive.

WEINBERG: For example it's been published by a number of people that dust from the atmosphere is an effective nucleating agent. Could you comment about that, please?

TURNBULL: Well, it's certainly an effective *condensation* nucleating agent. I will give you a demonstration some time on it if you don't believe it. But the experience indicates that the proportion of dust that is effective in crystal nucleation is rather small and that the conditions required for a crystal nucleation are very much more stringent than those required for condensation nucleation.

MOSS: Do I gather from the crystallization studies that there is no simple way of deciding between the amorphous cluster models such as Michael Hoare describes and the continuous random dense packing of spheres?

TURNBULL: It's not evident to me that the crystallization resistance favors one or the other of the two models. It simply indicates that the short-range order must be essentially reconstructed in order for crystallization to occur.

MOSS: Would you care to comment on auxiliary evidence that leads you to favor one over the other? It's a leading question I'm sure.

TURNBULL: Intuitively I favor the dense random packing, but I suppose that because I've been thinking along those lines for a long while I could be prejudiced about that. It's not obvious to me that you could come up to the appropriate density with the amorphous cluster models. With the microcrystallite model, there is the connective tissue problem, and it seems that the connective tissue configurations should show up somehow in the structural studies.

MACEDO: You mentioned in passing a spinodal crystalization, could you mention what thoughts you have about it?

TURNBULL: Well, you recall that Kauzmann was very much concerned with the vanishing of the entropy and to resolve the problem he supposed that the glass would tend continuously toward a crystalline arrangement. In structural or mechanistic terms it might be imagined that in the melt microcrystallite clusters are forming all the time and that the number and extent of these clusters increase with cooling until at a spinodal point all the clusters would impinge. This situation would be unstable and would give rise to the normal topological sequence that we find in normal grain growth.

ANGELL: I just want to continue that point a little bit further remembering the publication by Alder and Wainwright for two-dimensional hard discs in which they found a region in which the pressure-area relationship corresponded to mechanical instability. In point of fact in the unstable region they saw large fluctuations in the pressure in this system rather than the collapse of the system to separate phases, which of course you would see in an infinite system: but the fact that the van der Waals-like loop exists even under these somewhat artificial conditions is a little bit worrying. It does raise a question about the ultimate mechanical stability of random close packed assemblies.

TURNBULL: I think that we would agree that there is an important distinction between two-and three-dimensional crystallization behavior. In two dimensions the preferred cluster is a triangle which by itself can be replicated to fill space. On this basis it has been thought, but perhaps not proven, that a two-dimensional random system would collapse upon compression into a crystalline arrangement.

HELFAND: I would like to pursue further the question of whether one would expect, at some temperature, a spinodal crystallization. I don't believe that the answer is necessarily yes because of the Kauzmann paradox. When, and if, the entropy falls to zero it does not imply that there is only a single state for the system, but merely that in a system of N particles the number of states does not grow as fast as e^{aN} as N goes to infinity. There can still be an extremely large number of states of which only an insignificant one is the crystal. The answer to whether a spinodal crystallization occurs is to be found by determining whether there is a mode of mechanical instability of the glass leading to the crystal. It is still not obvious what that mode might be.

TURNBULL: Well, I think we'd agree that the resolution of the entropy problem doesn't demand a spinodal crystallization. This was shown by the work of Gibbs and DiMarzio. Microscopically there is much correlation in the atomic arrangements in the so-called random models, which will reduce their configurational entropy to very small values. I think that Zachariasen probably put it right when he spoke of the random network as a solid with an infinite unit cell. The point is that the correlations in the random network, subject to the constraints that are used in building it, greatly reduce the entropy while not leading to crystalline order.

RAVECHÉ: Perhaps it's a matter of semantics whether one has a spinodal type of decomposition or not, but I find it hard to believe that there isn't a limit to supercooling especially simple fluids. By a limit I mean a state in which every density fluctuation would in fact lower the free energy and drive the system to the other phase.

TURNBULL: This question hinges on the mechanical stability of the dense random packed structure; there is some evidence that this structure can be stable against shear. The melt-crystal interface developed by Spaepen and Meyer may imply a vanishing of the nucleation barrier at 0 degrees Kelvin since it is a purely entropic model. However, the applicability of the model under conditions that are very far from equilibrium is not clear.

DIMARZIO: I'd like to point out that one can classify molecules into two classes, those whose lowest energy shapes *do pack* in regular array and those whose lowest energy shapes *do not pack* in regular array. And it's this latter class for which the question of crystallization is irrelevant. There's no crystal and yet these molecules form glasses.

An example of this latter class is given by *atactic* polymers. The lowest energy shapes don't pack in regular array and, consequently the lowest free energy situation is the glassy state.

TURNBULL: Your statement is true provided we disallow the breaking of chemical bonds. If we may break and reform bonds then the lowest energy state is crystalline even for the initially atactic polymer. A fully connected random network of Si or SiO_2 is uncrystallizable in the same sense.

Dr. Hoare, I'm still not clear on the number of atoms at which the energy of the most stable amorphoid becomes greater than that of the same mass in a crystalline close-packed configuration. I gather it's 115 or higher, is that correct?

HOARE: It's certainly higher—if what we have in mind is a recognizable microcrystallite, perhaps of Gibbs-Wulff polyhedral type. But, as you know, there are some very competitive structures in the $N < 100$ size range if one is willing to include multiply-twinned structures and the like. For example the Mackay structure of 55 atoms. This structure seems to hold the record for both binding energy and free energy at all relevant temperatures and moreover gives very satisfactory comparison with the cluster-beam scattering patterns in that size range. Of course it should always be remembered that there will be quite large fluctuations of structure in such small systems and that relative stabilities of isolated clusters can only be a rough guide to whether they are viable in the glassy matrix. However, to answer your original question, if we take crystallinity more loosely as being marked by the first appearance of vestigial close-packed planes, this could occur around some 40 atoms; if we require well-formed crystallites, the answer would have to be in the hundreds of atoms or higher. The diffraction work on argon clusters by Farges, Raoult, and Torchet due to be published soon should answer this question quite definitively.

BURTON: There are extensive electron-microscopy studies of small particles. The indication is that at least in platinum the normal cubic material is never seen in particles below 70 or 80 Å. This is of the order of 10,000 atoms.

HALPERIN: I'd like to probe the question of what the energies involved in these structures are. For example how do they compare with crystallographic energies when you look either at the whole structure or perhaps at the typical energies of central atoms?

HOARE: I think—I'm sorry I haven't got the figures to show you—they are probably marginally less stable in potential energies than one or another crystallographic structure if you're willing to assume multiple-twin structures.

HALPERIN: I really want to get quantitative. I mean, how do the energies compare with kT on a per atom basis?

HOARE: How do they compare with kT?

HALPERIN: Well, you know, typical temperatures associated with liquidlike structures of the Lennard-Jones type.

HOARE: Of course the binding energies of isolated clusters, whether of crystallographic or other structures, cannot possibly reach the lattice energy per atom until one is up into the thousands of atoms range. How they may compare in a solidlike matrix remains a matter of conjecture, though the binding energies of the isolated structures should be some guide. This is, of course, a matter of statics. In dynamic calculations one can put in as much kinetic energy as the model will bear without inducing some sort of melting transition. From the computer simulations of Burton, Cotterill, and others it would seem that disorganization of a 50–100 atom cluster sets in at about kT equal to some 0.2 to 0.3 of the Lennard-Jones well depth per atom. At higher energies than this the solid like models will be literally inappropriate, though they may retain some validity in the spirit of the cell theory of liquids.

MOSS: To what extent are noncentral forces important in the stabilization of your structures?

HOARE: I don't know. I wish we could find a realistic three-body force. We have the feeling that most unusual effects such as that are amplified in small structures if anything but that's all I'd really say.

MOSS: Because most of the metals that one knows about are not well characterized by central force models.

J. A. BUCARO (*Naval Research Labs, Washington, D.C.*): Prof. Cargill made the point—I think I understood him correctly—that in attempting to distinguish between possible microcrystal structures (one in which the crystalline units are together but oriented differently and the second in which the crystals are spaced by some fluidlike region) scattering experiments cannot tell the difference, i.e., could not see scattering from such differences.

In such scattering experiments it is my understanding that there are two conditions in which one can get sufficient scattering intensity to see such effects. One is that the radiation probe wavelength be comparable to the size of the microstructure units. The second is that the local differences in the dielectric constant (or electron density, etc.) be large. An example of the first case is optical scattering from phase-separated glasses where although the dielectric constant differences are only several percent, the microstructure size is close to the optical wavelength. An example of the second is optical scattering from anistropic molecules in a liquid. Here, the molecular dimensions are only angstroms but one gets a large scattering of light at wavelength 6000 Å because the local dielectric constant changes by factors of 2 and 3 when the molecule rotates.

There is small-angle x-ray scattering work in silica, which probes down to about 80 Å. This agrees with the computed intensity values based on a liquidlike model almost perfectly. This I would think precludes any microcrystal models with structure as large as this even if such units had only small percentage differences in electron density.

CARGILL: The point which I wanted to make was *not* that x-ray scattering couldn't tell the difference between two structural models, one of which had void regions and the other which did not, but rather that the amount of scattering and its angular dependence would depend on details of the joining together of the microcrystals or of the amorphous clusters. You are quite right that if the electron density difference is large enough and if the spatial distribution of this electron density difference is well defined, one can calculate what the scattering should be, and you can look and see if you find it.

The problem is in dealing with models in which this connective tissue, its electron density and its spatial distribution, are not well specified. I quite agree that scattering measurements are important, and that one can distinguish between a pail of water and a pail of ice cubes, but when you get down to a closer comparison you must carefully specify the model structures that are involved.

BRAWER: Just a kind of detail, when you did the x-ray scatterings of these clusters did you average over all possible configurations of them when you did them, considering them as just a sort of ensemble of randomly oriented clusters or was this the x-ray scattering of one particular cluster?

CARGILL: Yes, the scattering patterns that I showed for microcrystals and those which Dr. Burton has shown for noncrystalline clusters were for isotropic scattering, which involves taking all possible orientations of the microcrystal or of the cluster.

BRAWER: If you sort of assume these things were in some way oriented, could these scattering patterns be changed significantly?

CARGILL: Some thought has been given to such intercrystal interference effects. The calculated scattering patterns that I have shown ignore them. Other calculations, which include several microcrystals, indicate that, if the microcrystals are randomly oriented with respect to one another, the only effect of intercrystalline contributions is removing or reducing the small-angle scattering. If there are small misorientations between adjacent microcrystals, then you get something that looks like a strained microcrystal of larger size. These things have been considered to some extent, but I think it's fair to say that one could grind through with more detail than has been done. I don't think it would improve agreement between the microcrystal scattering patterns and experimentally observed patterns appreciably, but the calculations haven't been done.

A. P. DEFONZO (*Brown University, Providence, R.I.*): What about other properties? Are there other properties that have been investigated that would distinguish between these?

CARGILL: I think that some of the properties which Prof. Turnbull discussed yesterday, including the crystallization behavior of various types of amorphous solids, i.e., whether it is grain growth or nucleation-and-growth, might give indirect support to the amorphous or noncrystallographic structures over the microcrystalline ones. Certainly, for each type of amorphous material there are many properties that have been measured and for which explanations have been attempted using the various structural models. And I tried to separate the usefulness of the models for explaining these sorts of properties from the more direct comparisons with specific structural data like distribution functions and densities. Perhaps this is an artificial separation; I hope to discuss applications of some models in calculations of vibrational properties and of elastic constants for some of these materials later in the discussion period.

RAVECHÉ: I'd like to ask Dr. Cargill whether he has considered the possibility that if one does what is just a single scattering experiment to measure the structure factor, one might not be able to tell the difference between the several possible models. That is, one may have to investigate higher order correlation functions.

CARGILL: This "possibility" is certainly true. However, even a single scattering experiment can demonstrate that many types of models are not appropriate for a given material. Such comparisons with scattering measurements greatly reduce the number of competitive model structures.

ANGELL: I think this is a question of clarification. One sees always as a characteristic of these dense random packings the splitting in the second peak of the RDF, and I wonder if it would be possible for either Dr. Hoare or Dr. Cargill to give us a short and succinct geometrical picture of where this splitting originates? In asking, I have in mind the fact that you see this also in Woodcock's radial distribution function for "glassy" ionic KCl where the charge ordering requires that the coordination numbers be somewhat different than for hard sphere packing.

CARGILL: Well, I can reproduce what both John Finney and Charles Bennett proposed as origins for the peak splitting.

These explanations are already preserved for posterity in the very nice papers of Finney and Bennett. We have a distribution function where, in terms of sphere diameters, the second maximum is split into two components of about the square root of three and at about two. Both Finney and Bennett suggested that the peak at two diameters was associated with collineations, which were found to be frequently occurring in the Bernal structure, and in fact Bernal commented on the occurrence of such collineations before detailed distribution functions had become available. The peak at the square root of three one can associate with configurations of four balls in contact. That somewhat begs the question of why these configurations are particularly frequently occurring in the dense random packings.

BRAWER: Dr. Moss, in the packing of spheres with molecules in them, even though the spheres themselves are correlated, the molecules within the spheres are presumably not correlated, so why should this packing lead to a long-range order?

MOSS: There are two sets of correlations: intramolecular and intermolecular. We were primarily concerned with the sharpness of the first diffuse peak in As_2S_3, which clearly came from intermolecular distances. Naturally the intramolecular correlations are also important in the bulk glass.

BRAWER: If you smear the electron density over the whole molecule you should get essentially the same kind of thing you get in dense hard-packed fluids. But if I understand correctly, you attribute that first sharp peak to some atomic separation, sulphur, arsenic, or whatever, and I don't see why that particular atomic separation should be correlated by the random packing of spheres.

MOSS: My only addition to my previous comment would be that there is, in most dense sphere packings, correlation out to about $6d$ where d is the hard sphere diameter. It was this that caught our attention.

MACEDO: I think the results that have been done at The Naval Research Laboratories on silica are extremely interesting and really very important. The big problem is that I, not being an x-ray man, didn't know whether to consider it for real or not. If it is for real, it really has to have a major impact on our modeling because there is so much more order there than anybody thought.

CARGILL: Dr. Moss, do you think it's significant in their reduction of the data that they assumed a Gaussian shape for the Si—Si distance, where earlier work (Mozzi and Warren, 1969) had suggested that a Gaussian distribution in the Si—O—Si bond angle would lead to a very asymmetrical distribution of Si—Si distances?

MOSS: Yes. I think that what Konnert and Karle have shown is that there are interesting longer range correlations in SiO_2 than have previously been discussed. But I do not think that their handling of the first few neighbors was as rigorous as Mozzi and Warren and still believe that it is especially the breadth and shape of the Si—O—Si contribution that rules out a microcrystalline interpretation.

J. P. DE NEUFVILLE (*Exxon Research and Engineering Co.*): Dr. Boyer, is the presumption that each coil corresponds to just a single chain wrapped up within itself? If there are instead a series of interpenetrating coils, then it is not necessary that the short-range correlations occur between sections of the same molecule in those short-range models you presented? Finally is the dimension of the coil simply measured as the distance of the chain from one end to the other? Or what is the specification of that?

BOYER: The current opinion is that the amorphous solid state consists of interpenetrating randomly coiled polymer chains. Thus, correlations of molecular orientations will mostly be between different polymer chains. It is possible that a given chain can turn back and interact with itself. A common measure of coil dimensions is the root mean square end-to-end distance, which is proportional to the square root of molecular weight. Only in special situations such as extended chain crystals does the contour length of the molecule become involved.

PATTERSON: There are short-range correlations in orientation between molecules in most liquids. These correlations occur because the molecules are geometrically anisotropic and must pack in a finite volume. There are short-range correlations in orientation between polymer molecules in the liquid state as well. The question of the chain length dependence of the angular correlations in *n*-alkane liquids was raised by Dr. Boyer. Experimentally, such correlations can be determined from depolarized Rayleigh scattering. If the depolarized intensity, I_{HV}, is plotted against chain length n at 160°C, its value rises linearly with n for short chains, as shown by Dr. Boyer. However, the depolarized intensity starts to approach an asymptote in the range $n = 20–30$ and is essentially constant for $n > 30$. If the value of I_{HV} measured for the longer *n*-alkanes is compared to the intensity calculated for the scattering by isolated chains, it is found to be approximately 4 times as large. Thus, there are significant correlations in orientation between *n*-alkane molecules in the liquid state and these correlations would be expected to persist for polyethylene. This has been confirmed for polyethylenes of 1000 and 2000 molecular weight. The question might be asked whether these results imply a high degree of parallelism between alkane chains? The magnitude of the angular correlations observed in the alkane liquids is comparable to that observed in liquid chloroform or acetonitrile. Thus, there is a tendency for neighboring chains to be parallel, but this effect is no stronger than that observed in liquids composed of small molecules. There is no indication of longer range liquid crystalline type order in the *n*-alkane liquids or the low molecular weight polyethylenes discussed above.

SIMHA: In his paper Dr. Moss referred to a correlation length of 15 Å in selenium at room temperature, I believe, i.e., some 10 degrees below T_g. Considering the size of the Se atom, this represents a respectable distance. It would be most interesting, if the distribution function could be determined over a temperature range which permits a reasonable comparison between polymer and monomer fluid.

MOSS: Yes, I agree but I do not know of any diffraction results that seriously attack the question of the structure of the pure monomeric fluid.

DE NEUFVILLE: I would just make a comment that in selenium what we know about the liquid is that the chain length does decrease with increasing temperature, but your question was, what if you were now to take those seleniums and freeze them and do the x-ray diffraction? People have tried desperately to look for differences among those seleniums. Actually one of the things Adi Eisenberg did years ago, was to measure T_g and indeed irrespective of the quenching temperature, he got the same T_g. Since he had the idea that the ring and chain fractions were changing with temperature, he interpreted the null result as an exact cancellation of the effect of the shortening of the chains at high temperature and the reduction of the monomer ring component at high temperature. We probably do not know enough about selenium to say anymore.

MOSS: Yes, correct.

STERNSTEIN: There appears to be some confusion regarding what is meant by order in an ostensibly structureless glassy polymer. In part, the difficulty arises from the baseline definition of what represents complete disorder. A linear polymer molecule does not behave as if it were a freely jointed, freely rotating chain. It follows that inferences drawn from such a model as regards orientation correlations are not very realistic. It is well established that a linear polymer molecule obeys a one-dimensional (at least) Ising model, the cooperative interactions of which come from the *inter*dependent rotational energies of the segments of the chain.

If one considers a "simple" polymer chain such as polymethylene, then there are three rotational states available to each segment of the chain, namely, a trans state (†), and left (g^-) and right handed (g^+) gauche states. If independent statistical models are used, then adjacent pair rotational isomer probabilities (g^+, g^+), (g^-, g^-), and (g^+, g^-) are all equal. However, the cooperative (Ising) model treatment shows clearly that (g^+, g^-) has a very small probability of occurrence, and may be ignored frequently. Thus, a considerably different picture of local chain conformation arises from the two models.

If we recognize that the occurrence of a triplet such as (g^+, g^+, g^+) represents a single complete helix of the chain, it is apparent that the local helicity and longer range "order" depend on the distributions of rotational isomers. Thus, the Ising chain represents a more realistic picture of the disordered state of a chain molecule than does an independent statistical model. I maintain that detailed knowledge of pairwise and higher ordered interactions and the resultant rotational isomer sequence probabilities provide the necessary theoretical base from which "order" in glassy polymers should be measured.

GOLDSTEIN: Dr. Hoare, Slade Cargill showed this morning some information about pure metal amorphous materials that were prepared I believe by vapor deposition: these were pure metals, lacking small amounts of nonmetallic materials which presumably stabilize structures. And the striking thing about them is that these amorphous metal deposits crystallize at quite low temperatures. You prepare them I suppose, at 4° and then about 15° they begin to crystallize. I wonder if you can rationalize this in terms of the stability of the amorphous clusters that you discussed?

HOARE: Well I'll say two things. First, in talking about simple pure soft-sphere packings I take it for granted throughout that, where mixtures are concerned, they will tend to imitate the pure structure with the second component relieving the strain in the manner suggested by Polk, Dixmier, and Sadoc, and others—allowing such structures not only to form more easily but also perhaps to develop larger and less strained local motifs than would otherwise be possible.

Secondly, I can't emphasize enough that it should be quite sufficient to have a vague statistical tendency to form locally structured motifs. So long as they have sufficient identity in their shape and dynamics to give a differentiation into clusterlike regions with connective regions having appreciably lower resistance to shear, it might be enough to give a glass transition.

But a direct answer to your question would have to include some geometrical account of the nature of the nucleation barrier to crystallization. Along these lines I can only speculate. It does seem, however, that one important feature may be the tendency for small icosahedra of 13 atoms to collect a full shell of octahedra about their surfaces in a way that prohibits the growth of the lattice (FIGURE 6a). If one could demonstrate this convincingly by free-energy calculations, one might have a definite picture of the nucleation barrier, i.e., of the type of fluctuations required for the lattice to form. Difficult as this would be, the "packing amorphon" approach would seem to offer some hope of explaining the glass transition and crystallization as a few-body problem (even if "few" might imply some hundreds), thereby uncoupling it from the mysterious and *essentially* long-range problem of the true phase transition.

As to the specific effect of removing impurities, this can only serve to *de-*

stabilize the resulting structure in the manner generally accepted. I would, however, introduce a note of caution where vapor-deposited glasses are concerned. It seems to me that they may well differ essentially from those glasses which have experienced a glass-transition during formation, lacking that element of cooperative rearrangement into local structures.

HELFAND: If we examine the question of how far out one expects order to appear, given a certain degree of short-range order, there is a technique which liquid-state people use. They convert their correlation functions into direct correlation functions, the Ornstein-Zernike idea. In that way they take out of the correlation function that part which merely arises by reproducing the short-range order over and over. It may be worthwhile to look at such direct correlation functions in addition to the correlation functions we saw today.

GOLDSTEIN: I pointed out that the configurational entropy difference between glass and crystal and between two samples of glasses of different fictive temperatures does tend to diminish as you go to lower temperatures, and at least one possible explanation, which I can't say definitively is right, is that the entropy decrease is associated with what we've been calling the beta relaxational degrees of freedom. If this could be confirmed, what it would mean is that at least a large part of the entropy in the amorphous phase at T_g is associated with the "connective tissue" if the beta relaxations can be identified as belonging to the connective tissue.

F. SPAEPEN (*Harvard University, Cambridge, Mass.*): Dr. Hoare, in reference to the slide we just saw, somewhere on there a Grigorovici-Polk hybrid structure was mentioned. The point I want to make is that nobody has actually made such a structure. People have imagined mixing up amorphons and a random network, but physically it doesn't exist yet. The whole issue of putting these clusters together to make a continuous structure boils down to how exactly do you make this binding tissue? We have some preliminary evidence that this is not a simple matter. As an extention of the interface work mentioned yesterday, we have tried to create an interface between a germanium single crystal and an amorphous random network structure and it turns out to do that quite a bit of excess distortion energy must be supplied in order to link them up. For this reason, if these clusters are connected by random network tissue, both the clusters and the random network will be highly strained.

HOARE: It's true that I did draw parallels between packing amorphons in atomic glasses and the Grigorovici-type structures in germanium. But the energetics and steric properties in the two cases differ considerably. Generally speaking the degree of strain to be expected in the "connective regions" of a simple packing is considerably less than that in a bonded network, where the angle-dependence in the potential imposes far more stringent conditions. The problem of "dangling bonds" doesn't worry us in the metallic structures, though the element of misfit and strain is still there.

ANGELL: To the extent that we're interested in random networks I think it was very appropriate for Professor Moss this morning to mention "amorphous" ice, or "vitreous" ice, which is currently being given much attention. It is of particular interest because of the extensive analogy between the polymorphs of ice and those of silica. However, there was one statement of fact which he made incorrectly. The actual situation is even more interesting, so I am making the correction. He said that the open network is obtained upon depositing water molecules from the vapor at 10 K, whereas in point of fact you only get the open network upon depositing at 70 K. If you deposit at 10 K you get a network in which each water molecule is still four coordinated but in which the density is something like 20% greater than for the open network. The explanation which has been given by Narten, Rice, and Venkatesh, and others working on it, is that depositing at very low temperatures, when you don't give the system adequate time to sort out the best network, you actually get interpenetration of networks, i.e., you get a sort of a mixing in some of the short range orders typical of the higher pressure polymorphs of ice. I don't know whether this is appropriate except in a case like water where you are putting down individual molecules, but do you think it is possible in the case of random networks like vitreous silica to occasionally throw up interpenetrating local structure elements as a higher energy form? Some of the questions opened up by this amorphous ice work are intriguing and ought to be kept in mind when considering other types of random networks.

CARGILL: That's a very interesting question which you have raised. I think it brings forth questions of the extent to which one can see differences by structure sensitive techniques, like neutron or x-ray scattering, in amorphous materials which have been prepared in different ways or which have been subject to various mistreatments after they've been prepared. For example, the irreversible densification of silica by high-pressure treatments. I'm not very familiar with the extent to which densified silica has been examined by x-ray scattering, I believe that this had been looked at in France and that no discernable differences were found in the radial distribution functions.

DE NEUFVILLE: I was just going to comment on Dr. Angell's remark about amorphous H_2O. In most of the random network materials that I'm familiar with such as germania or silica or the chalcogenide glasses, deposition at low temperatures results in a greater density deficit, consequently I think there's something weird about this dense glassy water, and I'd like to hear some other thoughts on it. I don't think it's a general feature at all.

ANGELL: Let me clarify that. If you do the deposition at 10 K and then you warm it up progressively towards 77 K, then progressive changes in structure occur with increasing temperature which are irreversible and which lead you ultimately to the same x-ray density and the same distribution function that you get in the material deposited at 77 K. [Correction added later: Reference to the current reports on this subject (S. A. Rice, Topics in Current Chemistry, Vol. 60: 109) show this latter statement to be incorrect. Warming a 10 K deposit to 77 K produces some changes but does not produce the same structure as obtained by depositing at 77 K: a peak indicative of close-packed or interstitial molecules, which is characteristic of the low-temperature deposit is retained. The low temperature deposit can be understood either as a network with predominantly ice II or ice III-like (bent bond) local geometry, or as an Ice I-like open network containing interstitial molecules in numbers amounting to 19% of the total molecules present. The former but not the latter could have an analog in the case of silica, germania or BeF_2. It is thought to represent a static model for warm water whereas the 77 K deposit seems to resemble strongly supercooled water.]

DE NEUFVILLE: So is this dense a-H_2O something like an analog to densified silica?

ANGELL: Not necessarily; as far as we've analyzed our own computer simulation work on silica, it appears that you get densified silica just by twisting tetrahedra without actually causing any interpenetration of elements of the network, whereas, the only way (as I understand it from listening to the people who have done the work), the best way to interpret the vitreous ice result is actually to allow some network interpenetration to occur. [Later note: For other possibilities, see correction to preceding statement.]

Brawer: Generally one finds that glasses prepared by different methods with somewhat different properties have identical x-ray patterns, at least at the smaller values of k. This indicates that the long-range order is similar for glasses prepared by quite different methods. It may be interesting to look at the scattering at large k to see if in fact the short-range order is dependent upon the method of fabrication.

Also, if it's true that the x-ray pattern of silica is unchanged when the glass is densified, then this is remarkable because the infrared absorption in this case changes considerably.

Leadbetter: I can comment some more on that. You can densify silica in at least two ways: one, by squeezing it, and the other, by irradiating it in a reactor. Some years ago we looked by x-ray diffraction at silica which had been pile irradiated. This is densified by 2% or 3%. There was an enormous change in the first diffraction peak: it drops in intensity by about 30% and broadens considerably. This first diffraction peak is the clear measure of the extent and the nature of the long-range order; so this result means that the long-range order has very considerably decreased.

When you Fourier transform these data you can also see an extra peak coming into the radial distribution function, which can be associated with interstitial atoms in the structure. This whole thing impinges on the point that Pete Macedo raised about Konnert and Karle. Their detailed conclusions may be open to discussion, but it's irrelevant to the point at issue. The fact that you have a strong sharp first peak in the diffraction pattern directly reflects that you have long range order and what they are essentially doing is trying to fit that by a model in detail. Whether you need a tridymite model I don't know but the fact is that to fit that first diffraction peak well you have to consider order out to quite long distances and that's an inescapable fact. This shows up more particularly in some of the chalcogenide glasses where you have a sharp peak at even lower scattering vectors than in silica. A final point relating to Steve Brawer's comment just now about preparing glasses in different ways is that as Simon Moss showed this morning you can get enormously different structures by vapor depositing chalcogenide glasses and by preparing them from the melt. Their diffraction patterns are completely different.

Macedo: I'm going to change the subject a little bit but get back to the point. There's been a lot of discussion about this business of some structure being hung up very tightly, and some structure being loose that can wiggle about in the material. I want to point out you don't even have to use a β relaxation to do the things that Goldstein has been talking about. The α relaxation itself is in every material at least a factor of a thousand in breadth; there are relaxation times which are 1,000 times shorter than the average relaxation. In some materials it may even be a million times shorter, so just looking at the α relaxation in detail there must be areas in the material where the molecules are a lot looser than in other areas, and looser by factors of a million in some materials; at least a factor of a thousand in any material.

Johari: Such a distribution of relaxation times as you described would not produce a bi-modal distribution function, it would not produce two relaxation peaks, one above and one below T_g; it will simply produce one relaxation peak that is highly smeared out.

Macedo: If you have a structure in which some molecules are looser than others, statistically you would predict a smeared out distribution, which in fact is always seen. There is also a β relaxation in certain materials. It may have separate molecular origins or may be just part of the α relaxation.

GOLDSTEIN: I think we are all aware of the fact that the α and the β relaxations merge at a higher temperature and only separate gradually on cooling. And it is sometimes not really clear, depending on the experimental technique and the substance, whether you are seeing one or two processes. Macedo's point is well taken; things are rather spread out around T_g and below, whether you regard it as two relaxations or one.

JOHARI: The spreading out of the relaxation time spectrum need not be due to the existence of a multiplicity of molecular environments or a distribution of activation energies associated with them. G. Williams, among others, has shown that, if the dipole correlation function is not exponential in time, one can find a very broad relaxation spectrum. A distribution of activation energies is not needed. So the breadth of the α or β regions does not quite indicate that some molecules are jumping at rates that differ by factors of millions from others.